Advance Praise for
Spirituality and Health Research

"Simply stated, Dr. Koenig's book is as close to a one-stop research reference as you will find on the market today. Students *and* established scholars of religion and health will benefit from excellent chapters concerning the development of important research questions, the selection of appropriate research designs, measurements, and analytic strategies, and publishing, research funding, and grant writing. All disciplines should have such a comprehensive *and* practical *and* accessible reference."

—Terrence D. Hill, Department of Sociology,
Florida State University

"Religious principles rest on faith—belief even in the absence of evidence, whereas scientific principles rest on skepticism—disbelief even in the presence of evidence. Beliefs can have significant effects on health whether or not the beliefs are true (e.g., placebo effects). Science, therefore, is especially well-suited for testing the effects of people holding religious beliefs or engaging in religious behaviors on health outcomes. In *Spirituality and Health Research*, Koenig provides a valuable guide for designing and executing such scientific investigations. The result is a worthwhile read for students and faculty alike."

—John T. Cacioppo, Tiffany and Margaret Blake Distinguished
Service Professor, The University of Chicago

"Research methods are best learned within the context of a substantive field that is near to your heart. This impressive volume is indispensible for those who want to learn more about research methods on religion, spirituality, and health. This comprehensive survey of the field is unprecedented: it contains everything from finding funding to selecting a journal for publication. What a stellar accomplishment!"

—Neal Krause, Marshall H. Becker Collegiate Professor,
University of Michigan

SPIRITUALITY AND HEALTH RESEARCH

SPIRITUALITY & HEALTH RESEARCH

Methods, Measurement, Statistics, and Resources

Harold G. Koenig, MD

TEMPLETON PRESS

Templeton Press
300 Conshohocken State Road, Suite 550
West Conshohocken, PA 19428
www.templetonpress.org

Figures 17.1, 17.2, and 17.3 used by permission of
Oxford University Press

Designed and typeset by Gopa & Ted2, Inc.

Printed in the United States of America

11 12 13 14 15 16   10 9 8 7 6 5 4 3 2 1

Library of Congress
Cataloging-in-Publication Data

Koenig, Harold G. (Harold George), 1951-
  Spirituality and health research : methods,
measurements, statistics, and resources /
Harold G. Koenig.
    p. ; cm.
  Includes bibliographical references and
index.
  ISBN 978-1-59947-349-9 (pbk. : alk. paper)
1. Qualitative research. 2. Medicine—
Research—Methodology. 3. Spirituality.
I. Title.
  [DNLM: 1. Health Services Research.
2. Religion and Medicine. 3. Research Design.
4. Spirituality. W 84.3]
  R853.Q34K64 2011
  610.72'1—dc23

                                    2011021826

To Bob, Martha, Katherine, and Allison Haley

Contents

Preface

THIS BOOK IS for investigators at all levels of training and experience who wish to conduct research on religion/spirituality (R/S) and health. Researchers early in their careers and those who have only recently switched focus to this topic will want to read the chapters sequentially. Experienced researchers may wish to skip some of the more basic chapters and focus on the technical chapters involving measures, modeling, statistical analyses, and sources of funding support, as well as the chapter that provides an agenda of highest-priority research areas. Regardless of whether the reader is a novice or a seasoned investigator, this volume—based on nearly 30 years of experience conducting research—will provide invaluable information to increase the investigator's likelihood of success in developing, getting funding for, executing, and publishing research in this area.

> This book is for investigators at all levels of training and experience who wish to conduct research on religion, spirituality, and health.

The future of the field of R/S and health depends on at least two things: ideas and the testing of those ideas through research. Ideas, particularly novel ones, often come from careful, thoughtful reasoning by a single investigator deeply immersed in the subject. However, such ideas also often arise from discussion and debate within the research community, since they must withstand scrutiny and criticism from peers. Ideas, however, cannot verify themselves—regardless of how much agreement there is about them. Only careful, objective observation can test whether ideas correspond to reality. These ideas form and inform the hypotheses that research studies test through systematic observations and experiment.

There are practical reasons that research in this area is so important, is likely to have a high payoff in the years ahead, and is worth the investment by government and private funding

> Given the role that R/S could play in preventing illness, speeding recovery, and motivating individuals to care for one another in the community (thereby reducing the need for expensive health services), research in this area will be of critical importance in addressing the escalating health-care costs in the United States and countries around the world.

agencies. As people in countries around the world are living longer due to medical advances, this has created a real quandary for government-funded health programs that will soon become swamped by the health-care needs of their aging populations. Given the role that R/S could play in preventing illness, speeding recovery, and motivating individuals to care for one another in the community (thereby reducing the need for expensive health services), research in this area will be of critical importance in addressing the escalating health-care costs in the United States and countries around the world. Because we still know very little about how R/S affects health in different situations or interacts with existing treatments, there is almost endless opportunity for novel research that could substantially impact public health.

In medicine and all segments of health care, research drives decision-making. Where to invest resources and time, what kinds of treatments to provide, and what approaches to health care to take—all are determined by scientific research. This is the day of *evidence-based* medicine. Research, then, will be an essential factor in determining what contributions (if any) R/S can make to the health and well-being of individuals and populations. This is one of the reasons that I chose to devote my academic career to conducting research in this area, and why I am so committed now to preparing others to do the same.

Acknowledgments

THIS BOOK WOULD not have been possible without the help and assistance of some very dear colleagues of mine, who reviewed and commented on several of the chapters. A sincere thanks to (in alphabetical order) Nancy Blasdell, Terrence Hill, Maragatha Kuchibhatla, Jason Newsom, Rene Oscarson, David Rosmarin, Lisa Satanovsky, Harold Scarbro, and Michael Sheridan. This does not mean, however, that all of these individuals have endorsed everything in this book.

SPIRITUALITY AND HEALTH RESEARCH

Introduction

IN THIS INTRODUCTION I describe the audience for the book and the contents of each chapter so that the reader will get a sense of the material covered in this volume. Each of the twenty-one chapters is short, highly focused, easy to read, and full of practical information designed to build the reader's knowledge base. The target audience for this book is anyone interested in conducting research on religion/spirituality (R/S) and health, or learning about how such research is done. This book is based on five-day research workshops that I've been teaching at Duke University during the summer for the past eight years. This workshop has now been taken by nearly five hundred individuals interested in learning about or conducting research on this topic.[1] Participants have ranged from interested laypersons to clergy and chaplains to students to tenured research professors at Harvard and Johns Hopkins. To my knowledge, this is the only place in the world where researchers can obtain formal training on how to conduct research on R/S and health. Many individuals who cannot take the time or cannot afford to attend the workshops have contacted me asking how they can get ahold of the material that I present in these workshops. This book is a response to those requests, and is now required reading for anyone attending the workshops.

> The target audience for this book is anyone interested in conducting research on religion, spirituality, and health, or learning about how such research is done.

As I indicated in the preface, those likely to get the most out of this book are graduate students, young faculty members (where young is anyone under seventy), and seasoned researchers who are interested in conducting R/S-health research. Much of the information presented here cannot be obtained in undergraduate or graduate courses on research methods, study design, or statistics. Rather, I present practical, basic informa-

> Much of the information presented here cannot be obtained in undergraduate or graduate courses on research methods, study design, or statistics.

tion to help the researcher design a research study, obtain funding for the research, manage the project to completion, analyze the results, and publish it in an academic journal—all tailored to research on R/S and health. Others, particularly teachers and educators, will also find this book useful—perhaps even to teach courses on research methods more generally. Specific chapters can be taken out and used for instructing students on research design, statistics, or grant writing. Finally, I suspect that even the nonresearcher may find this book accessible and of interest. Be forewarned, though, that it doesn't read like a novel but rather like an almanac, full of facts and information.

Chapter 1 begins with an overview of the research on R/S and health. This is a concise review of what the nearly three thousand published quantitative studies to date have found. The majority of research so far has reported a positive relationship between R/S and both mental and physical health, although about 10 percent of studies suggest the opposite and about 25 percent indicate no association. So a lot remains unknown.

Chapter 2 examines the strengths and weaknesses of the research thus far. Among the strengths are the many different research designs used to examine these relationships, long observation periods in some studies, large random population-based samples, many different populations studied in geographical locations around the world, many different investigators reporting similar results, and improvements in research methodology during the past few years. There are also many weaknesses in the existing research, indicating much more work is needed. Valid concerns exist about the cross-sectional nature of much of this research, use of small nonrandom samples, poor methods, inadequate control for confounders, incorrect modeling of variables, overinterpretation of results, lack of clinical trials, lack of certainty about mechanism, lack of appreciation for the complexity of the R/S-health relationship, lack of consistency in the findings, relatively weak associations, failure to consider the time frame necessary for R/S to affect health, and failure to consider lifetime exposure. No doubt, there is plenty of room and opportunity for research that addresses these problems.

Chapter 3 identifies and prioritizes a future research agenda for the field. Research should focus on high-priority, high-pay-off studies with public health impact, common disorders influenced by psychosocial and behavioral factors, evaluation of disease detection and health promotion within faith communities, effects on use of health services, and effects of addressing R/S needs in clinical practice on patient and clinician outcomes. Low-priority studies and dead ends are also discussed, and researchers are encouraged to avoid them.

Chapter 4 is the first of six chapters on research design, and appropriately focuses on identifying a research question. The research question and accompanying hypothesis determine all aspects of a research study, including the background for the study, the preliminary research and pilot work, the choice of research design, the type and size of sample, the size of the research team, and the funding requirements, all of which must flow naturally and logically from that primary question. Investigators are encouraged to identify a research question that captures their interest and passion, and is feasible, novel, ethical, and relevant. I also point out that ethical concerns are often used to justify not doing research on R/S and health. Lack of a clear understanding of what is and is not ethical can serve as a barrier to doing important research.

Chapter 5 discusses how to choose a research design specific to the research question. Research designs are divided into observational and experimental, which in turn can be divided into qualitative and quantitative for observational studies and controlled and uncontrolled for experimental studies. Other factors that influence choice of design include the investigator's experience with a particular design, the funding support, the availability of subjects, and the participation of consultants with expertise in that design.

Chapter 6 examines the different types of research samples, describes how to identify the right sample for a research question, reviews methods for selecting a sample, and discusses issues related to response rate for observational studies. For intervention studies, inclusion and exclusion criteria are addressed, and the challenge of finding a right balance between the homogeneity and heterogeneity of subjects is discussed.

Chapter 7 provides an overview of qualitative methods. This design is often ideal for R/S and health research, where relationships cannot be fully described by relying on quantitative methods alone. Qualitative research seeks to answer questions related to social experience, how it is created, and how it gives meaning to life. This approach is crucial early on in a research program to obtain a deeper and richer understanding of a phenomenon. It is also important later on when the results of quantitative studies need interpretation and application to clinical practice. The different kinds of qualitative research are described, and the differences between qualitative and quantitative methods are outlined.

Chapter 8 focuses on observational designs such as case-control, cross-sectional, retrospective cohort, and prospective cohort studies. The strengths and weaknesses of each design are discussed, with an emphasis on cross-sectional and prospective studies. Cross-sectional designs are the easiest and least expensive, but emphasis must be placed on systematically or randomly identifying a sample, use of reliable and valid measures to assess variables, and efforts to maximize response rate and account for all nonresponders. Prospective cohort designs are more expensive and time-consuming, but almost always preferred over cross-sectional studies. In prospective designs, the emphasis is placed on using validated measures, ensuring interviewer consistency, maximizing follow-up of all enrolled subjects, minimizing contact between interviewers and subjects that affect health outcomes, and accounting for all dropouts. How to conduct an observational study is reviewed from start to finish, and then a specific example of a prospective study is provided and the challenges involved in executing that study discussed.

Chapter 9 examines the randomized clinical trial, a powerful design capable of determining whether an R/S intervention actually causes changes in a health outcome. The strengths of this design are discussed along with the many weaknesses that can result in misleading findings. Basic features of clinical trials are then discussed, including the standardization of the intervention, choosing a control group, selecting subjects, measuring outcomes, types of informed consent, types of randomization, types of blinding, and statistical methods for analyzing results.

Chapter 10 provides examples of randomized clinical trials involving R/S interventions, demonstrating that such studies are quite possible. Clinical trials are described in subjects with mental disorders (depression and anxiety) and physical disorders (breast cancer, congestive heart failure, malignant melanoma). Both Western and Eastern religious interventions are discussed, along with studies examining the efficacy of chaplain interventions. Many lessons can be learned from the experiences of investigators who have attempted studies of this kind. Those that have been successful teach us a lot. Those that have failed due to lack of funding support, difficulty recruiting subjects, or inadequacies in design teach us even more.

Chapter 11 is the first of three chapters dealing with measurement. This first chapter addresses the thorny topic of definitions. First discussed are the optimal criteria for definitions of terms such as religion, spirituality, and secularism when used in research settings vs. clinical settings. The definitions of these terms depend on the unique needs of the setting. Issue is taken with the now popular and widely used definition of spirituality (especially dominant in academic circles) that views it as much broader than religion and that even includes those who are completely secular. Examples are provided of what happens when there is definitional confusion, in particular the development of spirituality measures contaminated with health outcomes that lead to tautological relationships. Finally, definitions for religion, spirituality, and secularism are provided and suggestions made on when to use them.

Chapter 12 discusses various approaches to quantitative measurement that include self-administered scales, interviewer-administered scales, and novel methods of measurement that seek to increase objectivity and accuracy. Sixteen dimensions of religion or religiousness are first presented and then reduced into three basic categories of religious belief and activity. Then examined are religion-specific scales developed for studying religious groups including Jews, Muslims, Hindus, Buddhists, and members of New Age religions.

Chapter 13 describes the most commonly used scales today and discusses their strengths and weaknesses. Nineteen scales are reviewed, and recommendations are made on the best scales to use depending on the investigator's need—the best overall measure, the briefest measure, the most comprehensive measure, and the best combination of measures. The chapter is rounded out with a discussion of how to develop a scale from scratch if none exists that assesses what the researcher wants to measure.

Chapter 14 is the first of five chapters that focus on statistical analyses, including the development of statistical models and the separation of confounders from mediators and explanatory variables. This chapter covers the fundamental rules of statistical methods, presents guidelines on how to take a systematic approach toward analyzing data, and discusses the steps involved in preparing a data set for analysis. Recommendations are made on how to analyze R/S variables in statistical models and on ways of addressing the problem of multiple comparisons.

Chapter 15 provides a detailed guide on statistical tests for most every situation and describes when a test is indicated, illustrated with examples of R/S research questions that these tests can answer. The chapter starts out by examining the different forms that response categories can take (levels of measurement) that determines choice of statistical test: categorical, continuous, and ordinal. Based on level of measurement and study design, the chapter describes specific statistical tests for analyzing data in observational and experimental studies, depending on whether samples are independent or matched. Included here is a review of statistical methods for longitudinal studies, which is a priority now in R/S-health research. The chapter ends with a discussion of situations when a statistician is needed.

Chapter 16 is a key chapter that describes the different classes of variables (predictors, outcomes, confounders, mediators, moderators) and focuses on the widespread problem of confusing confounders and explanatory variables. The importance of carefully separating confounders from explanatory variables is emphasized and contrasted with the common practice of lumping them all into a single category. This practice can lead to an underestimation of the relationship between R/S variables and health outcomes. Also addressed is the challenge of distinguishing confounders from explanatory variables, and baseline physical health is used as an example.

Chapter 17 prepares the reader for a discussion of statistical modeling by presenting hypothetical causal models for explaining how R/S might affect health. Having such a model is important for specifying research questions, designing research studies to address them, and setting up statistical analyses that fully capture the effects that R/S may be having. A model is developed from a Western religious perspective that explains how R/S may directly and indirectly influence physical health through psychological traits, lifestyle choices, health behaviors, mental and social health, and basic physiological functions. That model is then adapted for Eastern religious and secular humanistic perspectives. An emphasis is placed on the effects that genetic, environmental, and epigenetic factors have on constructs at every level, underscoring the tremendous complexity of the R/S-health relationship.

Chapter 18 presents several examples of published research where investigators did not model their variables appropriately, resulting in an underestimation of the effects that R/S factors had on a health outcome and a misinterpretation of the results. Also provided are examples of published studies where investigators modeled their variables correctly, and considered both the direct effect of R/S on the outcome and the indirect effects through intervening explanatory variables, while appropriately recognizing R/S as the source of the effect. Also provided are illustrations of how to model the effects of an R/S predictor on a health outcome, first with a single explanatory variable and then with multiple explanatory variables.

Chapter 19 focuses on why publishing research is so important, provides resources on how to improve writing and grammar skills, discusses how to structure a research report, describes how to submit a research report to a journal, provides detailed instructions on how to respond to journal reviewers, makes recommendations on what to do when a paper is rejected, suggests academic journals in which to publish R/S-health research, describes how to publish via online Open Access journals, and suggests other ways of getting research findings into print. Getting research published is a skill that can and must be learned, and this chapter provides the details of that process.

Chapter 20 explores ways of obtaining external funding for conducting research, beginning first with how to do research without such support. Lack of external funding should not stop anyone from doing R/S and health research. This chapter describes what it takes to get external research funding, emphasizing that while external funding support is hard to get, it is not impossible. Provided here are many possible sources of external funding, from government programs to private foundations to individual donors. Ways of maximizing success are described based on experience learned over the past eighteen years raising more than $10 million for research on R/S and health.

> This book will be an invaluable resource for those wanting to use the methods of science to discover how and why R/S and health are connected, and for those wanting to develop and test R/S interventions that utilize those connections.

Chapter 21 provides details on how to write a grant to obtain research support. Described here are the preliminary steps that researchers need to take before starting to write a grant, and the importance of making the grant easy to read using a plain and direct writing style with simple short sentences. A detailed description is provided on how to structure a grant, section by section, referring to the results of a survey of grant reviewers on the most common weaknesses in the grants they reviewed. Applicants are encouraged to ensure that each grant section contains the content and detail that reviewers expect and are warned about what happens when reviewers are surprised or irritated. Grant writing is brutal business and time-intensive, but necessary for sustaining a research program.

The book concludes with some final thoughts on the needs of this growing field and the challenges that investigators will face when conducting research in this area. Despite these obstacles, all should be encouraged by the tremendous opportunity that exists for research on R/S and health and the tremendous need for well-trained researchers in this area. This book will be an invaluable resource for those wanting to use the methods of science to discover how and why R/S and health are connected, and for those wanting to develop and test R/S interventions that utilize those connections.

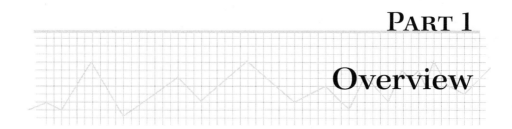

PART 1

Overview

CHAPTER 1

Overview of the Research

FOR THOUSANDS OF years, as far back as historical records go, people around the world have held religious beliefs and engaged in religious practices. Why would humans spend their time and energy on such activities? Why would such beliefs and practices persist and even flourish in some of the most developed countries of the world and among well-educated and informed people? For example, recent national polls of the United States by the Gallup and Pew organizations have found that 55 to 65 percent of Americans indicate that religion is an important or very important part of their daily life.[1] What function does religion serve that keeps people believing and practicing? One possibility is that it helps to preserve health.

In this first chapter I briefly review research on the relationships between religious involvement and mental, social, and physical health. That research has been rapidly increasing in volume, especially over the past twenty years. Figure 1.1 shows the number of peer-reviewed articles on religion/spirituality (R/S) and health appearing in Medline and PsychINFO from 1965 to 2009. Note that the figures are noncumulative, referring to the number of articles published during each five-year period. Although only about 5 to 10 percent of these articles are research related, the number of research studies is rapidly accumulating. Overall, there now exist about three thousand quantitative original data-based studies on R/S and health. The review in this chapter sets the stage for the remainder of this book, which focuses on a critique of the research and, in particular, on a discussion of how to conduct, analyze, interpret, publish, and fund research on religion, spirituality and health.

Mental Health

The majority (70 to 75 percent) of research on R/S and health has focused on mental health (Figure 1.2). I summarize this research by dividing it into studies on positive emotions and studies on negative emotions. The summaries presented here (see Table 1.1 on page 19) are from systematic reviews of the literature contained in the appendices of two editions of the *Handbook of Religion and Health*; all studies referred to below are reviewed there in detail.[2]

Positive Emotions

R/S has been linked to a number of positive psychological emotions that represent the opposite of the negative emotions and mental disorders that I discuss in the next section.

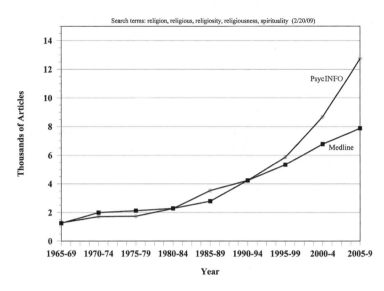
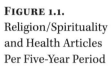

FIGURE 1.1.
Religion/Spirituality and Health Articles Per Five-Year Period

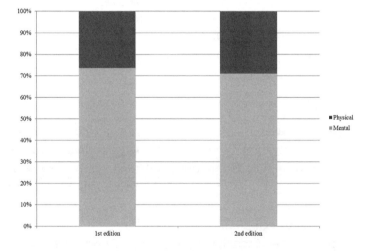

FIGURE 1.2.
Percentage of Studies on Mental and Physical Health. Compiled by Dr. Wolfgang v. Ungern-Sternberg; based on studies reported in the first and second editions of the *Handbook of Religion and Health.*

Well-Being

As of early 2010 at least 326 quantitative studies had examined relationships between R/S and well-being, with 256 (79 percent) finding greater happiness, satisfaction with life, or overall sense that life is good in those who were more R/S. All of these studies reported statistically significant findings, except for eight studies in which results were at a trend level ($0.05 < p < 0.10$). Of the

120 studies judged as the methodologically most rigorous, 98 (82 percent) found greater well-being among those who were more R/S (two at a trend level). Less than 1 percent reported lower well-being in the more R/S.

Hope and Optimism

At least 40 studies have examined relationships between R/S and hope, with 29 (73 percent) finding greater hope among the more R/S (two at a trend level). Likewise, at least 32 studies have examined relationships between R/S and optimism, and of those, 26 (81 percent) reported a significant positive relationship.

Meaning and Purpose

Having meaning and purpose in life is a positive aspect of mental health that is not only strongly correlated with well-being but also associated with resilience in the face of difficult circumstances. Of the 45 studies that have now examined relationships with R/S, 42 (93 percent) reported greater meaning or purpose among the more R/S. Of the 10 best studies in terms of methodological rigor, all 10 (100 percent) reported significant positive relationships.

Self-Esteem

Low self-esteem is often associated with an emotional disorder such as depression. In contrast, high self-esteem is strongly correlated with positive emotions and good mental health. Of 69 quantitative studies examining the relationship between R/S and self-esteem, 42 (61 percent) found significantly higher levels of self-esteem in those scoring higher on R/S; only 2 studies (3 percent) reported that R/S persons had lower self-esteem. Of the 25 methodologically most rigorous studies, 17 (68 percent) reported greater self-esteem in the more R/S.

Sense of Personal Control

Persons with a high internal locus of control (LOC) believe that events in life are a result of their own actions; in contrast, those with an external LOC believe that powerful others or external events control their lives. Of the 21 studies we identified in our systematic review that examined relationships between R/S and LOC, 13 (62 percent) reported that those who were more R/S scored significantly higher on having a sense of personal control.

Negative Emotions

In contrast to these positive indicators of mental health are negative emotional states, which when they interfere with an individual's functioning are called "mental disorders." These include depression, suicide, anxiety, alcohol abuse, and drug abuse.

Depression

Depression was the leading cause of disability in the world (measured by years of life lived with disability) in 1990[3] and is expected to be the world's second-leading cause of disability in 2020, surpassed only by cardiovascular disease.[4] The lifetime prevalence of depression in the United States is 20 percent in women and 10 percent in men.[5] At least 444 studies have now quantitatively examined relationships between R/S and depression, and 272 (61 percent) of those found less depression, faster remission from depression, or a reduction in depression severity in response to an R/S intervention (ten studies at a trend level). In contrast, only 6 percent reported greater depression in those who were more R/S. Of the 178 methodologically most rigorous studies, 119 (67 percent) found inverse relationships between R/S and depression.

Suicide

Strongly linked to depression is suicide. Nearly 10 percent of those with severe depression end their lives by committing suicide,[6] and depression is the most common cause of suicide.[7] We identified 141 studies that had examined relationships between R/S and some aspect of suicide (completed suicide, attempted suicide, or attitudes toward suicide), and 106 (75 percent) reported significant inverse relationships; 80 percent of the best designed studies reported this finding.

Anxiety

Anxiety is a negative emotion that may present as an isolated problem by itself or in combination with depression. Of the 299 studies we located that examined relationships with R/S, 147 (49 percent) reported inverse relationships. Of the 67 best-designed studies, 38 (55 percent) reported inverse relationships. Of 33 studies reporting greater anxiety among the more R/S, all but 2 studies were cross-sectional in design, leaving open the possibility that anxiety led to greater R/S as individuals turned to religion to cope with whatever was making them anxious (as the saying goes, "There are no atheists in foxholes"[8]). Interestingly, of the 40 experimental studies or clinical trials, 29 (73 percent) reported that an R/S intervention was effective in reducing anxiety.

Alcohol Use/Abuse

We identified 278 studies that examined relationships between R/S and alcohol use or abuse, and 240 (86 percent) of those found less alcohol use or abuse among the more R/S (eleven at a trend level). Of the 145 best-designed studies, 131 (90 percent) reported significant inverse relationships with R/S. Less than 1 percent reported a positive relationship.

Drug Abuse

At least 185 studies have examined relationships between R/S and drug abuse, and 155 (84 percent) of those found less drug abuse among those who were more R/S. Of the 38 prospective cohort studies, clinical trials, or experimental studies, 36 (95 percent) found that R/S predicted less drug use or reported that R/S interventions reduced drug use.

Thus, there is a lot of evidence indicating that R/S beliefs and behaviors are associated with more positive emotions and fewer negative emotions, emotional disorders, or substance use problems.

> There is a lot of evidence indicating that R/S beliefs and behaviors are associated with more positive emotions and fewer negative emotions, emotional disorders, and substance use problems.

TABLE 1.1.

Summary of Findings on Religion, Spirituality and Specific Health Conditions[a]

	All Studies[b]			Best Studies[c]		
	Negative	Positive	Total	Negative	Positive	Total
Positive Emotions						
Well-being, % (n)	1% (3)	79% (256)	326	1% (1)	82% (98)	120
Hope	0% (0)	73% (29)	40	0% (0)	50% (3)	6
Optimism	0% (0)	81% (26)	32	0% (0)	73% (8)	11
Meaning and Purpose	0% (0)	93% (42)	45	0% (0)	100% (10)	10
Self-Esteem	3% (2)	61% (42)	69	8% (2)	68% (17)	25
Personal Control	14% (3)	62% (13)	21	33% (3)	44% (4)	9
Negative Emotions/Disorders						
Depression	6% (28)	61% (272)	444	7% (13)	67% (119)	178
Suicide	3% (4)	75% (106)	141	4% (2)	80% (39)	49
Anxiety	11% (33)	49% (147)	299	10% (7)	55% (38)	67
Alcohol Use/Abuse	1% (4)	86% (240)	278	1% (1)	90% (131)	145
Drug Use/Abuse	1% (2)	84% (155)	185	1% (1)	86% (96)	112
Human Virtues						
Forgiveness	0% (0)	85% (34)	40	0% (0)	70% (7)	10
Altruism	11% (5)	70% (33)	47	10% (2)	75% (15)	20
Gratefulness	0% (0)	100% (5)	5	0% (0)	100% (3)	3
Social Connections						
Social Support	0% (0)	82% (61)	74	0% (0)	93% (27)	29
Marital Stability	0% (0)	86% (68)	79	0% (0)	92% (35)	38
Social Capital	0% (0)	79% (11)	14	0% (0)	77% (10)	13
Delinquency/Crime	3% (3)	79% (82)	104	2% (1)	82% (49)	60
Health Behaviors						
Exercise	16% (6)	68% (25)	37	10% (2)	76% (16)	21
Diet	5% (1)	62% (13)	21	0% (0)	70% (7)	10
Cholesterol	13% (3)	52% (12)	23	11% (1)	56% (5)	9
Weight	39% (14)	19% (7)	36	44% (11)	20% (5)	25
Risky Sexual Activity	1% (1)	86% (82)	95	0% (0)	84% (42)	50
Cigarette Smoking	0% (0)	90% (123)	137	0% (0)	90% (75)	83
Disease Detect/Prevention						
Screening	18% (8)	64% (28)	44	22% (6)	52% (14)	27
Compliance	15% (4)	56% (15)	27	40% (2)	60% (3)	5

continued on next page

	All Studies[b]			Best Studies[c]		
	Negative	Positive	Total	Negative	Positive	Total
Physiological Functions						
Immune Function	4% (1)	56% (14)	25	0% (0)	60% (6)	10
Endocrine Function	0% (0)	74% (23)	31	0% (0)	69% (9)	13
Cardiovascular Function	6% (1)	69% (11)	16	8% (1)	69% (9)	13
Medical Diseases and Mortality						
Coronary Heart Disease	5% (1)	63% (12)	19	8% (1)	69% (9)	13
Hypertension	11% (7)	57% (36)	63	13% (5)	62% (24)	39
Cerebrovascular Disease	11% (1)	44% (4)	9	12% (1)	67% (4)	6
Dementia	14% (3)	48% (10)	21	21% (3)	57% (8)	14
Cancer	12% (3)	56% (14)	25	6% (1)	65% (11)	17
Mortality	6% (7)	68% (82)	121	4% (4)	66% (61)	92
				6% (1)	76% (13)[d]	17

a. See Appendices, *Handbook of Religion and Health*, 1st and 2nd eds., for all studies above.

b. "Negative" indicates worse health, "positive" indicates better health. *Not included here* are studies that found no association, mixed (positive and negative) findings, or complex results that were too hard to decipher; "total," however, includes all studies (positive, negative, no association, mixed, complex).

c. "Best" studies are those studies whose research methodology we rated a 7 or higher out of a possible 10 points maximum.

d. Very best studies (i.e., quality ratings of 9 or 10 out of 10).

Social Health

Social health is known to influence physical health and disease susceptibility on the individual level[9] and to affect resiliency in response to trauma or disaster on the individual and community levels.[10] Under social health I include human virtues (prosocial positive psychological traits), social support, marital stability, social capital, and delinquency/crime.

Human Virtues

Among the human virtues (or prosocial positive psychological traits), I include forgiveness, altruism, and gratefulness. These virtues enhance and maintain social relationships. With regard to forgiveness, at least 40 studies have now examined relationships with R/S. Of those, 34 (85 percent) found that R/S was significantly correlated with being more forgiving (one at a trend level). Similarly, at least 47 studies have examined relationships between R/S and altruism (volunteering, donating money to the needy, etc.), of which 33 (70 percent) reported more altruistic activities among the more religious. Finally, we located 5 studies that examined relationships between R/S and gratefulness, and all five found significantly higher levels of gratefulness among the more religious.

Social Support

We identified 74 studies that examined relationships between R/S and social support, and 61 (82 percent) found significant positive associations, especially the more methodologically rigorous studies, where 93 percent (27 of 29 studies) reported this finding. An important aspect of social support is having a marital partner available to provide support in time of need. Of 79 additional studies that examined relationships with marital satisfaction, marital commitment, relationship cohesion, marital sexual fidelity, divorce/separation, spousal abuse, couples' problem solving, or forgiveness in marriage, 68 (86 percent) found significant positive relationships with R/S (one at a trend level). Of the higher-quality studies, 92 percent (35 of 38) reported positive relationships.

Social Capital

Social capital is defined as community participation, volunteerism, trust, reciprocity between people in the community, and membership in community-based, civic, political, or social justice organizations. Social capital reflects the overall social health of a community. In contrast, crime and delinquency rates reflect the opposite. A number of studies have now examined relationships between R/S, social capital, and its converse, delinquency and crime. At least 14 studies have examined relationships between R/S and social capital, and 11 (79 percent) found significant positive associations. At least 104 studies have now examined relationships between R/S and antisocial behaviors, crime, or delinquency, and 82 (79 percent) found lower rates among those who were more R/S (two at a trend level). Another aspect of social capital is performance by youth in school. Of the 11 studies that examined relationships between R/S and school performance (assessed by grades, GPA, or likelihood of graduation), all 11 (100 percent) found significant positive relationships.

Thus, R/S involvement is strongly associated with prosocial traits, greater social support, and higher social capital, all of which could influence relationships with physical health.

> R/S involvement is strongly associated with prosocial traits, greater social support, and higher social capital, all of which could influence relationships with physical health.

PHYSICAL HEALTH

In this section I begin by examining studies on R/S and health behaviors known to affect physical health (exercise, diet, weight, risky sexual activity, cigarette smoking), and then go on to explore more direct relationships between R/S and specific physical health conditions (heart disease, hypertension, cerebrovascular disease, dementia, immune dysfunction, endocrine dysfunction, cancer, and overall mortality).

Health Behaviors

Exercise
At least 37 studies have examined relationships between R/S and exercise, and 25 (68 percent) of those found positive relationships, 6 (16 percent) reported negative relationships, and the remaining studies found no association. Of the 21 methodologically most rigorous studies, 16 (76 percent) reported that those who were more R/S were more likely to exercise.

Diet
We identified 21 studies that examined relationships between R/S and overall diet quality, and 23 studies examining relationships with cholesterol level. Of those examining overall diet, 13 (62 percent) found that those who were more R/S were more likely to consume a higher-quality diet (i.e., greater intake of

fruits and vegetables, vitamins, fish, overall better nutritional status or lower risk). Of those examining cholesterol levels, 12 (52 percent) reported inverse relationships with R/S or a reduction in cholesterol in response to R/S interventions.

Weight

Relationships with weight, however, go in the opposite direction compared to other health behaviors. Of 36 studies that examined these associations, 14 (39 percent) found that R/S was associated with greater weight, whereas only 7 (19 percent) found lower weight among the more religious. Many of these studies controlled for race and gender, so it looks like greater weight is a problem among the more religious.

Risky Sexual Activity

Sexual activity that involves multiple partners, premarital sex, or extramarital sex increases the risk of sexually transmitted diseases such as HIV infection, gonorrhea, chlamydia, trichomoniasis, bacterial vaginosis, lymphogranuloma venereum, human papillomavirus, genital herpes, and syphilis. We identified 95 studies that examined relationships between R/S and risky sexual behaviors. Of those, 82 (86 percent) found such behaviors less common among the more R/S (84 percent of the methodologically most rigorous studies reported this). Of the 9 prospective cohort studies in this group, all 9 (100 percent) found that R/S predicted less risky sexual activity over time.

Smoking

Cigarette smoking is known to cause chronic obstructive lung disease, heart disease, atherosclerosis, hypertension, stroke, and cataracts, as well as 87 percent of all lung cancers and 30 percent of all cancers in general, according to the American Cancer Society. At least 135 studies have now examined relationships between R/S and cigarette smoking, and 122 (90 percent) of those reported significant inverse relationships (three at a trend level). Of the 83 best-designed studies, 75 (90 percent) reported less smoking by the more R/S.

> Those who are R/S live a healthier lifestyle that lowers their risk of physical illness.

In general, then, those who are R/S live a healthier lifestyle that lowers their risk of physical illness. I now examine relationships between R/S and specific diseases and physiological states.

Physical Disorders

Heart Disease

At least 19 studies have examined relationships between R/S and coronary artery disease (CAD). Of those, 12 (63 percent) reported significant inverse associations (69 percent of studies with the best designs). In an additional 16 studies, R/S or spiritual interventions (primarily meditation) resulted in better cardiac surgery outcomes, lower cardiovascular reactivity, greater heart rate variability, or other positive cardiovascular functions in 11 (69 percent) of those studies.

Hypertension

At least 63 studies have examined relationships between R/S and blood pressure (BP) or hypertension, and 36 (57 percent) of those reported lower BP or less hypertension in those who were more R/S or received R/S interventions. Of the 39 best studies, 24 (62 percent) reported this finding. In contrast, 7 of 63 studies (11 percent) reported higher BP or more hypertension in the more R/S (6 of those 7 were cross-sectional).

Cerebrovascular Disease

We identified 9 studies that focused on relationships between R/S and stroke, transient ischemic attack (TIA), or carotid artery thickness, or examined the effects of an R/S intervention on these outcomes. Four (44 percent) of those studies reported that R/S was related to significantly less disease, 4 found no association, and 1 found greater carotid artery thickness in those who were more R/S (but no difference in stroke or TIAs).

Dementia

We located 21 studies that examined relationships between R/S and dementia or cognitive impairment. Of those, 10 (48 percent) reported significant inverse relationships, 3 (14 percent) found significant positive relationships, 2 reported mixed findings, and

6 (29 percent) found no association. Of the 14 most rigorously designed studies, 8 (57 percent) reported inverse relationships with R/S, whereas 3 reported significant positive relationships. Of the 7 prospective cohort studies, 5 (71 percent) found that R/S involvement at baseline predicted significantly less cognitive decline over time.

Immune Dysfunction

At least 25 studies have examined relationships between R/S and some aspect of immune function. Of those, 14 (56 percent) found better immune functions among those who were more R/S or reported positive effects of R/S interventions on immune functions (60 percent of the most rigorously designed studies found this).

Endocrine Dysfunction

We identified 29 studies that examined relationships between R/S and cortisol levels or reported the effects of R/S interventions on cortisol. Of those, 19 (66 percent) found lower cortisol levels or a decrease in cortisol. We could locate only 6 studies that examined catecholamines (epinephrine or norepinephrine) levels, and 4 of those studies reported that R/S was inversely related to or that R/S interventions reduced these levels. When studies that measured both cortisol and catecholamines were considered as a single study, this resulted in 31 studies that had examined endocrine functions; of those, 23 (74 percent) found a relationship between R/S and either better cortisol or better catecholamine levels or reported that an R/S intervention reduced those levels.

Cancer

At least 25 studies examined relationships between R/S and either the onset of cancer or its progression over time, and 14 (56 percent) of those found inverse relationships; 2 found that R/S was associated with a higher cancer risk. Of the 17 studies with the most rigorous designs, 11 (65 percent) reported lower risk or greater survival among those who were more R/S.

Overall Mortality

Perhaps the most powerful evidence for an effect of R/S on physical health comes from mortality studies. At least 121 studies have now examined that relationship, with 82 (68 percent) finding that greater R/S involvement predicted greater longevity, and 7 studies (6 percent) reported shorter longevity. Among studies with the most rigorous methodology, 13 of 17 (76 percent) found that R/S predicted greater longevity.

RELATIONSHIPS WITH HEALTH

Figure 1.3 illustrates the findings from each edition of the *Handbook*. In that figure, the first edition (published in 2001) reviews research conducted prior to the year 2000, and the second edition (published in 2012) reviews research conducted between 2000 and 2010. To understand Figure 1.3, the reader should know what the terms in the legend mean. "Complex" means that it was difficult to decipher whether the findings were positive or negative based on the investigators' description of results. "Negative" means there was either a trend toward (0.05 < p < 0.10) or a significant (p ≤ 0.05) relationship between R/S and *poorer*

FIGURE 1.3. Findings in the First and Second Editions of the *Handbook on Religion and Health*, Compiled by Dr. Wolfgang v. Ungern-Sternberg.

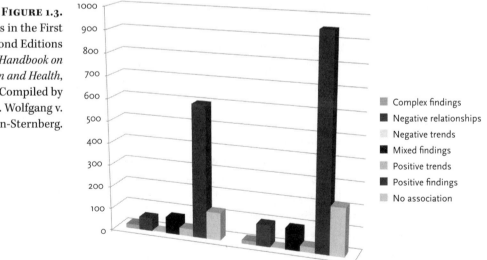

health. "Positive" means that there was either a trend toward (0.05 < p < 0.10) or a significant (p ≤ 0.05) relationship between R/S and *better* health. "Mixed" means that findings were both significantly positive and significantly negative between R/S and health, depending on R/S variable assessed. Figure 1.3 indicates that a majority of the studies published thus far on religion, spirituality, and health have found that R/S is related to better mental health, better social health, and better physical health. The more methodologically rigorous studies are just as likely, if not more likely, to report such findings. The fact is, however, that 4 percent of studies examining mental health and 8.5 percent of studies examining physical health find that R/S is associated with worse health, and many of those studies were methodologically rigorous as well.

Among studies with the most rigorous methodology, 13 of 17 (76 percent) found that R/S predicted greater longevity.

The majority of the research conducted to date has found a positive relationship between R/S and both mental and physical health, whereas less than 10 percent of studies suggest the opposite and about 25 percent indicate no association.

Summary and Conclusions

The majority of the research conducted to date has found a positive relationship between R/S and both mental and physical health, whereas less than 10 percent of studies suggest the opposite and about 25 percent indicate no association. Although a lot has already been learned about the relationship between R/S and health, the research conducted thus far only scratches the surface of what needs to be known about this complex relationship. In the remaining two chapters of this overview, I examine the strengths and weaknesses of the research, and then point out the kinds of studies most needed to advance scientific knowledge in the field.

CHAPTER 2

Strengths, Weaknesses, and Challenges

IN THIS CHAPTER I discuss the strengths and weaknesses of the research reviewed in Chapter 1. How credible are the findings thus far reported, and what aspects of the research leave room for improvement? What are the challenges that this new field faces now and that must be overcome if the field is to grow and flourish?

STRENGTHS

The strengths of the existing research include the sheer number of studies, the many different research designs, the long periods of observation, the large random samples, the many different population groups studied, the wide range of geographical locations, the many different groups of investigators reporting similar findings, and the emergence of findings even when researchers were not looking for them. Based on theoretical grounds alone, the findings reported from these studies fit a pattern that would be expected if R/S did indeed have a positive impact on health.

Large Number of Studies

The findings from more than 1,800 quantitative studies support a positive association between R/S and better health. How could all of these studies be wrong? Even if only 10 percent of those were true, that would still represent a lot of evidence. Where there is smoke, there is usually a fire, and there is a lot of smoke here.

Different Research Designs

Every type of research design imaginable has examined relationships between R/S and health. Although excluded from the review in the last chapter, hundreds—perhaps thousands—of qualitative studies have now been done, where researchers interviewed people in different circumstances (healthy and well, mentally ill, psychologically stressed, physically ill, dying, victims of natural disasters, victims of war, abuse, rape, etc.) asking about the role that R/S has played. The overwhelming majority of these reports indicate that R/S beliefs provide comfort and hope, and assist people in coping with their circumstances. These reports have justified the many quantitative studies that have now examined relationships between R/S and mental, social, and physical health. Several thousand observational studies (using cross-sectional or prospective designs) have now measured R/S involvement and various aspects of health, with two-thirds reporting positive relationships. Finally, many experimental studies and clinical trials have tested whether R/S interventions improve health (mostly mental health), and a majority of these also reported positive effects. Thus, regardless of research methodology, the results are often similar and suggest that R/S is related to better health.

> For observational studies (the vast majority of research on R/S and health), the sampling method is important for generalizing results.

Long Observation Periods

A significant proportion of the research on R/S and health involves a prospective cohort design with follow-up periods ranging in length from a few months to over fifty years. For example, a study by Strawbridge and colleagues reported on a twenty-eight-year follow-up of over five thousand participants in the Alameda County Study.[1] Likewise, McCullough and colleagues followed over a thousand members of the Terman cohort for 65 years from their teen years to older age.[2] Both studies examined effects of R/S on longevity, both reporting positive results. Length of follow-up is clearly a strength, although only a few studies have followed subjects for more than twenty-five years (also discussed below among weaknesses).

Large Random Samples

For observational studies (the vast majority of research on R/S and health), the sampling method is important for generalizing results. Every method of selecting a sample has been used in R/S-health studies, from convenience samples (anyone willing to fill out a questionnaire) to systematic samples (consecutive patients admitted to the hospital or seen in a clinic) to random, population-based samples (where a method is used to randomly select a representative subsample of a population). While use of small, unrepresentative samples is frequent in R/S-health research, there have also been hundreds of studies that utilized large random samples and reported positive relationships.

Different Population Groups

Many populations have been studied, including people of different ages (young, middle-age, old), races (Caucasian, African, Chinese, Indian, Jewish, Arabic, Hispanic), gender, education level, socioeconomic status, and physical or emotional health. Positive relationships have been reported in each of these population groups, and when findings have varied, this has usually been in groups where it would be expected (e.g., lack of relationships between R/S and health in young, healthy males with low stress levels).

Different Geographical Locations

Studies have been conducted in many geographical locations all over the world, including the United States, Canada, Mexico, Central and South America, Africa, the Middle East, Australia, Western and Eastern Europe, the Far East—and in almost every country. The positive findings have been reported in most areas, although tend to be stronger in developing countries where material resources are less abundant. Political forces influence the findings in some parts of the world where atheistic philosophies of government have suppressed religious freedoms. Here, relationships with health outcomes may be affected by the fear that revealing religious beliefs and practices may have negative consequences on subjects or family members.

Different Investigative Groups

Perhaps one of the greatest strengths of the research done thus far is the number of different investigators and investigator teams that have reported positive findings. Not only are Duke investigators reporting findings between R/S and health, but so are many, many other research teams at universities scattered across the United States and worldwide. Furthermore, many of these investigators have not previously published on R/S and health, and are reporting for the first time on this relationship. Reviewing the tremendous variety of authors among the citations in the *Handbook* makes this abundantly clear.

Findings Present When Not Looking

When research reports first started appearing that indicated a relationship between R/S and health, such findings often emerged from the data even though investigators were not looking for them. Recurrent positive relationships between R/S and health kept appearing in correlation tables of papers that were focused on other subjects. Eventually, researchers started to take note of these findings and then intentionally started looking for them. This is clearly a strength of the research and suggests that the findings are real.

Findings Where Expected

In explaining criteria that need to be met in a causal relationship between two variables, Austin Hill includes plausibility and coherence.[3] *Plausibility* means that an association is consistent with the currently accepted understanding of psychological or pathological processes—that is, there is a logical connection between the two variables. *Coherence* means that the association is compatible with existing theory and knowledge. Based on what we know about psychological, social, behavioral, and physiological processes, the relationship between R/S and health is both plausible and coherent. Therefore, a positive relationship between R/S and health should be expected (and, in the majority of studies, is what is found). Chapter 17 provides a logical, rational theoretical model that explains how R/S might influence health.

WEAKNESSES

Besides the strengths, there are also weaknesses in the existing research, which critics are anxious to point out,[4] and these too must be acknowledged. Some of these concerns are completely valid and must be addressed in future research. Other concerns, however, have been exaggerated by those who have set standards higher than expected for other kinds of research in the social and behavioral sciences. Valid concerns include that many studies linking R/S and health are cross-sectional, employ small convenience samples, use sloppy methods, assess R/S using faulty measures, report analyses that do not control for potential confounders, model variables incorrectly, and overinterpret the findings that result.

Cross-Sectional Design

Approximately 80 to 90 percent of studies on R/S and health are cross-sectional. What this means is that even if an association is found, there is no way to determine if it is R/S influencing the health state or the health state affecting R/S. For example, a positive association between religious attendance and good physical health could have two interpretations: either religious attendance causes better physical health, or good physical health enables people to attend religious services. If R/S is related to physical or mental health in a cross-sectional study, then, researchers cannot conclude that R/S caused the good physical or mental health. Cross-sectional data can only determine whether two variables are related, not whether one causes the other. Much of what we know about the R/S-health relationship is based on cross-sectional findings.

Small, Unrepresentative Samples

Lack of funding support for R/S and health has made it difficult to design studies that involve large, random samples (see Chapter 20). As a result, many reports on the R/S-health relationship involve small, nonrandom samples. Even if a relationship is found among such participants, nothing is known about what this relationship might be in those not participating in the study. Participants in R/S-health studies are often people who are interested in the topic—that is, those who are more R/S or are more likely to volunteer. As a result, this impairs researchers' ability to generalize the results to anyone other than those who participated in the study itself.

Interestingly, this problem should actually make it more difficult to find a positive relationship between R/S and health for at least two reasons. First, the sample may not be large enough to have adequate "power" to detect an association if present.

Second, there is a ceiling effect in terms of R/S—that is, since many participants are R/S (since this is what attracted them to the study), they all score high on R/S measures. Consequently, there may not be enough nonreligious people in the sample to allow for adequate variability (particularly if non-religious people have worse health). This reduces the likelihood of detecting an association between R/S and the health outcome. Some investigators have sought to overcome this problem by oversampling nonreligious subjects.

Poor Methods

Again, lack of funding is an issue. Most R/S studies were not designed from the start to examine the R/S-health relationship. Instead, many researchers analyzed data from studies designed for another purpose that happened to include R/S measures (usually for demographic purposes). These researchers are then stuck with whatever methods were used by the original investigators, who had little or no interest in R/S and health. Again, poor methods would be expected to lower the likelihood of detecting significant relationships, since as noted earlier, poor methodology adds variability to the predictors and outcomes being measured. Recall that in reviewing the research on R/S and health in Chapter 1, we found that studies with more rigorous methodology tended to be *more likely* to report positive findings.

Poor Measures

Many studies include only one or two superficial questions about R/S involvement. Again, this is often because the research was not intended to study the R/S-health relationship, and the original researchers did not want to take up much interview space with questions on this topic. The fact that relationships with health are often found when only one or two global measures of R/S are used is pretty remarkable. Multi-item measures with high internal reliability that assess different dimensions of R/S would be expected to increase the likelihood that relationships with health would be found, or at least to improve our understanding of the way that different aspects of R/S influence health.

One concern over R/S measures is more serious than simply their superficial nature, however, and this needs to be recognized immediately and corrected. Some R/S measures (especially measures of spirituality) contain items that assess the health outcomes that they are trying to predict, resulting in the reporting of tautological relationships. I address this more fully in Chapter 11 on definitions and raise the issue again in several other chapters as well.

Inadequate Controls

A number of early studies on the R/S-health relationship did not control for confounders that could have explained the relationship. For example, gender, age, race, or socioeconomic status were not taken into account in some of these studies. Thus, the finding of a positive relationship between religious attendance and longevity might simply be explained by the fact that women attend religious services more often and women live longer, rather than that religious attendance itself actually causes an increase in longevity. Findings of this type that did not control for gender in the analysis, then, would be suspicious. Interestingly, failure to control for confounders such as age, race, and socioeconomic status could reduce the likelihood that an association between R/S and health will be found, since religious involvement is more common among older adults, minority groups, and the poor—groups that are also at higher risk for health problems than the general population.

Incorrect Modeling

When examining R/S variables in statistical models along with other predictors where the goal is to determine if R/S predicts a health outcome, it is important to consider the *direct effects* of R/S variables on the outcome and the *indirect effects* that occur through intervening variables in the model (i.e., mediators). Investigators often simply control for these intervening variables and then report the direct effects. If those direct effects are not robust, then they conclude that the relationship between R/S and the health outcome is weak or nonexistent. Failure to consider indirect effects through mediators (which may be considerably larger than direct effects) results in an underestimation of the effects of R/S on health (see chapters 16, 17, and 18 for an in-depth discussion of this issue).

Overinterpretation of Results

Some researchers may make claims that go beyond the data—that is, interpret results in ways that are not scientifically appropriate. For example, as noted above, finding a cross-sectional relationship between R/S and better health does not automatically mean that R/S caused the good health outcome, but only that the two factors are associated. A claim that R/S resulted in better health, without also discussing the possibility that better health may have enabled R/S participation, would be an overinterpretation of results. Likewise, in prospective studies where R/S involvement is measured at baseline and found to predict better health over time, this does not "prove" that R/S was responsible for the positive health outcome. Other unmeasured factors could have been correlated with both R/S and the health outcome, explaining the finding. While prospective studies add the element of time and new methods of analysis of longitudinal data can contribute information toward causality (see below), only a randomized clinical trial (RCT) can definitively show that R/S actually improves health.

Miscellaneous Weaknesses

Other weaknesses of the existing research include the following: (1) there are not nearly enough studies on clinical applications, which are needed to inform practitioners how to apply research findings in patient care (see Chapter 3); (2) there are not nearly enough RCTs (so the findings are often simply dismissed as being "correlational"); (3) there remains uncertainty about the mechanisms by which R/S influences physical health, especially the underlying basic biological and physiological processes involved; a better understanding of such mechanisms is needed before relationships between R/S and health will be more widely acknowledged; (4) the complexity of the relationship (see below); (5) failure to consider time frame during which R/S effects are likely to occur (see below); and (6) failure to consider lifetime exposure to R/S influences (see below).

Relationships between R/S and health are extremely complex, often involving variables and relationships between variables that are dynamic and changing over time. Failure to appreciate this affects study design as well as interpretation of results. This complexity may help to explain the lack of consistency in findings, including results that appear to conflict with one another (e.g., religious attendance associated with better physical health; private devotional activities such as prayer associated with worse health). Complexity may also account for the relatively weak relationships reported in some studies; correlations between R/S and health often range from 0.10 to 0.20 and explain only a small proportion of the variance in health outcomes.

Failure to consider length of time before effects are evident and length of exposure to the R/S predictor are other weaknesses. While a number of long-term studies have been conducted over many decades, these are still relatively few as noted earlier. This is problematic since it may take many decades before the effects of R/S involvement on health become detectable with current methods. Finally, no studies have quantified R/S exposure throughout the lifetime of the individual and examined degree of exposure as a predictor of health outcomes. Almost all studies have measured R/S beliefs and practices only in the present (ignoring the effects that past involvement may have had on health). Failure to assess exposure results in underestimation of the effects that R/S involvement may have on health outcomes, especially when researchers consider baseline physical health a confounder variable in statistical analyses (see Chapter 16).

EXAGGERATED CONCERNS

While many concerns about R/S-health research are valid, critics have also exaggerated or overemphasized some concerns. Furthermore, some critics make demands of R/S research that are sometimes not made of other types of behavioral science research. I discuss the following below: emphasis on the correlational nature of the findings, the quality of R/S measures, the adequacy of analyses, the interpretation of results, the bias of investigators, and the high standards that R/S-health researchers are expected to meet.

> While many concerns about R/S-health research are valid, critics have also exaggerated or overemphasized some concerns.

Correlational Findings

As noted above, some critics say that relationships between R/S and health are simply correlational (observational), and dismiss the findings on this basis. The fact is that many important findings in medicine have been correlational, including the finding that cigarette smoking causes lung cancer. No study has ever randomized people to smoking vs. not smoking. Furthermore, new methods of analyzing longitudinal data are now being developed (for example, inverse probability of treatment weighting and marginal structural modeling)[5] that produce findings even more reliable and generalizable than RCTs. Indeed, RCTs have their own problems (see Chapter 9).

Quality of Measures

Critics and researchers within the R/S field often voice concerns about the inadequacy of R/S measures or that the current measures developed in Christian populations don't apply to persons of non-Christian faith traditions or to persons living in secular areas of the world (such as Europe). Admittedly, many measures used today were developed in Protestant Christian populations and in English-speaking countries, primarily the United States and Great Britain. Admittedly, since different faith traditions emphasize different aspects of R/S belief and practice, some measures may not give adequate weight to all R/S expressions, which affects the accuracy by which R/S commitment is assessed. For example, Catholics tend to stress the importance of attending religious services weekly, whereas Baptists tend to highlight reading the Bible, which Catholics emphasize less. Therefore, measuring R/S in Catholics by frequency of Bible reading might not accurately assess level of commitment, nor might the measurement of religious attendance in Baptists fully capture the intensity of their R/S involvement. Similarly, cultural factors in different areas of the world may influence the expression of R/S belief. For example, in secular areas of the world like Europe, where the dominant culture provides little support for R/S activities, this atmosphere could influence the expression of R/S belief and its use as a coping behavior.

These problems with measurement, however, may be exaggerated beyond the effects they actually have, and the result may be that good measures of R/S are avoided or replaced by inferior measures. In reality, R/S beliefs and practices are a lot more alike than they are different, especially in monotheistic countries around the world, and these beliefs and practices can usually quite accurately distinguish persons for whom R/S is important from those who are secular or only marginally interested in R/S.

Inadequate Controls

This is a common complaint that critics often use to invalidate research findings on R/S and health. While inadequate controls may have been a problem in the past, it is much less of a problem today. If studies submitted to peer-reviewed journals do not adequately control for confounders, then they are unlikely to be published, which has been the situation for at least the past ten to fifteen years. In fact, some R/S-health studies have actually proven exemplary in this regard. The twenty-eight-year study by Strawbridge and colleagues mentioned above not only controlled for baseline covariates in their prospective analysis but also controlled for time-varying covariates (changes in covariates that occurred during the follow-up period). As noted above, statistical models used in R/S-health research are sometimes "overcontrolled," a situation that occurs when investigators fail to distinguish confounders from explanatory variables.

Overinterpretation of Results

While some findings may have been overinterpreted, there has also been a problem with underinterpretation. For example, when a positive relationship is found between R/S involvement and poor health in a cross-sectional study or longitudinal study with a short follow-up period, investigators may interpret this finding to indicate that R/S is the cause of poor health. Given the role that R/S often plays in people coping with serious health problems, researchers may not consider that such a finding may have been due to participants turning to R/S to cope as their health worsened. Likewise, failure to consider indirect effects in models that include mediators, or failure to accurately measure and fully control for the effects of race, age, education, and socioeconomic status, may also produce results that underestimate the true association.

Bias of Investigators

Another common complaint is that R/S-health researchers are themselves religious and therefore want to find an association between R/S and health, leading to bias in the results that they report. These claims are sometimes made in a way suggesting that nonreligious researchers do not have this problem. The fact is that *all* researchers are biased—that is, they have their hypotheses that they are trying to confirm. Sometimes entire research programs and even academic careers rest on confirming such hypotheses. Likewise, consider the bias that drug companies or companies producing other medical interventions have as they investigate the usefulness of their products. Millions of dollars may already be invested in certain treatments. These companies put tremendous pressure on researchers to confirm that such treatments work. Thus, bias is everywhere in scientific research. The code of scientific ethics, however, requires that researchers design studies so that their own biases do not enter into the ways the study is run, the data is analyzed, or how the results are interpreted.

Higher Standards

Besides claiming investigator bias, critics may also hold R/S-health research to higher research standards than is usual for other areas of behavioral science research. Such concerns are mainly raised in order to undercut the research that has been reported showing links between R/S and health. Just because the subject is religion, somehow this means that ethical standards should be higher than for other psychosocial and behavioral research. R/S-health researchers should be held to the *same* standards as everybody else; the bar should not be higher or lower. Accusations that R/S-health researchers are "dredging" their data or burying research findings that do not agree with their hypotheses is nothing new or unique to R/S-health research. R/S researchers should always follow an analysis plan, report all statistical tests done, and seek to publish their findings regardless of whether they support or contradict their hypotheses, but the temptation to not do this faces all those conducting scientific research, not just R/S-health researchers. As noted above, the success of dissertations, research programs, and academic careers all rest on obtaining significant results, and no one is immune from such pressure.

CHALLENGES

Helping to explain the weakness in R/S-health research described above are recognized barriers to conducting rigorous, well-designed studies, which include lack of funding, lack of trained investigators, and lack of trained investigators with sustained research programs.

Lack of Funding

The usual sources of research funding—that is, the National Institutes of Health (NIH) and National Science Foundation (NSF)—have often been reluctant to support research on R/S and health. The usual explanation given by these funding bodies is that they seldom receive solid, well-designed proposals in this area. However, the real explanation usually goes much deeper. Reviewers on study sections are typically highly talented, mainstream scientists who, while extremely knowledgeable in the social, psychological, and behavioral sciences, usually know almost nothing about R/S and health research, methods, or measures. The long-term antagonism between R/S and science, and concerns over church-state separation, often influence reviewers' attitudes toward R/S-health proposals. Unfortunately, few funding organizations besides NIH and NSF provide the kind of support needed to design and carry out studies focused on the R/S-health relationship, particularly research that has the potential to produce groundbreaking findings. The only exception, to my knowledge, is the Templeton Foundation, and it cannot support all the research that needs to be done in this area (see Chapter 20).

> At least partly responsible for weakness in R/S-health research are recognized barriers to conducting rigorous, well-designed studies, which include lack of funding, lack of trained investigators, and lack of trained investigators with sustained research programs.

Lack of Trained Investigators

There is some truth in the complaint by funding bodies that they seldom receive solid, well-designed proposals in this area. The fact is that those who are interested in R/S-health research are not usually highly trained scientists, and highly trained scientists are not usually interested in R/S-health research. There are no PhD programs on R/S and health. This does not mean that motivated students cannot do a PhD dissertation in another area such as psychology, sociology, nursing, or public health with a focus on R/S and health, but they usually have difficulty finding advisors in this area. In fact, advisors who are available may even discourage students from pursuing such research. Research faculty may also find it difficult pursuing research in this area for similar reasons—that is, lack of support by colleagues, lack of institutional funding for pilot work, and lack of specific training on R/S-health research (especially training in areas related to measurement and familianty with the dynamics that affect study design).

Lack of Sustained Research

Sustained research programs usually require trained investigators interested in R/S-health research, stable leadership, and adequate research funding to build and maintain research teams. Only a few research groups have consistently published research on R/S and health over time. This presents a major challenge for any scientific field that advances through a stepwise discovery of findings, where each new finding builds on what has been discovered previously. Infrastructure to support research teams over time is usually necessary for major discoveries in any field, discoveries that are not usually made by researchers working in isolation or as a result of single studies. This is a major barrier that stands in the way of research advances in R/S and health.

SUMMARY AND CONCLUSIONS

Research published thus far on R/S and health has numerous strengths. These include the sheer number of studies, the different research designs used to examine these relationships, the long observation periods involved in some studies, studies of large random population–based samples, the many different population groups studied in different geographical areas around the world, similar reports from different investigators unknown to each other, significant findings often emerging even when not being looked for—all of these testify to the strength of the research already done.

There is also, however, much room for improvement, and weaknesses in the research need correction to arrive at a more accurate picture of whether and how R/S may be affecting health. These weaknesses include valid concerns about the cross-sectional nature of much of the research, poor samples (nonrandom, small), poor methods, inadequate control for confounders, incorrect modeling of variables, overinterpretation of results, few studies on clinical applications, few clinical trials examining physical health outcomes, lack of certainty concerning the mechanisms by which R/S influences physical health, lack of appreciation for the complexity of the R/S-health relationship, lack of consistency in some of the findings, relatively weak associations, failure to consider the time frame necessary for R/S to affect health, and failure to consider lifetime exposure to R/S on outcomes.

However, critics have exaggerated some of these concerns and have overemphasized weaknesses as though they were specific only to R/S-health research and not to all social and behavioral science research. These criticisms include the correlational nature of the findings, the quality of the measures, the inability to apply R/S measures to certain groups, inadequate control for confounders, overinterpretation of results, and the religious bias of R/S-health researchers. Many challenges also influence the growth of R/S-health research, including a lack of funding for such research, a lack of trained investigators, and a lack of sustained research programs on R/S and health. The strengths of the research should encourage further study, the weaknesses should represent opportunities, the exaggerated criticisms should provoke confrontation, and the challenges should produce determination.

CHAPTER 3

A Research Agenda for the Field

OUTLINE

I. Mental Health
1. Common Emotional Disorders
2. Emotional Disorders in the Elderly and Chronically Ill
3. Caregiver Coping and Adaptation
4. Chronic Mental Disorders
5. Prevention of Substance Abuse
6. Human Virtues
7. Positive Emotions
8. Interactions with Conventional Treatments
9. Negative Effects on Mental Health
10. Understanding Religion-Specific Effects

II. Physical Health
1. Stress-Related Physiological Functions
2. Stress-Related Diseases
3. Neurological Diseases
4. Immune System Disorders
5. Lifestyle-Related Disorders
6. Physical Disability and Chronic Pain
7. Aging Process
8. Genetics, Epigenetics, Inter-generational Transmission

9. Interactions with Conventional Treatments
10. Faith-Based Disease Detection and Prevention Programs

III. Use of Health Services
1. Emergency Room Use
2. Rehabilitation
3. Acute Hospitalization
4. Long-Term Hospitalization
5. End-of-Life Care
6. Outpatient Care
7. Medication Use

IV. Clinical Applications
1. Spiritual History Taking
2. Addressing Spiritual Issues
3. Chaplain Interventions
4. Religious Volunteers
5. Effects of Religious Atmosphere
6. Training of Health Professionals

V. Low-Priority Studies / Dead Ends

VI. Qualitative vs. Quantitative Research, Collaboration

VII. Summary and Conclusions

THIS CHAPTER SEEKS to identify the studies on religion, spirituality, and health that should be at the top of anyone's research agenda in this field. Having such a research agenda enables investigators to focus their efforts on the highest-priority studies. Quantitative and qualitative studies in many areas are needed. Important in the design and implementation of these studies is collaboration between researchers, as no single research group has all the resources necessary to fully explore the R/S-health relationship. Besides identifying high-priority studies, however, it is also important to designate low-priority studies and dead ends that should not be pursued and would only waste scarce resources. There are limitations in funding support and limitations in the time that researchers have to spend on R/S-health research, especially when research on R/S and health is not directly related to a researcher's primary field of expertise or to what the researcher's supervisors feel is an appropriate use of time. Thus, there is no need to expend limited time and financial resources on research that does not advance the field or provide new information.

> Having such a research agenda enables investigators to focus their efforts on the highest-priority studies.

I examine high-priority topics below in categories of mental health, physical health, use of health services, and clinical applications (see Table 3.1 on page 55). My emphasis here is on quantitative research, although I will also address the need for qualitative studies.

MENTAL HEALTH

Because the health benefits of R/S are likely to involve psychological, social, and behavioral pathways (see Chapter 17), these factors could be considered either as health outcomes themselves or as mediators on the pathway leading to physical health outcomes. Research is needed on the effect of R/S factors on the development and course of common emotional disorders (depression, anxiety), chronic mental disorders, and substance abuse problems, especially as these conditions occur in special populations such as children/adolescents or the chronically ill. Research is also needed on positive psychological states and prosocial attitudes and behaviors (called "human virtues") that lead to a happy and fulfilling life and may serve to prevent mental disorders. Research on how R/S interacts with treatments for mental disorders, both biological and psychological treatments, is another high-priority area. Studying the specific effects of different religions, while perhaps politically unpopular, is nevertheless an important area for research study. We also know very little about the negative effects of R/S on mental health or the extent to which such negative effects are dependent on or determined by an individual's temperament or personality. Finally, intervention studies of all kinds are a high priority.

> **Research is needed on the effect of R/S factors on the development and course of common emotional disorders (depression, anxiety), chronic mental disorders, and substance abuse problems.**

Common Emotional Disorders

Emotional disorders, especially depression and anxiety disorders, need study because they are so prevalent. As noted in Chapter 1, 10 percent of men and 20 percent of women will have a significant depressive disorder at some time during their life, and depression is among the most disabling health conditions worldwide. Research is needed in special populations such as children and adolescents (who represent our future) and middle-aged working adults (who face the burden of supporting their families and paying taxes to fund social and health-care programs), given that almost no information exists on the role of R/S in prevention or treatment of emotional disorders in these groups.

While hundreds of cross-sectional studies have examined relationships between R/S and depression and anxiety, fewer prospective studies have considered how R/S affects depression over time. Furthermore, as emphasized in Chapter 2, observational studies can say nothing definitive about the causal relationship between R/S and mental health (even when using lagged analyses in prospective studies or more sophisticated methods of analyzing longitudinal data). Clinical trials are required for that. Thus, there is a particular need for intervention studies that examine the effects of R/S interventions on affecting the development and course of emotional disorders, especially in patients who indicate that R/S is important to them. While expensive to implement, difficult to execute, and sometimes misleading, intervention studies can help determine whether R/S involvement actually affects mental health, rather than simply being correlated with it.

Emotional Disorders in the Elderly and Chronically Ill

Depression and anxiety may be particularly problematic among baby boomers in the United States as they age, since rates of these disorders in this population group are already quite high. What will happen when this 76-million-member cohort develops chronic illness and disability that will likely challenge the independent lifestyles that this generation so cherishes? Might rates of depression and anxiety increase even further? Emotional disorders are also likely to become more and more of a problem in developing countries as health-care practices improve and life span increases, yet with accompanying chronic illness and disability. Very little research exists on the role that R/S plays in preventing or shortening the course of depression (or possibly exacerbating it) in those struggling with disabling medical or neurological diseases. I would include here studies on the development and course of emotional disorders in those with dementia, given projections of a dramatic increase in dementia rates during the next thirty years.

Caregiver Coping and Adaptation

As we face a rapidly expanding older population living with chronic illness and disability, studying the role of R/S in the adaptation and well-being of family caregivers is of key importance. Anything enabling caregivers to care for loved ones at home may help prevent admissions to acute or long-term-care institutions where quality of life is much lower and the cost of care much higher. This issue, the care of the chronically ill elderly, has huge public health importance since the costs of caring for this group will soon overwhelm the financial solvency of health care and other social programs.

Chronic Mental Disorders

Research is needed on how R/S affects the development and course of chronic mental disorders. A huge gap is present here due to past avoidance of the topic by conventional mental health researchers. By "chronic mental disorders" I mean schizophrenia, schizoaffective disorder, bipolar disorder, other psychotic disorders, and severe personality disorders (antisocial, borderline, etc.). Such research is needed in persons of all ages, ethnic backgrounds, and geographic locations. More information is needed on the role of R/S in children and adolescents on the cause, longitudinal course, and capacity to cope with mental disorders. For example, besides a few small studies teaching patients meditation practices, to my knowledge there is only one published study on R/S and attention deficit hyperactivity disorder in the entire research literature.[1]

Prevention of Substance Abuse

Alcohol abuse and drug abuse are widespread and increasing, often tracking along with emotional disorders and criminal activity. Because substance-use disorders (SUD) are common and costly to society, understanding the role of R/S in their prevention and treatment is important. As noted in Chapter 1, 85 to 90 percent of over four hundred studies suggest that R/S beliefs and activities are inversely related to alcohol and drug use and abuse, with the vast majority of these studies conducted in children, adolescents, or college students. This suggests a role for R/S involvement and faith-based programs in the early prevention and in the later treatment of SUD. While Alcoholics Anonymous and similar drug treatment programs are widespread and reportedly successful, more research on these programs is also needed to document their effectiveness.

Human Virtues

There is need for research on the effects of R/S on the development and maintenance of virtuous attitudes and behaviors (gratefulness, humility, forgiveness, generosity, altruism, self-discipline, etc.), which may help in the prevention or treatment of emotional disorders, substance abuse, and other mental disorders or social problems. The degree to which R/S sources successfully promote these virtues must be compared to secular sources of these positive psychological traits. There may also be physiological consequences of human virtues that could help to explain the mechanism by which R/S affects physical health. Although there have been initial attempts to begin research programs on such topics, much more work remains.

Positive Emotions

Because of the role that R/S could play in generating positive emotions (joy, happiness, meaning, purpose, hope, optimism), longitudinal and interventional studies are needed that compare R/S activities to humanistic, secular forms of social or psychological involvement. As with research on the human virtues, studies on positive emotions could be particularly important if future research finds that these are linked to physiological functions (immune, endocrine, cardiovascular) and physical health outcomes. Major government funding bodies such as the National Institute of Mental Health have been primarily focused on mental disorders, and have tended to ignore the positive aspects of mental health as reflected by indicators of human thriving and flourishing. The possibility that positive emotions may actually help to prevent the development of mental disorders, or assist in recovery from those disorders, has not been adequately investigated.

Interactions with Conventional Treatments

Studying interactions between R/S and conventional treatments for mental and emotional disorders is also a high priority. This applies to biological treatments such as electroconvulsive therapy and psychotropic medications (antidepressants, anti-anxiety drugs, antipsychotics), many of which are now being tested in huge clinical trials supported by government and industry funding. Biological treatments may be more or less effective in persons who rely on religious beliefs to cope with environmental stressors that biological treatments may not be able to change. This also applies to conventional psychological therapies, since there is evidence that those who are more R/S respond more quickly to such therapies.[2]

Negative Effects on Mental Health

Also important to study are the negative effects of R/S on mental health, including more subtle effects such as the promotion of psychosocial strains. Such strains may result from struggles that individuals face when trying to live up to the high standards set by their faith traditions. Short-term and long-term effects need to be examined. Do the short-term guilt and emotional turmoil that result from trying to be more forgiving, honest, generous, or self-sacrificing ultimately result in better mental health, greater psychological stability, and stronger social relationships over the long term? This is what many religious traditions claim. Does the baseline psychological state of the person influence what effects R/S may have? In other words, might R/S exacerbate emotional disorders over time in those who are predisposed to them because these vulnerable individuals are not able to tolerate the short-term psychological strains that R/S expectations cause? For example, certain R/S beliefs may induce severe guilt and ruminative preoccupations in persons with obsessive-compulsive traits. Alternatively, in those with antisocial traits, the same R/S beliefs may help to constrain self-destructive or other-destructive behaviors and enhance self-control. This level of detail is necessary in future studies to help determine why R/S may be beneficial for some but not for others.

Understanding Religion-Specific Effects

Another high priority is investigating the effects that different religious belief systems have (Christian, Jewish, Hindu, Buddhist, Muslim) on mental health. Do different religions, with varying beliefs, doctrines, and practices, influence mental health in different ways? Are such effects environment- or culture-specific? What effects do different forms of religious involvement (i.e., individual-oriented vs. community-oriented types of R/S) have on mental health? For example, in the United States, do Eastern forms of R/S practice (transcendental or mindfulness meditation) that are individual-oriented, often performed alone or in private, and often divorced from the religious traditions out of which they emerged have the same mental health benefits as R/S practice that are rooted within Western religious traditions and promote community involvement? What about in China, Japan, or India? What effect on mental health do individual vs. community-focused R/S practices have, and does it make a difference whether they are rooted with the religious traditions common to those geographical areas?

PHYSICAL HEALTH

In chapter 1, I noted that only slightly more than a quarter of the studies on R/S and health focus on physical health outcomes. Consequently, much work is needed to acquire a better understanding of whether R/S beliefs and activities affect the onset and course of physical illnesses and how this comes about. Of particular importance are studies that examine basic physiological functions that protect against or influence the course of common medical illnesses, especially physiological functions influenced by psychological or social stressors.

Stress-Related Physiological Functions

Studies are needed on R/S and indicators of immune functions such as natural killer cell activity, lymphocyte proliferation, t-lymphocyte cell numbers, cytokine levels (anti-inflammatory and pro-inflammatory), and other immune indicators. Both cross-sectional and prospective studies are needed in this area, although more definitive research involving the effect of R/S interventions on these immune functions is even more vital so that causal mechanisms can be established. Immune functions are thought to be located at a central position along the pathway that leads from R/S involvement to physical health and greater

TABLE 3.1.

Proposed Research Agenda[a] for the Field of Religion, Spirituality, and Health

Mental Health

1. Common emotional disorders (depression, anxiety) [MC][b]
2. Emotional disorders in the chronically ill or disabled [MC]
3. Caregiver coping and adaptation [MC]
4. Chronic mental disorders (schizophrenia, bipolar, etc.) [MC]
5. Prevention of substance abuse (alcohol, drugs, smoking) [HC]
6. Human virtues (forgiveness, gratefulness, generosity, altruism) [MC]
7. Positive emotions (joy, happiness, meaning, purpose, hope, optimism) [MC]
8. Interactions with conventional treatments (medication, psychotherapy) [LC]
9. Negative effects on mental health [MC]
10. Understanding religion-specific effects [MC]

Physical Health

1. Stress-related physiological functions (immune, endocrine, cardiovascular) [HC]
2. Stress-related diseases (cardiovascular, gastrointestinal, infectious) [MC]
3. Neurological disorders (Alzheimer's, vascular dementia, Parkinson's) [MC]
4. Immune system disorders (AIDS, autoimmune) [HC]
5. Lifestyle-related disorders (cardiovascular, metabolic, pulmonary, venereal) [MC]
6. Physical disability and chronic pain [MC]
7. Aging process [HC]
8. Genetics, epigenetics, intergenerational disease transmission [HC]
9. Interactions with conventional treatments (medications, surgery, radiation therapy) [LC]
10. Faith-based disease detection and prevention programs [HC]

Use of Health Services

1. Emergency-room use [MC]
2. Rehabilitation [MC]
3. Acute hospitalization [MC]
4. Long-term hospitalization (nursing home) [MC]
5. End-of-life care (including hospice) [MC]
6. Outpatient care [MC]
7. Medication use [MC]

Clinical Applications

1. Spiritual history taking (physicians, nurses, social workers, etc.) [LC]
2. Addressing spiritual issues [LC]
3. Chaplain interventions [MC]
4. Religious volunteers (visiting in hospital/nursing home) [LC]
5. Effects of religious atmosphere (hospital/nursing home) [MC]
6. Training of health professionals [MC]

a. Listed in order of priority (1= highest). Based on the author's experience and knowledge in the area.
b. MC = moderate cost, LC = low cost, HC = high cost (in terms of funding support needed)

longevity, so such functions need to be investigated thoroughly using a host of research methodologies.

Since neuroendocrine functions are likely responsible for immune system changes during psychological and social stress, more information is also needed on relationships between R/S and stress hormones such as cortisol, epinephrine, norepinephrine, growth hormone, prolactin, and neurotransmitters such as serotonin and dopamine. Little research has explored these relationships to date, resulting in a pressing need for cross-sectional, prospective, and experimental studies.

More information is also needed on relationships between R/S and other physiological markers related to cardiovascular functions, including C-reactive protein (predictor of coronary artery disease and myocardial infarction), endothelial function (predictor of a wide range of cardiovascular diseases), heart-rate variability, blood pressure reactivity (predictors of myocardial infarction, hypertension, and stroke), and carotid artery thickness (predictive of stroke and dementia). Results from such studies could help explain why cardiovascular diseases are less common among those who are more R/S.

Research is also needed to examine physiological changes in the body during R/S activities performed in a group setting during religious services, including prayer, singing of religious hymns, or religious rituals such as Holy Communion (receiving the Eucharist), activities that over 40 percent of the U.S. population participate in at least weekly. Likewise, what effect might private R/S activities such as prayer or scripture reading have on physiological functions? While many studies have examined the effects of Eastern meditation, little research has focused on Western forms of prayer or other private religious rituals. Likewise, studies are needed on physiological changes that occur with spiritually inspired acts of altruism or volunteering. We know very little about the changes in immune, endocrine, and cardiovascular function that occur as a result of such activities, especially when inspired by R/S motivations. The development of new technologies that allow the measurement of physiological functions with less and less invasive methods has now increased the feasibility of such studies.

Stress-Related Diseases

This category includes all of the cardiovascular diseases (coronary artery disease, cardiac arrhythmias, peripheral vascular disease, hypertension, renal disease, stroke, vascular dementia), perhaps certain types of cancer (breast, colon), musculoskeletal disorders related to inflammation (chronic fatigue syndrome, fibromyalgia), gastrointestinal disorders (irritable bowel syndrome, peptic ulcer disease, Crohn's disease, inflammatory bowel disease), and other illnesses known to be affected by psychosocial stressors (asthma, etc.). These are by far the most common, disabling, and deadly illnesses affecting humanity, so research that links R/S to such conditions will have enormous public health significance in the United States and around the world. As with mental disorders, R/S *interventions* are needed to determine effects on common stress-related diseases likely to be impacted by psychosocial and behavioral factors. Mainstream medical scientists often view intervention studies as the true test of whether a factor can prevent or treat disease, and findings from clinical trials are often taken more seriously than reports from observational studies.

Neurological Diseases

There is growing evidence from prospective cohort studies that R/S involvement may delay the progression of neurological diseases such as Alzheimer's disease.[3] Given the aging of the U.S. population and expected increase of dementia from 4 million to over 16 million over the next half-century, such research is critical. Psychological stress and depression are known to predict a faster progression of neurological diseases such as Alzheimer's disease, vascular dementia (due to small strokes related to hypertension and other cardiovascular risk factors), and possibly Parkinson's disease. The long-term cost of caring for persons with these progressive neurological disorders and the lack of curative treatments makes the identification of beliefs or behaviors that delay the onset or slow the progression of these disorders a high priority.

Immune System Disorders

Because R/S likely affects immune functions, studies are needed in immune system disorders such as rheumatoid arthritis, psoriasis, systemic lupus, and HIV/AIDS. These disorders are characterized by an immune system that is already disrupted, either underfunctioning (as in HIV/AIDS) or overfunctioning (as in autoimmune disorders). By reducing stress levels, R/S involvement may help return immune functions to a healthier balance.

Lifestyle-Related Disorders

Prospective studies show that attention to lifestyle choices and health behaviors can reduce mortality by over 50 percent during follow-up, may add at least fourteen years to the lifespan, and can reduce the risk of developing chronic disease by nearly 80 percent.[4] Illnesses affected by lifestyle include heart disease, diabetes, hypertension, stroke, kidney disease, gastrointestinal and lung cancers, chronic lung disease, venereal disease, arthritis, and dementia. Since there is such a strong, consistent relationship between R/S, healthy lifestyle choices, and positive health behaviors, there should also be relationships between R/S and health conditions affected by these choices and behaviors.

Physical Disability and Chronic Pain

As populations around the world grow older, physical disability will increase and affect demand for supportive care. Prospective studies are needed to determine the effects of R/S factors on ability to function (i.e., perform self-care activities involved in daily living), especially among those with serious health problems for which there may be no cure. There is preliminary evidence that R/S attitudes promote more hopeful, optimistic attitudes that could influence perceptions of disability and motivation toward recovery.[5] Likewise, studies are needed on the effects of R/S involvement on perceptions of chronic pain (severity, frequency, tolerability), since some studies indicate that R/S interventions may affect pain thresholds.[6]

Aging Process

There is evidence that physiological functions among those who are highly religious behave like those in persons who are younger in chronological age (i.e., cytokine levels[7] and cardio-vascular reactivity[8]). Furthermore, there is a vast amount of research indicating that religious involvement is associated with greater longevity (see Chapter 1). These findings suggest that R/S may help to slow the aging process. The basis for such a speculation is the known relationship between psychological stress and cellular aging.[9] Therefore, anything that reduces stress levels and increases social support may help to slow the aging process.

Genetics, Epigenetics, Intergenerational Transmission

Genetic factors are either responsible for or at least contribute to many mental and physical disorders. They may also influence the likelihood of R/S involvement through effects on personality. We know very little about the genetic basis for R/S experiences or whether such genetic factors overlap with those responsible for mental or physical illnesses. For example, polymorphisms of the serotonin transporter gene may increase susceptibility to stress and lead to depression, as well as to a greater (or lesser) likelihood of religious activity or a capacity for R/S experiences. The common personality trait here may be increased emotional sensitivity. R/S factors may also influence expression of genes that lead to medical conditions that are affected by the environment (epigenetics), including diabetes, cardiovascular diseases, cancer, or Alzheimer's disease. No studies have yet explored whether R/S factors might delay or prevent the switching on of genes that cause these diseases.

Research is also needed on whether R/S factors influence the transmission of diseases between parents and children. By enabling parents to cope more effectively with their cir-cumstances (family or job-related stressors) and health con-ditions (depression, disability, etc.), R/S may help prevent the transmission of disorders or delay their expression. While there is some research on depression suggesting this possibility,[10] no studies have yet examined R/S effects on the transmission of physical diseases between generations.

Interactions with Conventional Treatments

R/S factors may also influence response to medication, surgery, radiation therapy, and other biological therapies. Interactions with medications such as antibiotics, chemotherapy, cardiac medications, antihypertensive agents, and so forth have yet to be examined (with rare exceptions). Antibiotics and the immune system work synergistically to slow infections and eradicate them, providing a theoretical basis for a possible influence by R/S. Preliminary studies also suggest that R/S involvement may influence responses to chemotherapy or its side effects.[11] Thus, this promising area is wide open for research. Furthermore, such research would not require much funding support, since it would simply involve adding a few religious measures to baseline interviews administered in clinical trials testing the efficacy of these drugs.

> Interactions with medications such as antibiotics, chemotherapy, cardiac medications, antihypertensive agents, and so forth have yet to be examined.

Studies are also needed on the interaction between R/S and outcomes following surgery. There is tremendous potential for such studies based on the physiology of wound healing. Stress-related alterations in immune function are known to slow wound healing and increase rates of infection in younger and older adults.[12] If R/S relieves stress, then wounds ought to heal more quickly and complications should be fewer. Several studies have examined the impact of R/S on outcomes following cardiac surgery, and benefits have been reported,[13] underscoring the need for future research in this area.

> There is also a vast potential for research examining interactions between R/S and medical technologies such as radiation therapy for cancer, balloon angioplasties for narrowed arteries, gene therapies, laser treatments, and a host of other new and developing treatments.

There is also a vast potential for research examining interactions between R/S and medical technologies such as radiation therapy for cancer, balloon angioplasties for narrowed arteries, gene therapies, laser treatments, and a host of other new and developing treatments. Again, the hypothesis is that those who are more R/S will respond more quickly to these treatments, and those responses will last longer.

Faith-Based Disease Detection and Prevention Programs

Research is needed on disease detection and prevention programs that operate within faith communities (health ministries), studies that examine effectiveness and cost over time. Such ministries may improve detection of disease, increase compliance with medical treatments, and prevent hospitalization or long-term-care placement (by mobilizing support within the faith community). Given the impact that disease screening has on preventing the development and progression of physical illness, faith-based programs could influence community health through this pathway. Information is needed on effects that faith-based programs have on seeking regular medical care and obtaining disease screening procedures such as mammography, colonoscopy, blood pressure monitoring, blood glucose monitoring, and prostate and cervical cancer tests (prostate-specific-antigen blood levels and Pap smears). Several studies have found associations between disease-screening activities, level of R/S involvement, and faith-based screening programs. Research is also needed on whether ethnicity, age, education, or income level influences the effect that faith-based programs have on disease-screening practices.

Health education programs within congregations also have the potential to promote healthy diets, regular exercise, weight loss, compliance with medication, and adherence to other medical treatments, as well as transmit health information. Programs of this type may be particularly important in minority communities, where access to care is limited. People of all ages are involved in religious communities, providing a natural place where disease detection and health promotion activities could take place.

Finally, studies of parish nursing or congregational health

ministries are needed, including those that document the prevalence of such ministries, program content, reasons for and against such programs, and whether they improve congregational health or reduce the need for health services. Nearly one-third of congregations have health ministries, but little research has examined their costs and benefits.[14] Research is also needed on cooperative programs involving multiple faith congregations acting together to maintain community health and increase social capital (combat crime and murder, delinquency, teenage pregnancy, school dropouts, and other community problems).

USE OF HEALTH SERVICES

Throughout this chapter I have emphasized the need for studies on R/S and health outcomes that impact public health and have widespread applications. As people live longer, health-care costs are becoming a central concern for the United States and other countries around the globe, threatening to consume scarce resources needed for other purposes. In 2005, a time of economic prosperity in the United States, the director of the Congressional Budget Office commented, "There are no silver bullets. There is no single item—technology, disease management, tort law—that is likely to prove to be the answer to aligning incentives, providing high-quality care at reasonable costs, and financing it in a way that's economically viable. . . . Rising health-care costs represent the central domestic issue at this time. [Over the next 50 years, if nothing is done] the cost of Medicare and Medicaid will rise from 4 percent of the gross domestic product (GDP) to 20 percent—the current size of the entire federal budget."[15]

The economic situation has certainly not improved since 2005, especially with government bailouts and increasing national debt. Research that provides clues on how to stop this runaway train will likely get plenty of attention. Reducing health-care costs, then, is one of the highest-priority areas that R/S researchers should focus on. Research indicates that R/S

> **Reducing health-care costs, then, is one of the highest-priority areas that R/S researchers should focus on.**

is related to better mental health, better physical health, compliance with medical treatments, and engagement in disease-screening practices; therefore, those who are more R/S ought to utilize fewer health-care resources as well—especially when studied over the long term.

Emergency Room Use

Treatment in the emergency room (ER) is extremely expensive, and is often necessary for automobile accidents, gunshot wounds, and other major traumas commonly associated with drug or alcohol use or engagement in criminal activities. Another reason people use ERs is that they have no regular source of medical care. Consequently, medical conditions are allowed to progress until an emergency occurs. R/S involvement could affect lifestyle choices, health behaviors, and disease prevention practices, all of which might result in a reduction in the need for ER services (although socioeconomic factors may confound this relationship). No studies to my knowledge, however, have examined this possibility.

Rehabilitation

Short-term rehabilitative services help individuals regain their independence after their physical functioning has been affected by traumatic injuries, stroke, or other medical or surgical conditions that interfere with functioning. These services are staff-intensive and time-intensive, and thus can be quite expensive. With aging populations worldwide, rehabilitation services will be in greater and greater demand. Are R/S beliefs and practices related to shorter rehabilitation stays, faster recovery of physical function, and faster return to independent living? Given that R/S beliefs appear to promote optimism, hope, meaning, and purpose, one might expect R/S persons to have greater motivation to work hard to regain their independence, more so than people without such supportive beliefs. Few studies, however, have examined this possibility.

Acute Hospitalization

The most expensive form of medical care is acute hospitalization, which makes up the largest source of charges to Medicare and Medicaid, and accounts for 31 percent of all health-care expenditures in the United States. Despite evidence that R/S involvement may be associated with fewer acute hospital days,[16] little research has followed up on this. If R/S is associated with better health, then this should be reflected in how much time people spend in the hospital.

Long-Term Hospitalization

Nursing home care is also expensive, averaging about two hundred dollars per day (seventy-two thousand dollars per year in 2010). Medicare pays only a small proportion of nursing home care, so individuals must pay out-of-pocket for all charges until they exhaust their personal finances and become eligible for Medicaid. Again, as the population ages, more and more resources will be spent on long-term care. Few studies have examined whether R/S influences the need for nursing home care or affects the likelihood that families will place family members in a nursing home, rather than care for them at home. In a study at Duke Hospital, we found that during the ten-month period after hospital discharge, older African Americans who were highly involved in private devotional activities such as prayer and scripture reading during hospitalization spent only one-tenth the number of days in a nursing home (average five days) compared to those not involved in such religious activities (average fifty days).[17] More studies of this kind are needed.

End-of-Life Care

Approximately 30 percent of all Medicare expenditures pay for care in the last year of life, of which about one-third is spent in the last month of life. There is evidence that patients with advanced cancer who rely on R/S to cope are more likely to want expensive life-extending procedures (ventilator support, etc.) even when treatment is futile and of no use.[18] This appears to be true, however, only for those with R/S needs that no one is addressing.[19] Research is needed to better understand how R/S involvement influences end-of-life decisions regarding use of expensive technology and why this is so. Furthermore, how does R/S influence decisions on whether to go into hospice care and the quality of life and length of survival after hospice care begins?

Outpatient Care

How might R/S influence physician visits for preventive care and for treating existing conditions? There is some indication that R/S is related to continuity of care with a single physician, rather than bouncing from provider to provider.[20] How else might R/S influence the pattern of outpatient care (medical or psychiatric) that patients receive? Does this vary by religious denomination or level of religious commitment, and if so, why? How do such patterns of outpatient care influence likelihood of acute hospitalization or emergency room use?

Medication Use

We know that stressors, perceptions of disease severity, and chronic pain or other physical symptoms increase the use of medication (tranquilizers, sleeping pills, narcotic analgesics, etc.). We also know that R/S may influence stress levels, social support, and perceptions of disability and chronic pain levels. How, then, might R/S factors influence the use of medications? Factors such as objective disease severity, socioeconomic status, education level, age, gender, and ethnicity also influence medication use and will have to be considered. Given the cost of medication, of treating medication side effects, and of managing medication errors (both at home and in the hospital), the effects of R/S on medication use could have considerable economic impact.

Clinical Applications

Studies are needed to assess the benefits of clinical activities that apply the findings from research on R/S to the care of patients in health-care settings, and to determine the best method of training health professionals in this regard. Clinical applications include the assessment of spiritual needs as well as interventions to meet those needs.

Spiritual History Taking

The Joint Commission for the Accreditation of Hospital Organizations now strongly encourages that a spiritual history be taken on all patients admitted to hospitals, nursing homes, or home health care.[21] Likewise, physicians have been encouraged to take a spiritual history.[22] We also know that 35 percent of physicians sometimes inquire about patients' religious or spiritual issues (10 percent often or always do so).[23] However, very little research exists on patient receptiveness to health professionals (doctors, nurses, social workers, rehabilitation specialists, etc.) initiating a spiritual history. Does it make a difference in patient outcomes if a physician, a nurse, or a chaplain does the spiritual history? How acceptable is this to patients, depending on the particular health professional asking the questions? What effect do such activities have on the clinician-patient relationship? How might such activities affect satisfaction with care from both the patient's and the health professional's perspective? Might there also be effects on mental health, ability to cope with illness, or quality of life? How might a spiritual history influence physical health, medical outcomes, and physical functioning? What is the cost-benefit ratio of taking a health professional's time to identify or address spiritual needs? Studies could be designed to answer such questions, and some have already done so,[24] although much more is needed.

Addressing Spiritual Issues

Research is also needed on other R/S interventions that might be implemented by nonchaplain health professionals, including praying with patients or otherwise taking direct actions to meet patients' spiritual needs. Most physicians (93 percent) say that they encourage patients' own religious beliefs and practices, and nearly one in five physicians say that they at least sometimes pray with patients.[25] Again, this raises a number of questions: Do patients want this? How might this affect the clinician-patient relationship? How might such behaviors influence patients' ability to cope with illness or affect their physical health outcomes? We know almost nothing about such issues.

Chaplain Interventions

Between 1980 and 2003, 54 to 64 percent of all U.S. hospitals had chaplain services; the converse is also true—36 to 46 percent of hospitals had no chaplain services.[26] The Association of Professional Chaplains has argued that there should be a minimum chaplain/patient ratio of 1:100, and the ideal ratio is 1:30.[27] In 1997 (the latest data I could find), the chaplain/patient ratio in hospitals that had paid chaplains was 1:83 to 1:59 for nonreligious U.S. hospitals and 1:34 for religious hospitals.[28] A few studies have now examined the effectiveness and cost savings of chaplain interventions (see Chapter 10); however, these are relatively small and completely inadequate to determine the benefits and costs of chaplain services more generally. Many more studies are needed to determine the effectiveness of chaplain visits in meeting the emotional and spiritual needs of patients in various health-care settings (outpatient, hospital, nursing home). Since such visits could influence mental health, coping ability, use of hospital services (lengths of stay, nursing time, medication use), and physical health outcomes, studies are needed that examine these outcomes.

Research is also needed on the effectiveness of different chaplain activities (prayer, listening and support, reading scriptures, performing rituals, answer spiritual questions, providing psychological counseling, etc.). To my knowledge, we have no systematic information on chaplain activities that are most likely to benefit patients in terms of health outcomes.

Religious Volunteers

Since many U.S. hospitals (one-third to nearly one-half) don't have chaplain services, what do we know about visits from others who might help to meet patients' spiritual needs? Visitors might include community clergy, nonclergy church staff, members of the patient's congregation, or religious persons from outside the patient's congregation. How often do such visits take place, what are patients' perceptions of such visits, and how do patient outcomes vary depending on whether they receive such visits? Research of this kind is needed in both acute hospital and long-term-care settings. Of urgent need is research on who (if anyone) is addressing the spiritual needs of those in nursing homes, where there are usually no chaplains (except in religiously affiliated facilities) where community clergy seldom visit, and where many people spend the remaining days of their lives.

Effects of Religious Atmosphere

Does a religious or spiritual atmosphere in a hospital or nursing home make a difference? Does it affect patients' or families' satisfaction with care and feeling that their emotional and spiritual needs are being met? Are physical health outcomes and responses to medical treatments better? Some religiously affiliated hospitals and nursing homes make a real effort to define their spiritual mission and create an R/S atmosphere. Research is needed that compares health outcomes in institutions that provide such an atmosphere with institutions that don't. Such studies are difficult to conduct since hospitals and nursing homes affiliated with religious organizations often accept indigent patients with more than their share of social, mental, and physical health problems, and consequently poorer health outcomes. How can investigators identify and accurately control for such confounding factors? With rigorous attention to study design, such studies are possible and necessary. Finally, what exactly is an R/S atmosphere? What are the specific components of that atmosphere that actually lead to better health outcomes? To my knowledge, no systematic studies have tried to address such questions.

Training of Health Professionals

Research on health professional training programs (physicians, nurses, social workers, rehabilitation specialists, nursing aides) are needed to determine the best way to educate students on how to identify and address the spiritual needs of patients. When is the best time to include R/S curricula in the training of health professionals to maximize effectiveness? What are the most effective training approaches (lecture vs. workshop vs. case presentation vs. individual mentorship)? What are barriers that prevent training programs from including R/S in their curricula? Research has begun to address such questions,[29] but more studies are needed to guide educators.

LOW-PRIORITY STUDIES/DEAD ENDS

Of lowest priority are *cross-sectional* studies on R/S and positive emotions (well-being, life satisfaction), substance abuse, or other positive emotional states in Christian populations, since hundreds of studies now exist, with nearly 80 percent demonstrating significant associations. Little additional information is likely to result from repeating these studies over and over again. This does not, however, apply to studies in non-Christian populations, especially in other countries, where such research is greatly needed. Cross-sectional studies on depressive symptoms or anxiety are also of lower priority. The current need is for longitudinal studies and clinical trials (as discussed above).

Areas of research that should be considered dead ends are double-blinded distant intercessory prayer studies. After about two dozen such studies, it is now clear that continuing to repeat such research is a waste of valuable resources. There is no scientific rationale for such research and very little theological rationale. Recent studies from Duke University and Harvard University have clearly demonstrated that such studies are dead ends.[30] Likewise, any study that seeks to prove the supernatural, the paranormal, or any effect whose mechanism lies outside of known scientific (psychosocial, behavioral, or physiological) pathways should not be pursued.

> Areas of research that should be considered dead ends are double-blinded distant intercessory prayer studies. There is no scientific rationale for such research and very little theological rationale.

QUALITATIVE VS. QUANTITATIVE STUDIES, COLLABORATION

Qualitative studies are ideally suited for R/S-health research, as they have the potential to explain how and why R/S affects health in ways that quantitative studies cannot. Unfortunately, qualitative studies are often not given the same credit as quantitative studies by mainstream biomedical researchers due to concerns about objectivity. However, qualitative methods have dramatically advanced in recent years and funding agencies (such as NIH) increasingly encourage such methods, often as a complement to quantitative studies (see Chapter 7).

Whether qualitative or quantitative, priority must be given to collaboration. The "team approach" is essential to being competitive today. It is rare that any single research group has all the resources and expertise necessary to execute a significant research program. R/S research requires the collaboration of medical, biological, behavioral, and social scientists, as well as experts in religion/theology. Multicenter studies, because their results can be more easily generalized, are also preferred over single-site projects, further underscoring the need for collaboration.

SUMMARY AND CONCLUSIONS

Research on R/S and health should focus on (1) high-priority, high-payoff studies with public health impact, (2) common disorders influenced by psychosocial and behavioral factors, (3) disease detection and health promotion within faith communities, (4) use of health services, and (5) learning how R/S needs can best be addressed in clinical practice. Clinical trials are a priority in order to identify effective R/S interventions and to determine if and how R/S factors affect health. Qualitative studies have an important role that complements quantitative research, and can help to explain how R/S does what it does. I strongly encourage researchers to avoid cross-sectional studies on topics that have already been exhaustively researched, and to stay away from intercessory prayer studies or any study that seeks to prove the supernatural, which, even if true, likely operate outside the realm of the natural sciences and are therefore immune to conventional research tools. Finally, collaboration is essential for addressing research questions on R/S and health, which often requires expertise from multiple disciplines.

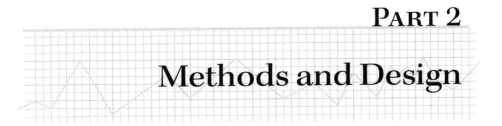

PART 2

Methods and Design

Identifying a Research Question

I N THE NEXT six chapters, I focus on more generic issues related to study design. In this chapter I describe the importance of the research question and how to go about identifying a research question that is relevant and can be answered. Getting this step right is the most important first step in designing a research project.

IMPORTANCE

The research question (expressed in research grant applications as the first "specific aim") is important because it directs everything that follows in a research study. All aspects of the project must flow naturally and logically from the research question. The research question protects against getting distracted and losing focus. The research question is like the conductor in an orchestra, whose job is to get all of the instruments to play together in order to create a beautiful piece of music. The conductor listens intently for any sounds that are out of tune and ensures that the many instruments play exactly at the right time and in the right combination to form the song's melody. This is what the research

> The research question is like the conductor in an orchestra, whose job is to get all of the instruments to play together in order to create a beautiful piece of music.

question accomplishes: it ensures that all aspects of the research are directed toward achieving a single goal and that all activities are in tune with that goal.

When adequately specified, the research question (and the hypothesis that answers it) determines the research design, the type of sample needed, the number of subjects needed, and, consequently, the size of the research team and the resources needed to conduct the study.

CHOOSING A RESEARCH QUESTION

How does one go about choosing the "right" research question? Because the research question may determine how investigators spend years of their lives, large amounts of financial resources, and enormous intellectual energy, plenty of time should be taken for making this decision. In choosing the research question, investigators want to consider several points: (1) what are they interested in, (2) what is feasible, (3) what is novel, (4) what is ethical, and (5) what is relevant.

Personal Interest

What is the researcher *passionately* interested in or want to understand better? Usually that passion comes from a personal experience the researcher has had in the past. The experience is usually, but not always, a negative one. For example, perhaps the researcher had a beloved child die of cancer, despite much prayer and reliance on God to heal the child. There is enough emotion here to sustain the researcher in conducting perhaps a long, difficult, and likely complicated research study to answer a question such as, "Does prayer by family members improve survival of children with cancer?"[1] If a research question does not have some emotion behind it, then the investigator may not have sufficient motivation to pursue the answer (bearing in mind that objectivity among researchers is an illusion).

Once a research question is decided on, the researcher should ask several related questions to determine if motivation is sufficient. First, is the researcher willing to devote the energy and time necessary to seek the answer to the research question? Identifying the right research question may take several months; writing of the grant usually takes at least twelve months;[2] a funding decision could take another twelve months (with revisions and resubmissions); and the research project could take many years to conduct before results are available (especially if an observational study). Second, how much is the researcher willing to give up in order to pursue the answer to the research question? No one has unlimited time and energy, so other activities must be sacrificed, especially if the researcher is at an early career stage. Simply writing a grant takes huge amounts of time, time that will have to be taken from somewhere else—weekends, late nights, holidays, vacations—time that could be spent with family and friends, or on hobbies and recreational activities. Third, is it really worth it? Will the answer to the research question make a difference that is worth the sacrifice and effort? If not, then the research question is the wrong one for this investigator.

Feasibility

Several factors should be considered when determining feasibility. First, is there a research design capable of answering the research question? Not all research questions can be answered using scientific methods. For example, there is no research design capable of answering the research question, "Does God exist?" or "Does God answer prayer?" Any research question that proposes a mechanism that exists outside of nature cannot be answered using scientific methods that are based within nature.

Second, is the research question feasible in terms of the funding support that can be raised to conduct the research? In other words, does the researcher have or can the researcher raise sufficient money to conduct the study? The researcher's academic position will affect the ability to secure sufficient funds. If not independently wealthy or funded by private sources, the researcher needs to be associated with an academic institution or university in order to obtain a research grant. This is true for both government funding agencies (with certain exceptions) and private foundations. This is especially true if the investigator does not have a long track record in successfully conducting research studies and publishing results, and may even be true if the researcher has such a track record.

Third, does the investigator have the time to carry out the research to answer the research question? What other administrative, research, teaching, and clinical responsibilities is the investigator being paid to do? Alternatively, does the investigator have time outside of regular work to devote to the project? If there is not enough time in the researcher's schedule to write the grant—and, if funded, to conduct the study—then the research question is not a feasible one.

Fourth, does the researcher have access to a large enough sample needed to answer the research question? Based on "power estimates" (see Chapter 21), how many subjects are necessary to answer the research question? Does the investigator have ready access to such individuals? Would the researcher have access to enough subjects to conduct the study if only 10 percent or 20 percent agreed to participate in the study? In other words, can the researcher acquire a large enough sample to have sufficient power to detect an effect?

Finally, does the investigator have the skills to recruit the subjects, measure the variables, manage the project, and analyze the data generated? The training necessary to conduct a successful research study is usually extensive and requires a period of mentorship (i.e., apprenticeship). This often involves obtaining a doctorate in the specific field (or a related field) that the investigator wishes to study. Unfortunately, those trained in clinical areas such as medicine, nursing, or chaplaincy often do not receive research training as part of their educational program. Even those with doctorate degrees in psychology, sociology, social work, nursing, or public health may need additional postgraduate training where they have a mentor and participate in that mentor's research, thereby obtaining the necessary skills to design, manage, and report research someday. Lacking any one of the five requirements above means that the research question is not feasible.

Novelty

Is the research question creative enough to capture the imagination and others and excite them to support the project with time, money, and other resources? Who would reference or cite this work (i.e., who is the intended audience)? The researcher needs to convince others that the research question is a novel one that will significantly advance knowledge in the field, and will ultimately impact the care of patients and improve public health.

If the research question is an old one and not yet answered, then the researcher needs to find out why. In other words, the investigator needs to conduct a careful background search to determine what previous research has tried to answer the question and why it was not successful. Perhaps no research design is capable of answering the question or the cost of answering the question is simply too great. Finding this out beforehand can save a lot of time. Related to research questions that are old and not yet answered are questions whose answers are taken for granted without any corroborating evidence. A generation or two ago everyone assumed that taking a tablespoon of castor oil each day kept people healthy. Asking this question, researchers found that castor oil is rich in ricinoleic acid, which inhibits the growth of many viruses, bacteria, and yeasts, helping to explain why castor oil is good for health.

Even if the research question has been previously studied and answered, the researcher may still argue that additional research is needed to buttress the earlier work. The goal may be to improve on that research in order to arrive at more definitive conclusions. Again, this requires identifying the previous research and learning what was done, what was found, and what weaknesses were present that the proposed study would address.

Ethical

Can the research question be answered by research that is ethical? Can the research be designed in a way that does not violate the rights or well-being of participants? This can be especially important in studies involving R/S interventions.

I have found that clinicians, especially chaplains, often give ethical reasons for not doing important research. Objections such as "We can't make subjects more religious" or "We can't allow subjects to be in the control group without an intervention" often stand in the way of research that needs to be done. Is it really unethical to make persons more R/S—if after being fully informed they consent to participate and the intervention is in line with and supportive of subjects' preexisting R/S beliefs? Is it really unethical to have subjects randomized to a "usual care" control group, when there is currently no definitive research showing that an R/S intervention (for example, a chaplain visit) improves health or medical outcomes? Bear in mind that there probably won't be any such evidence until someone compares those who receive the intervention to those who don't. The result of oversensitivity to ethical concerns is that the experts in R/S interventions—chaplains and clergy—end up not doing research on R/S and health, and instead leave that research to those without R/S training or theological expertise. Whether a research project is ethical always involves weighing the benefits vs. the costs, and if the benefits far outweigh the costs and people are willing to take the risks, then even some very dangerous research projects are sometimes deemed ethical.

Chaplains and other clinicians should recognize that if the research involves any *real* ethical concerns, the Institutional Review Board (IRB) will quickly point these out and not allow the research to be done. This is why it is important for investigators to check with their IRB early when deciding on a research question and the best research design to answer it. Today's regulations are so strict that most ethical concerns must be taken care of before the IRB even considers approving a research proposal (and chaplains are often members of the IRB).

Relevance

Will answering the research question provide new information that is relevant to the health of others—that is, improve individual health or public health more generally? Will the research results advance the health-care field? Will the results improve the care that patients receive? Will it reduce the costs of services? Will it influence health-care policy? Funding organizations, whether NIH, NSF, Templeton, or an other private foundation, require that the researcher describe the relevance of the project's outcomes before they will provide support. For Templeton proposals, both the "outputs" (i.e., number of publications, presentations, media contacts, etc.) and the "outcomes" need to be described. By outcome, the foundation means the impact the study results will have on humanity and, more broadly, on changing the culture of health care. The researcher is obligated, then, to explain in the proposal how answering the research question will make a real difference in the world. Unless the investigator can clearly articulate what impact the research will have on improving health and well-being, the research question is not a good one.

General Issues

Before deciding on a research question, the investigator needs to conduct a comprehensive review of the literature to identify other studies that may have asked the same question (as noted above). Research usually builds on what has already been learned, and a good research study always adds something to existing knowledge. The investigator, then, must have a thorough understanding of what that existing knowledge is. Finally, the researcher should discuss the research question with colleagues and especially with knowledgeable experts in the field to get their sense of whether the research is feasible, novel, ethical, and relevant.

Specifying the Research Question and Hypothesis

Once the research question has been identified—one that the researcher is passionately interested in and is feasible, novel, ethical, and relevant—then the research question must be stated. This is called "specifying" the research question and

> Once the research question has been identified—one that the researcher is passionately interested in and is feasible, novel, ethical, and relevant—then the research question must be stated.

involves stating the question in a focused and specific manner. For example, let's say that an investigator in interested in studying whether R/S involvement is related to blood pressure. An *incorrect* way of specifying the research question is, "What is the relationship between religion and blood pressure?" Stating the question in this manner is too general. The way it is written, the research question is not specific enough to guide the design of the research study to answer the question. The researcher needs to indicate what type of religious activity, what aspect of blood pressure, in what population, and in what location. A better way of specifying the question is, "What is the relationship between frequency of religious attendance and diastolic blood pressure in Southern Baptists from North Carolina?"

Besides specifying the research question, the investigator must also state a *hypothesis*—that is, what the research is expected to show. For the above research question, the hypothesis would likewise be stated in very specific and focused terms:[3] "We hypothesize that Southern Baptists from North Carolina who attend religious services weekly or more will have an average 5 mmHg lower diastolic blood pressure than those who attend services less than weekly." The hypothesis must be based on what is known from the existing research literature or from pilot data that the researcher has collected. The investigator must justify the hypothesis with a solid rationale based on existing theory and data. In the example above, the researcher does not necessarily have to show that previous research indicates that weekly attendance is associated with a 5 mmHg lower diastolic blood pressure (DBP). However, it does mean that other psychosocial activities like religious attendance have been shown to have an effect on DBP of this magnitude. Furthermore, the researcher must cite research documenting that 5 mmHg reduction in DBP is a clinically significant difference. If a difference of 5 mmHg of DBP has no health consequences, then the finding (and research question) would not be relevant.

The hypothesis stated above describes exactly how the research needs to be conducted. The study design would be observational and cross-sectional. The primary predictor would be religious attendance measured as weekly or more vs. less than weekly. The sample would be Southern Baptists from North Carolina. The average difference to be demonstrated would be 5 mmHg. This difference (or effect size), together with information from the existing literature on the likely standard deviation of that difference, can then be plugged into a power analysis (Chapter 21) to determine how large of a sample is needed to detect that difference at a p-value < 0.05 and at a power of 80 percent or higher (the standard). The sample size, then, will determine the size of the research team and the funding necessary to conduct the study.

There should be only *one primary* overarching research question. This single research question must "sell the grant."

NUMBER OF RESEARCH QUESTIONS

There should be only *one primary* overarching research question. This single research question must "sell the grant" (if part of a funding proposal). The power analysis that determines the size of the sample is required only for the primary research question. This underscores the importance of the primary research question, the accompanying hypothesis, and the way these are stated.

Although additional research questions are allowed and usually expected, there should probably be no more than two or three highly focused *secondary* questions, and those questions (and accompanying hypotheses) need to be directly related to the primary research question and *flow naturally from it.* For the primary research question stated earlier, the following secondary questions would be appropriate: "Does gender moderate the relationship between religious attendance and diastolic blood pressure in Southern Baptists in North Carolina?"; "Does race moderate the relationship between religious attendance and diastolic blood pressure in . . . ?"; and "What psychosocial factors mediate or explain the relationship between religious attendance and diastolic blood pressure . . . ?"

Summary and Conclusions

The primary research question and accompanying hypothesis determine all aspects of the research study, including the background for the study, the preliminary research and pilot work, the choice of research design needed, the type and size of sample, the size of research team, and the funding requirements, all of which must flow naturally and logically from it. Researchers should take time to identify a primary research question that captures their interest and passion and is feasible, novel, ethical, and relevant. A thorough background review of the literature should guide selection of the research question and, once selected, it should be discussed with colleagues and experts. The way the researcher specifies the research question and accompanying hypothesis helps to protect against lack of focus and directs the power analysis. As many as two or three additional research questions are allowed, but they must be directly related to the primary research question. Always remember that the primary research question must convince others that the research is worth doing.

CHAPTER 5

Choosing a Research Design

CHOOSING A RESEARCH design, like all other aspects of a research study, depends on the research question.[1] Choice of research design also depends on other factors (experience of investigator, research funds available to do the research, etc.), but these are less important than choosing the best design to answer the primary research question. Research designs can be divided into two major categories: observational and experimental. Each of these, in turn, can be broken down into subcategories, which can themselves be divided into further categories (see Table 5.1 on page 88). Before proceeding, however, I'd like to briefly discuss how the choice of study design affects causal inference.

CAUSAL INFERENCES

David A. Kenny discusses the following three criteria that must be met before concluding that one variable A (e.g., religion/spirituality) causes changes in another variable B (e.g., a health outcome): (1) a significant association between the two variables, (2) the relationship is not "spurious" (i.e., there is no alternative cause or third variable that explains the relationship), and

> Choosing a research design, like all other aspects of a research study, depends on the research question.

> Qualitative research is indicated early in a research program when very little is known about a subject or how it exists and operates in the real world.

(3) variable A precedes variable B in terms of timing.[2] Observational studies (cross-sectional and longitudinal) suffer from the inability to establish criterion #2, since there is no way that researchers could know or measure all of the possible causes of variable B. Cross-sectional studies only fulfill criterion #1 and so are the weakest designs in terms of establishing causation. Longitudinal studies fulfill criteria #1 and #3, and so add information toward establishing causality. Only experimental studies—that is, randomized clinical trials with a control group—however, are capable of fulfilling criterion #2 and therefore establishing causation (since the process of randomization equalizes the groups in terms of other causal factors and therefore eliminates their influence on the outcome). With these considerations in mind, I now describe the different types of research design.

Observational Designs

Qualitative

Qualitative research is discussed in greater detail in Chapter 7. Here, however, I discuss when a qualitative study would be the design of choice for a research question. The most common qualitative methods include in-depth interviews and field observations (i.e., interviewing participants or participating in a group with participants) in order to obtain a better and deeper understanding of a phenomenon. Qualitative research is indicated early in a research program when very little is known about a subject or how it exists and operates in the real world. Qualitative research can also be useful for developing quantitative measures (knowing which questions to ask on surveys) and for interpreting data collected using quantitative methods (as in a "mixed-methods" design). There are five basic approaches, each using a different method of collecting and analyzing the data and interpreting results: phenomenology, grounded theory, ethnography, historical analysis, and discourse analysis. A sixth approach, triangulation, uses a combination of two or more of the other five approaches.[3]

For example, if a researcher wants to learn more about the role that R/S beliefs and practices play in the experience of patients dying with cancer, and there has been little previous research on this subject, then a qualitative research design might be chosen (perhaps using a grounded theory approach). The researcher would interview patients in a hospice program at different stages before death to determine how R/S beliefs and coping behaviors differ and identify the purposes they serve as death approaches. Patients could describe, in their own words, their experience with religion and its personal meaning to them. The information collected might be itself useful to health professionals caring for dying patients and could be valuable for informing the design of future quantitative studies (i.e., hypothesis-generating) that could later collect information to determine if the results from the qualitative study applies to other individuals in similar circumstances (i.e., to determine if the findings from the qualitative study can be generalized).

Another example of when a qualitative design would be appropriate is if the researcher wanted to develop a valid and reliable quantitative measure for assessing R/S involvement in children with severe physical disabilities. Children with severe physical disabilities would be identified and interviewed individually and together as part of a focus group. The researcher would ask questions about the children's experiences with severe disability and as part of the focus group would encourage members of the group to share their experiences with others and reflect on others' experiences. In this way, close-ended questions for the measurement tool would be generated. The researcher would then clarify those questions by presenting them back to the group, and eventually a set of questions would be identified that adequately reflected the children's R/S experiences. These questions would then be administered in a quantitative study to a much larger group to obtain estimates of reliability and to determine how the items hold together.

TABLE 5.1.

Types of Research Designs

Observational		
Qualitative design	Phenomenology	
	Grounded theory	
	Ethnography	
	Historical	
	Discourse analysis	
	Triangulation	
Quantitative design	Cross-sectional	
		Case-control
		Classical cross-sectional
	Longitudinal	
		Retrospective cohort
		Prospective cohort
Experimental		
Interventions without a control group		
Interventions with a control group (i.e., randomized clinical trials)		

Quantitative

Quantitative observational designs are discussed in greater detail in Chapter 8. I discuss them here with respect to choosing a research design to answer a research question. Research questions that seek to determine the strength of relationships between R/S and health usually require quantitative methods. Quantitative observational designs include cross-sectional (case-control and classical cross-sectional) and longitudinal (retrospective and prospective) cohort studies.

A *case-control design* is optimal for research questions pertaining to subject characteristics that might be etiologically responsible for rare conditions. For example, consider the research question, "What role does intensity of religious belief play in cancer patients who report a spontaneous remission of their cancers?" Spontaneous remission of cancer is a relatively rare phenomenon. The investigator might advertise or otherwise seek to identify individuals whose cancers have spontaneously remitted (cases) and then compare their average level of religious belief with

that of nonremitted cancer patients (controls) matched by cancer type, stage, age, gender, race, and other relevant characteristics. If differences are found (i.e., more intense religious belief among those reporting spontaneous remissions), then the investigator might conclude that an association existed between intensity of religious belief and spontaneous remission of cancer.

Classical cross-sectional study designs are used to determine whether one characteristic is associated with another characteristic at one point in time. An example of a research question that might call for such a design would be, "Is frequency of religious attendance associated with level of depressive symptoms in Catholics living in New York City?" As with case-control studies, such a study can only answer research questions on whether certain characteristics are correlated or associated with one another, not whether one causes the other.

In contrast, *longitudinal studies* (which assess the same group of people several times over time) add the element of time to the relationship, so it now becomes possible to go beyond simple association or correlation and allows the establishment of causal order (i.e., that R/S preceded the health outcome). Retrospective cohort designs are only useful for research questions pertaining to records that have been collected at some time in the past. For example, consider the research question, "Do patients receiving a chaplain visit during acute hospitalization have a lower hospital readmission rate during the five years after their hospital discharge?" If the hospital happened to keep records of everyone receiving a chaplain visit and information on frequency of hospital readmission was also available for the five-year period after discharge, then an investigator could use these records to compare readmission rates between patients receiving a chaplain visit (vs. not) during that period. Records would already be available, and all the researcher has to do is identify those with and without a chaplain visit and then examine the hospital records during the next five years to determine the average number of hospital readmissions in the two groups. The researcher knows that the chaplain visit came first and hospital readmissions occurred during the five years after the chaplain visit. Thus, this research design adds the element of time, but all the information on both predictor (chaplain visit) and outcome (hospital readmissions) has already been collected in the past (hence, retrospective).

Prospective cohort designs also add the element of time (and thus provide evidence for, but not proof of, causality). Instead of having to depend on existing records, however, the researcher assesses participants in the present and then follows them forward in time, assessing outcomes at different time points during the follow-up period. Such a design is useful for research questions similar to those for which a retrospective cohort design might be chosen. Consider the same research question above: "Do patients receiving a chaplain visit during acute hospitalization experience a lower hospital readmission rate during the five years after hospital discharge?" Using a prospective cohort design, the researcher assesses patients admitted to the hospital in the present and determines whether they receive a chaplain visit during that admission. The researcher then follows these patients over the next five years and compares readmission rates of those who did and did not receive a chaplain visit.

Prospective cohort designs have many advantages over retrospective cohort designs: researchers can measure the exposure variable (chaplain visit vs. not) more accurately since they determine this in the present. They can also measure whatever other subject characteristics they wish to (both at baseline and follow-up). In contrast, investigators who use a retrospective cohort design must rely entirely on what others have collected in the past (i.e., how they measured the predictor, controls, and outcome variables) and there is often no way of checking whether this information is accurate; these are the limitations of examining existing records in retrospective studies.

EXPERIMENTAL DESIGNS

Without a Control Group

Experimental studies with and without control groups are discussed in Chapter 9. Again, I focus here on when such designs would be chosen to answer a specific research question.

An experimental study that does not involve a control group can provide preliminary evidence that an intervention is effective. This would be the design of choice if the investigator didn't have the financial resources to conduct a clinical trial that included a control group, since a single-group design is simpler and less expensive (although much less powerful) than a randomized two-group design.

> An experimental study that does not involve a control group can provide preliminary evidence that an intervention is effective.

For example, consider the research question, "Is religious cognitive-behavioral therapy (CBT) effective in reducing depressive symptoms in older adults with chronic pain?" When using an experimental design without a control group, the researcher would simply identify a group of older adults with chronic pain and then administer religious CBT to all of them over twelve weeks, comparing depressive symptoms before the intervention (at baseline) with depressive symptoms after the intervention (at twelve weeks). A significant reduction in depressive symptoms would provide preliminary evidence that the religious CBT was efficacious. This is also called a one-group pretest/posttest design. The weakness of this design is that the depressed patients receiving the intervention might have improved anyway during the twelve weeks due to the natural course of depression. Alternatively, subjects may have improved because they were involved in a study (making them feel better about themselves because they were contributing to scientific knowledge) and were actively engaged with study personnel (providing human interaction and support). Thus, the benefits may have had nothing to do with the religious CBT, but were due instead to simply the passing of time or their participation in a study.

With a Control Group

As noted in chapters 2 and 3, a randomized clinical trial (RCT) is indicated when a research question involves testing whether an intervention is truly efficacious in causing a change in health among those receiving the intervention compared to control subjects without the intervention. When subjects are randomized to either the intervention or control groups and followed over time, any change in the intervention group above and beyond that in the control group can be attributed to the intervention (assuming that randomization was effective and subjects in both groups were similar in all relevant characteristics at baseline). An RCT, however, is much more expensive and difficult to manage than an experimental study without a control group.

> A randomized clinical trial (RCT) is indicated when a research question involves testing whether an intervention is truly efficacious in causing a change in health among those receiving the intervention compared to control subjects without the intervention.

Consider the same research question above, "Is religious cognitive-behavioral therapy (CBT) effective in reducing depressive symptoms in older adults with chronic pain?" This time, subjects are randomized to either the religious CBT intervention or a control group that receives the same evaluations and engages with research staff in exactly the same way as subjects randomized to the religious CBT intervention. Both groups are assessed before and after the intervention. Instead of simply assessing subjects receiving the religious CBT before and after the intervention (as in an experimental study without a control group), the researcher now compares subjects receiving the religious CBT at baseline and follow-up with subjects not receiving the religious CBT to see if there is any difference. If depressive symptoms are reduced significantly more in the religious CBT group compared to the control group, then the investigator can conclude that the religious CBT caused the greater improvement (in this particular example, however, improvement may be due simply to the time spent with therapists delivering the religious CBT; thus, a better design would have those in the control group receiving a comparable intervention but without religious consent).

OTHER CONSIDERATIONS

There are other considerations in choosing a research design besides the best design for the research question. While less important, they are nevertheless relevant to a researcher's choice of design. One consideration has to do with the prior experience of the investigator. Another has to do with the availability of resources to conduct the study.

Investigator Experience

A researcher with experience only in qualitative research would probably not wish to choose a research question that required a quantitative design. Each design is literally a specialized area in itself, with its own terminology and research methods. Qualitative research involves a technical language, a way of collecting data, and a method of analysis that would be foreign to most researchers whose expertise is in cross-sectional and prospective cohort designs, and vice versa. Likewise, the randomized control design involves procedures for identifying subjects and monitoring intervention fidelity that may overwhelm an expert in qualitative or observational designs. Thus, the investigator needs to have training and expertise in the design chosen. If the research question requires a design other than that which the investigator is familiar, then another research question should be chosen—one that can be answered using a design that is familiar to the investigator.

Available Resources

By resources, I mean not only financial ones but also access to subjects and availability of consultants with expertise in the design of choice.

Financial

The amount of funding support available to conduct a study helps determine whether a cross-sectional design with a single assessment or a prospective design with multiple assessments is feasible. A cross-sectional study that involves sending a questionnaire and collecting responses by mail might require little or no support. In contrast, a prospective study would likely require hiring interviewers to administer a questionnaire and then readminister it during follow-up assessments. Locating subjects for such interviews and keeping them motivated and interested in participating also involves personnel time. All of this increases the cost of the study. Likewise, finances determine whether a randomized clinical trial with a control group might be the choice of design vs. a single-group experimental design without controls. As noted earlier, adding a control group complicates the study in an exponential fashion, requiring more personnel and greater monitoring. Thus, a small cross-sectional or qualitative study may be conducted without any funding support at all, whereas a cohort study or experimental study would not usually be possible without support.

Subjects

Even with ample resources, the availability of subjects to participate in the research may affect choice of design. For example, after obtaining NIH support to conduct a prospective study of depression in patients with congestive heart failure, our team was not able to carry out the study as planned since congestive heart failure patients at Duke Hospital were involved in other studies being conducted by their own cardiologists. The cardiologists had no problem with our assessing their patients only once (i.e., using a cross-sectional design), but not if multiple assessments were required that would take up a lot of their time (which was necessary for our prospective design). We could have been forced to conduct only a cross-sectional study because of the lack of available subjects, despite having plentiful NIH funding. A prospective design, however, was our only option, so in order to execute the study as funded, we decided to forget about Duke Hospital and instead enroll CHF patients at another hospital in a different city where the competition for patients was less intense.

Consultants

Choice of design may also depend on the availability of consultants with expertise in that design. We once proposed a study to examine the effect that genetic factors had on depressed patients' response to religious psychotherapy. In order to do the study, we needed consultants both in psychiatric genetics and in managing psychotherapy clinical trials. Consultants were difficult to find, especially those with expertise in genetics, nearly causing us to scrap the entire project and instead do an observational study using an existing data set.

Another factor that may influence design choice is the availability of a statistician with expertise in the particular design. Prospective studies that are competitive for grant funding today require sophisticated methods of longitudinal data analysis as part of the research plan (e.g., analysis of individual subject trajectories over time or use of random effects models). Unless the investigator has access to a statistician with the ability to conduct such analyses, another research design should be chosen.

SUMMARY AND CONCLUSIONS

The choice of research design first and foremost depends on what the investigator's research question is. There are two basic types of design: observational and experimental. These can be further divided into four categories: observational-qualitative, observational-quantitative, experimental without controls, and experimental with controls (e.g., RCT). Research questions having to do with acquiring an in-depth understanding of a phenomenon, identifying an association between two variables, or determining whether an intervention has an effect on a health outcome require different types of design. Other factors also influence choice of design. These include the investigator's experience with a particular design, having adequate funding support, availability of subjects, and availability of consultants.

These latter factors, however important and influential, should not determine the choice of study design. If a design cannot be found that naturally fits the research question, then the investigator needs to consider whether that research question is the right one to be asking.

Selecting a Sample

"SAMPLE" IN CLINICAL research means those who participate in the research and provide data relevant to the study's aims. Deciding on what sample to use and choosing the method of selecting that sample are crucial both for observational and experimental studies. As with choosing a study design, the kind of participants selected to make up a sample depend on the research question. In this chapter I examine the types of samples that are required for different kinds of research questions and then discuss the different ways that participants may be selected for a sample.

TYPES OF POPULATIONS

A *population* is the total membership of a defined group of people. A sample is any subset of a defined population. Depending on the research question, a researcher might choose several kinds of populations, including community-dwelling individuals, individuals being seen in health-care settings (clinical), or those with a specific illness.

Community-Based

Community-based means individuals who are living in the community at the time they participate in the research study. In general, community-based populations include people who are relatively healthy. Community-based populations generally do not include people who are institutionalized—that is, prisoners, nursing home residents, those in mental asylums, or those who are acutely hospitalized. Examples of community-based samples are those included in the General Social Survey, National Survey of Black Americans, Gallup polls, or Pew Foundation surveys.

Research questions related to public health usually involve a community-based population of people who start out relatively healthy and independent. For example, consider the research question we examined earlier in Chapter 4: "What is the relationship between frequency of religious attendance and diastolic blood pressure in Southern Baptists from North Carolina?" This research question requires a sample of community-dwelling persons in North Carolina with a Southern Baptist religious affiliation. Likewise, a research question such as, "Does frequency of prayer affect the likelihood of having a myocardial infarction in people without preexisting heart disease?" would require a community-based sample of people without a history of heart disease. These healthy individuals would likely be selected using a random or probability sampling method and followed over time to determine who developed a myocardial infarction. Frequency of prayer would be examined at baseline

> Depending on the research question, a researcher might choose several kinds of populations, including community-dwelling individuals, individuals being seen in health-care settings (clinical), or those with a specific illness.

as a predictor of those who developed a myocardial infarction. Such a study would involve "public health" because the results would apply to individuals in the general population.

Scandinavian countries are especially known for studies involving community-based samples that involve questions related to public health. The reason is that health information is collected on literally every person in certain geographic regions and is tracked over time as part of these countries' universal health-care system. Thus, entire populations involving tens of thousands of individuals can be studied to identify risk factors for disease.

Most studies involving community-based samples are observational, and usually cross-sectional or prospective in design. Qualitative studies would more likely involve only twenty to forty individuals with a condition of interest, not a general community-dwelling population. Experimental studies would usually select persons, either community dwelling or institutionalized, based on inclusion and exclusion criteria, and would not seek to generalize their findings to the broader population of largely healthy people living in the community.

Clinical

A clinical population consists of individuals with health problems. It may include those with medical problems seeking health care but living in the community (i.e., outpatients) or those residing in an institution (i.e., admitted to a hospital or residing in a nursing home). The key distinction is that these are individuals with health problems who are being treated by health-care professionals, not generally healthy individuals living in the community like a community-based population. There are two types of clinical populations: a population of individuals with a variety of health problems and a population consisting of patients with a specific illness.

General Clinical Population
Research questions related to disability, chronic pain, or chronic mental illness would require a more general clinical population of individuals with health conditions causing these problems.

Such individuals would most easily be identified in medical or psychiatric outpatient clinics or among those admitted to an acute care hospital, nursing home, or psychiatric facility. The investigator might likely select a sample from this population by recruiting consecutive patients seen in a medical/psychiatric clinic or consecutive patients admitted to a hospital. When acquiring a sample of subjects who are chronically institutionalized, such as nursing home patients, recruitment might involve approaching consecutive patients admitted to the facility, approaching the entire population of the facility, or identifying a random subsample of that population. An example of a research question that would require a general clinical sample might be, "What is the effect of religious coping on the course of disability in patients hospitalized with medical illness?"

Population with Specific Illness

This type of clinical population would be recruited if the investigator was interested in the effects of R/S on a specific medical or psychiatric illness rather than on more general physical or psychiatric symptoms. Subjects selected would only be those with the particular condition—for example, individuals with a diagnosis of congestive heart failure (CHF), or those with Alzheimer's disease, or men diagnosed with prostate cancer. The specific illness characterizes the population.

Obviously, such a population would be chosen if the investigator was interested in research questions related to the specific illness. For example, consider the research question, "What is the effect of centering prayer meditation on disease course in those with end-stage congestive heart failure who have a cardiac ejection fraction of less than 15?" This question would require an intervention study where participants with advanced heart failure would be recruited, taught to practice centering prayer, and then their heart failure monitored over time using echocardiograms that measure cardiac ejection fraction. Ideally, CHF patients would be randomized to either centering prayer or to a control group engaged in some other activity besides centering prayer, and then both groups would be assessed at baseline and compared over time.

Summary

The specific type of population the investigator chooses depends on the research question. For studies seeking to determine whether R/S involvement is related to the risk of developing an illness, a sample from a community population of healthy individuals without the condition (or perhaps those at high risk for the condition) would be chosen. For studies seeking to determine the impact of R/S on the course of disability or chronic pain, the investigator would choose a more general sample from a population of individuals with a variety of disabling, painful illnesses. For studies seeking to assess the effects of R/S on the course of a specific medical illness, then individuals with that illness would be chosen. Depending on the research question, there are also other populations besides population-based or clinical types, and these might include special populations such as incarcerated individuals, health-care professionals, police officers, and so forth.

SAMPLING METHODS— OBSERVATIONAL STUDIES

Having discussed different types of populations, I now examine the ways that researchers go about selecting subjects from a population to make up a sample. There are two basic sampling designs: *probability* (where a process of random selection is used so that each case in the population has an equal or known chance of being selected) and *nonprobability* (any process of nonrandom selection). There are four main types of probability sampling: simple random, stratified random, cluster, and systematic. There are four main types of nonprobability sampling: convenience or haphazard, purposive, quota, and referral or snowball. The key distinction is random versus nonrandom. The researcher can generalize with random samples because, under these sampling conditions, statistics can be applied to estimate parameters for the entire population. With nonrandom samples, the meaning of statistical tests is unclear.

> There are two basic sampling designs: *probability* (where a process of random selection is used so that each case in the population has an equal or known chance of being selected) and *nonprobability* (any process of nonrandom selection).

What statistical tests (p-values) really tell us is the probability that an association or difference is likely to exist in the population. With nonprobability samples, statistics are not interpretable in this way because the population is uncertain (however, this doesn't seem to stop researchers from using statistical methods to analyze data from nonrandom samples).

The sampling method chosen depends on the study design. For qualitative observational studies there are a variety of sampling methods used depending on the researcher's goals. These include such techniques as maximum variation sampling, theoretical sampling, convenience sampling, extreme or deviant case sampling, opportunistic sampling, and snowball sampling. For details on qualitative sampling methods, readers are referred elsewhere.[1] Deciding on how to identify potential respondents is important for qualitative research, although it is not clear that the sampling method is as important in qualitative research as it is in quantitative research.

For quantitative observational studies the sampling method is critical in cross-sectional and prospective cohort research designs, where obtaining generalizable results is a major goal. This is particularly true for R/S-health research since 90 percent of all quantitative research is of this type. I focus here on three general sampling methods used in quantitative observational studies: convenience sampling, systematic sampling (nonrandom and random), and random sampling (simple).

Convenience Sampling

A convenience sample takes the least amount of energy and fewest resources. Researchers recruit into the study anyone immediately available and willing to participate. For example, a researcher wants to examine the relationship between frequency of Bible reading and well-being. Not having much financial support or time to devote to the project, the researcher develops a questionnaire, prints one hundred copies, and creates a large sign that reads, "Please fill out my questionnaire." He then takes his questionnaires and sign, walks to the corner of the street, and holds up the sign so that anyone driving by can see it. As people drive by, they must decide on whether to stop and fill out the questionnaire. The researcher does this until one hundred people complete the questionnaire. The sample thus acquired is called a *convenience sample.*

With a convenience sample there is very little pressure on subjects to participate in the study. Those who do participate are likely to be nice people who want to help others and are interested in the topic of the research. In this case, participants would probably be those who are interested in religion (and are therefore more religious). Of course, these tendencies introduce tremendous bias into the results and affect to whom the results can be generalized (in this case, nice religious people who live or work near the researcher).

There is a difference between sample selection bias and generalization. Generalization is simply a function of sampling. If random sampling is employed, the researcher can generalize to a defined population. The problem raised in the previous example is one of nonprobability sampling (i.e., sampling bias). Convenience samples have a lot of special social, psychological, and biological features that make them unique, but these features are unknown because there is no defined population. With probability samples, researchers can compare characteristics of their sample with population estimates from the census or previous probability samples of the sample population. When characteristics of their sample deviate from population estimates, then researchers know that theirs is not a probability sample. Such comparisons are not possible with convenience samples.

The findings from the study described above will tell us very little about the relationship between Bible reading and well-being in the general population, even the general population of this particular geographic location. The reason is that the general population consists of religious and nonreligious persons, nice and not-so-nice people, and those who live in many different geographical locations, perhaps neighborhoods quite different from the neighborhood in which the researcher lives.

Many of the early studies reporting on the relationship between R/S and health consisted of students in classes that the researcher taught. First-year psychology or sociology undergraduates were especially likely to be recruited into such studies since they were readily available to researchers (i.e., their professors). In those days, there was no funding for this type of research so investigators had to get by with whatever was easiest and cheapest. There was good rationale for including students in such studies since this was one way to teach students how to do research. Students who participated would often get academic credit for doing so. Convenience samples can even result when a random sampling technique is used if the "response rate" is too low. The response rate is the percentage of persons approached who agree to participate (see discussion below). Technically, however, the response rate does not change the sampling method. Even with low response rates, researchers can do a decent job of estimating the population. Because the researcher has a defined population when using a random sampling method, she can see where the sample might over- or underrepresent certain groups, and then apply "weights" to better approximate the population.

Systematic Sampling

There are two types of systematic sampling. One involves nonrandom sampling and the other involves random sampling. An illustration of systematic nonrandom sampling would be consecutively admitted patients to a hospital. A list of all admissions to the hospital on a certain day would be obtained, and starting at the top of the list, the researcher would go down the list and approach every patient on the list in order of their admission. A systematic sample acquired using this method is considered better than a convenience sample since this procedure follows a system that can be described and replicated in other settings. Consequently, the results can be generalized (to some extent) to others not actually in the sample.

Recall the example presented earlier where a researcher printed out one hundred questionnaires and stood on the corner of the block holding up a sign requesting that people driving by stop and fill out the questionnaire. A researcher who wanted to recruit a more systematic sample might change tactics. Instead of simply standing on the corner and holding up a sign, the researcher might step out into the street and stop every car that comes by and ask motorists to fill out the questionnaire. The researcher would need to keep a record of the percentage of people approached who actually filled out the questionnaire (to calculate a response rate). This would be considered systematic sampling, and if the response rate was reasonable (see below), the sample acquired would be considered a systematic sample. Of course, there would still be plenty of problems with a sample acquired in this manner. First, all participants would have to own a car and be able to drive. Second, depending on the day or time of the day the study was conducted, the researcher might miss many working individuals who were already at their jobs. Third, participants would likely be those who lived or worked in the researcher's neighborhood and may not be representative of the socioeconomic distribution in other neighborhoods. Finally, those who did participate might still be nicer people than those who didn't, and they might also be more religious. Thus, the sample acquired in this manner would be biased in many ways that could affect the researcher's ability to generalize results to those who did not participate in the study. However, this method is still better than convenience sampling.

Systematic sampling should not be confused with *systematic random sampling*, a specific type of random sampling. In that case, the researcher would get a complete list of all members of a defined population. She would then calculate a sampling interval (the ratio of the number of cases in the population to the desired sample size). A sampling interval of twenty-five would mean that the researcher would select every twenty-fifth case on the original list. The key is to begin with a random start (randomly choose a case between person 1 and person 25), and then select every twenty-fifth person on the list.

Random Sampling (Probability Sampling)

One way to obtain a representative sample of a population is to approach and successfully recruit every person in the population. This, however, is usually impractical since the entire population may consist of thousands or millions of people and the researcher may not have sufficient resources to survey everyone. The best way of obtaining a representative sample for a study whose results can be generalized to the entire population—even those not participating in the study—is to collect a random subsample of individuals from that population. By "random," I don't mean haphazardly selecting people at random. The investigator must follow an established method for identifying a random sample. As noted above, there are four different methods, including simple random, stratified random, systematic (discussed above), and cluster sampling. When several different types are used in a single study, this is called multistage sampling. I discuss here the simple and stratified types, which are most commonly used in R/S-health research.

Simple Random Sampling

The first step in identifying a simple random sample of a population is to develop a list of all members of the population to which the researcher wishes to generalize. The researcher must then use an established method to identify a random subsample from that population. One method is picking numbers out of a hat. Let's say that the entire population consists of one thousand individuals. A unique identifying number ranging from 1 to 1,000 would be assigned to each person in the population, and these numbers would be written on separate pieces of paper. All one thousand pieces of paper would then be placed in the hat, shaken vigorously so that all pieces of paper become randomly distributed. The researcher would then reach into the hat one hundred times (or however large the researcher wishes the sample to be), picking out one piece of paper at a time. The numbers on the one hundred pieces of paper each correspond to an individual in the population. These individuals then represent a random subsample of the population. If all those selected agreed to participate, then the results from these one hundred participants could be generalized to the entire population of one thousand persons, even to the nine hundred who did not participate in the study. If all of the one hundred subjects do not agree to participate, then the question is whether there is any systematic nonresponse, which would make the sample systematically different from those who did not participate. If, however, the investigator could make the case that participants randomly refused to participate, then she could still generalize her results to the overall population.

A second method of random sampling uses a computer to generate a list of random numbers. This is easier than the above example and "looks better" than picking numbers out of a hat. Assuming again that there are one thousand people in the overall population each with a unique identifying number, the computer would generate one hundred random numbers between 1 and 1000. Those individuals to whom the random numbers were assigned would then be approached to participate in the study. Other methods of selecting a random subsample might use a table of random numbers to identify one hundred unique random numbers out of one thousand, or researchers might use a mechanical device like a ball machine with balls numbered between 1 and 1000 (quite popular in state lotteries). Using any of these approaches, the investigator could select a random subsample of one hundred individuals to participate in the study.

Stratified Random Sampling
(Proportional or Quota Sampling)

If certain characteristics of individuals are likely to influence the results of the study and the investigator wants to be sure that adequate numbers of persons with those characteristics are included in the sample, then stratified random sampling would be used. Random sampling is often stratified on the basis of characteristics such as gender, race, or socioeconomic status, especially in situations where, for example, gender influences the outcome and men are less likely to participate in a study than women, or race affects the outcome and blacks are less likely to participate than whites. In this case, investigators would divide the overall population of one thousand individuals into homogeneous subgroups (men, women, blacks, whites, etc.) and then take a random subsample from each subgroup until they acquired the number of subjects needed.

Response Rate

Once a random (or systematic) sample of individuals is identified, as noted above, this does not mean that everyone will agree to participate in the study. At this point, the response rate becomes important. Again, the response rate is the number of persons who participate in the study divided by the total number of persons that the investigator approaches (one hundred in our example here). Therefore, if only forty of those one hundred people agree to participate, then the response rate is 40 percent. The researcher may go back to those who did not agree to participate and try to convince them to change their minds in order to increase the response rate. While a few more individuals may agree, it is likely that even after going back two or three times, only about twenty more individuals will likely agree to participate, resulting in an overall response rate of 60 percent (sixty out of one hundred).

> The response rate is the number of persons who participate in the study divided by the total number of persons that the investigator approaches.

Replacement

If one hundred persons are really needed to participate in the study and only sixty out of one hundred have agreed, then the researcher may take another random subsample of forty persons from the population (those who were not selected in the first one-hundred-member subsample), and approach them to see if they would be willing to participate. It is likely, however, that only about 40 percent of those forty individuals are likely to agree, and even if the researcher goes back two or three times to convince them to participate, only about 20 percent more will likely agree. This procedure would increase the researcher's sample from sixty (obtained from the first random sample of one hundred persons) to eighty-four (i.e., an addition of twenty-four persons [$0.40 \times 40 + 0.20 \times 40 = 24$]). Thus, the researcher would still not have the one hundred participants needed. The process could be repeated several times over again until one hundred subjects were obtained. This procedure used for random sampling could also be used for systematic sampling to achieve the desired sample size. Replacement, however, would not be used for collecting a convenience sample, since the investigator will simply approach as many people as needed until he acquires the desired sample size.

When a replacement procedure is used, the likelihood that the sample obtained is truly representative still depends on the response rate. The response rate in the above example would be 60 percent, and this is what would be reported. The investigator would then need to carefully describe the replacement procedures in the methods section of the proposed study and any reports of the results.

Adequate Response Rates

Rather than replace nonparticipants when conducting random or systematic sampling to achieve a desired sample size, however, most investigators simply make every effort to enroll the initial subjects selected (by offering various enticements or making multiple attempts to convince subjects to participate) and then report the response rate. An adequate response rate for a sample to be considered systematic or random (vs. a convenience) depends on whether lack of response produces a "nonresponse bias," which happens when those who do not respond display characteristics that are systematically different from those who do respond. This then becomes the primary question. If the investigator has selected a random sample, then even a response rate of 5 percent would produce a representative sample. Generally speaking, a response rate of around 60 to 80 percent is probably needed for a sample to be representative of the entire population. The nonresponse bias is what researchers must worry about.

> Generally speaking, a response rate of around 70 to 80 percent is probably needed for a sample to be representative of the entire population. The nonresponse bias is what researchers must worry about.

For this reason, investigators should obtain as much information as possible about nonrespondents—that is, those who refused to participate in the study. Such information will be useful for arguing that those individuals who did agree to participate were representative of the total population and were not systematically different from nonparticipants in important ways that may bias the results. For example, if nonparticipant information can be obtained on age, gender, or race (especially if those factors are known to influence study outcomes), then the researcher can compare the characteristics of participants with those of the nonparticipants, and if there is no significant difference, the researcher can argue that nonparticipants were similar to participants. If individuals refuse to participate, however, it may not be allowable to use information about their age, race, or gender (even if readily available), since they did not give permission to use that information. The investigator should consult with the Institutional Review Board (IRB) to see if it will allow the use of data on nonparticipants if available. Even without information on nonrespondents, the researcher may use population data to compare the characteristics of their sample (those who did respond) to known population parameters (census) or previous studies of the same population.

Weighting

When either convenience sampling or systematic sampling is used, this introduces biases into the data that are often difficult to predict and can affect the researcher's conclusions. Most statistical tests assume that the sampling method is representative (i.e., random). Even when a random sampling method is used, as noted above, low response rates can affect whether the data collected are representative. Weighting techniques can be applied during the statistical analysis phase to convert an acquired sample into one that is more representative of the true population, at least in terms of demographics such as age, race, or gender. Almost all large epidemiological studies use weighting.

Final Considerations

Much thought should be given to the sampling method, especially for cross-sectional studies. The lowest-quality study is a cross-sectional study that uses convenience sampling. For a cross-sectional study to be funded or published today, random sampling is often needed. The sampling method determines if the sample chosen will be representative. Random sampling is less essential to identify subjects for a prospective cohort study, especially if the subjects followed have a specific medical or psychiatric condition (e.g., post-myocardial infarction or major depression) and the primary research question is to identify predictors of disease outcome or course. However, in large prospective surveys that track groups of the general population over time, such as the National Longitudinal Study of Adolescent Health or Establishing Populations for Epidemiological Studies of the Elderly, random sampling is usually employed to acquire the baseline sample.

SAMPLING METHODS— EXPERIMENTAL STUDIES

Unlike for quantitative observational studies, the particular sampling method (as described above) is less important for experimental studies, because the goal of experiments is to establish cause and effect, not to generalize. Furthermore, elaborate experimental designs (controlled settings) may not allow for probability sampling because it's not feasible. What is important, however, are the inclusion and exclusion (I/E) criteria that define the kind of participants researchers want in their study. While I/E criteria are also important for defining the sample for observational studies, they are particularly important for experimental studies since these will help to avoid including subjects who might be harmed by the intervention or for whom the intervention is not relevant. I/E criteria are equally important for experimental studies with and without a control group. Researchers often recruit subjects for experimental studies not by approaching subjects themselves (as in observational studies) but by posting advertisements in health-care facilities or in the local newspaper that seek volunteers or referrals from health professionals. Those advertisements often include the I/E criteria. Subjects who volunteer to participate or referrals from health professionals then undergo a rigorous evaluation to see whether they fulfill the I/E criteria. To illustrate how researchers use I/E criteria, I discuss below an experimental study where we sought to examine

> Unlike for quantitative observational studies, the particular sampling method (as described above) is less important for experimental studies.

> While I/E criteria are also important for defining the sample for observational studies, they are particularly important for experimental studies.

the effects of religious psychotherapy as a treatment for major depression in patients with chronic disabling medical illness.

Inclusion Criteria

Inclusion criteria are the primary characteristics that make subjects eligible for the study.[2] These criteria must be carefully defined and then assessed using an objective measure so that all subjects are recruited into the trial in the same manner. This is done in order to characterize the sample so that other researchers seeking to replicate the results of the present study will enroll similar subjects in their studies. In the psychotherapy study referred to above, the inclusion criteria were major depression (diagnosed with a structured clinical interview and fulfilling DSM-IV criteria), moderately severe depression (Beck Depression Inventory scores of 16 to 35), onset of depression within the past twelve months, and chronic disabling medical illness (six months or more of an ICD-10 medical diagnosis and difficulty functioning in six of twelve activities of daily living). In addition, subjects had to be ages eighteen to seventy-five, speak English, have adequate hearing and vision, be able to type fluently, and have access to the Internet or have a telephone (since intervention was to be delivered online by instant messaging or by telephone). Finally, subjects had to be religious in order to participate in a religious psychotherapy—that is, they had to indicate that religion was at least somewhat important to them.

Exclusion Criteria

Exclusion criteria make subjects ineligible for the study. In the psychotherapy study above, characteristics that excluded subjects were significant suicidal thoughts (assessed using a standard measure of risk), significant cognitive impairment (assessed using a standard measure of cognitive function), current treatment with antidepressant medication or psychotherapy, any ICD-10 medical diagnosis directly affecting the immune system or stress hormone levels (since these were a target of the intervention), and presence of other active psychiatric problems such as bipolar disorder, schizophrenia, alcohol or drug abuse/dependence, or posttraumatic stress disorder (all diagnosed using a structured psychiatric interview). The exclusion criteria were chosen based on the influence that these characteristics might have on subjects' response to the psychotherapy intervention. Our aim was to limit the influence of other factors likely to affect response so that we could detect the unique effect of the religious psychotherapy. Sometimes it may be difficult to decide whether a characteristic should be an inclusion or an exclusion criterion, because one may simply be the opposite of the other.

Homogeneous vs. Heterogeneous Criteria

Another purpose of I/E criteria is to enroll into a clinical trial subjects who are as similar as possible. The more homogeneous subjects that are in an experimental study, the easier it is to detect the effect of the intervention. If subjects are too dissimilar, these differences may affect the outcome being studied, increase variability, and reduce the likelihood of detecting an effect. The researcher's desire to achieve a homogeneous sample by instituting strict inclusion and exclusion criteria, however, must be balanced by the need to recruit sufficient subjects into the trial to reach the desired sample size. Too many inclusion and exclusion criteria make it more difficult to recruit subjects into the trial, reducing the sample size and the power to detect the intervention's effect. Achieving the target sample size is very important since many clinical trials end up having to be discontinued because researchers cannot recruit enough subjects. Desperate to enroll the necessary number of subjects, however, researchers may broaden their I/E criteria to increase enrollment. Unfortunately, this increases the heterogeneity of the sample. The more heterogeneous the sample, the greater the likelihood that differences among participants will have unpredictable effects on the outcome, reducing the study's ability to detect the intervention's effect. Thus, researchers must

> The more homogeneous subjects that are in an experimental study, the easier it is to detect the effect of the intervention.

> The more heterogeneous the sample, the greater the likelihood that differences among participants will have unpredictable effects on the outcome, reducing the study's ability to detect the intervention's effect.

walk a fine line when deciding on and sticking to I/E criteria for a study.

SUMMARY AND CONCLUSIONS

The sample that a researcher chooses for a study is determined by the research question. Basic population types (out of which samples are drawn) include community-dwelling healthy individuals and those with health problems in clinical settings (outpatients, patients acutely hospitalized, or patients living in long-term-care institutions). Populations of individuals with health problems may consist of those with different medical conditions (where disability, pain, or other general physical symptoms are the outcomes of interest) or those with specific illnesses (where the particular illness or course of that illness is the outcome of interest). The methods of selecting a sample include nonrandom and random sampling. The best way of choosing a sample is to use a random sampling method, because this will allow the results to be generalized beyond those individuals participating in the study (if nonresponse bias is not a problem). The sampling method is less important for experimental studies, since the goal of experiments is to establish cause and effect, not to generalize. In both observational and experimental studies, the researcher needs to specify inclusion and exclusion criteria to define the population to whom the results of the study will apply, and so that other researchers seeking to replicate the results of the study will enroll similar subjects in their studies. Choosing I/E criteria that achieve a balance between homogeneity and heterogeneity can be a real challenge in experimental studies.

Qualitative Research

Not everything that can be counted counts,
and not everything that counts can be counted.
Albert Einstein

I PROVIDE A BRIEF overview of qualitative research in this chapter. Admittedly, I am not an expert in qualitative methods and so will not try to provide an in-depth description of this group of research designs. However, religion/spirituality (R/S) health researchers—even those who only do quantitative research—need to know something about these methods and their unique contributions. Qualitative research is widely used not only in nursing, social work, and the social sciences, but also in marketing research, education studies, management studies, communication studies, and many other fields. Within medicine, qualitative studies may involve a single case report or a series of case reports, where researchers provide an in-depth description of a single case from beginning to end with follow-up information, or may do this for a series of cases, looking for common features between the cases.

> Qualitative methods fit remarkably well with the kinds of questions asked by R/S researchers, which may be difficult to answer using quantitative methods alone.

Until the 1970s, qualitative methods were limited to studies in anthropology and sociology. As qualitative methods began to expand into other disciplines in the 1980s and 1990s, they began to receive criticism from quantitative researchers, who claimed that this type of research was highly subjective, unreliable, and imprecise.[1] Over the last ten to twenty years, the field of qualitative research has responded with the development of new methods that have now addressed many earlier concerns.[2] Qualitative methods fit remarkably well with the kinds of questions asked by R/S researchers, which may be difficult to answer using quantitative methods alone. Those who are most interested in doing R/S-health research are often nurses, chaplains, social workers, and other social scientists who are trained in and familiar with this approach. I have found that investigators who tend to be people persons are naturally interested in the detailed life experiences and personal stories that are at the heart of qualitative research.

IMPORTANCE

> Qualitative studies are crucial for the development of hypotheses and for explaining findings from quantitative research.

Qualitative methods focus on the why and how. In R/S-health research, qualitative studies examine why R/S is related to health and how this relationship comes about in certain individuals and in certain contexts. Qualitative methods are ideally suited for answering such questions. However, they provide information only on the particular cases that are being studied and can make only partial generalizations and conclusions. Qualitative studies are crucial for the development of hypotheses and for explaining findings from quantitative research. A major strength of the qualitative approach is that it can provide rich, in-depth explanation and descriptions, which is usually not possible with quantitative research methods.

CHARACTERISTICS

Qualitative research focuses on answers to questions related to social experience, how it is created, and how it gives meaning to life. It allows multiple perspectives of the same reality to surface. There are seven basic characteristics:[3]

1. Belief that multiple realities exist and create meaning for the individual.
2. Belief that multiple realities require multiple approaches for collecting data.
3. Commitment to the participant's view of reality, rather than allowing the researcher's preconceived views to define reality.
4. Interviews take place in the natural context of the phenomenon (e.g., at the bedside of a dying patient or under the bridge where a person with schizophrenia sleeps).
5. Investigator is not separate from the research but considered an instrument of the study.
6. Participants determine the truth of the findings and give feedback to the researcher on whether findings reflect their lived experience.
7. Findings reported using a rich literary style that includes quotes and commentaries.

These characteristics distinguish qualitative research from quantitative studies. In *quantitative research* the emphasis is on objectivity, examination of a highly focused single reality, reductionism, control, and prediction. The predictors and outcomes must be measurable and quantifiable, and the parts must sum up to equal the whole. Statistical tests are used to analyze data that are context free, and researchers seek to generalize the results to other settings. The researcher is an outside observer who makes every effort to avoid influencing the data collection and so seeks to remain as separate from the research as possible. Those who participate in quantitative research are called "subjects" in order to objectify the entire process.

> In *quantitative* research the emphasis is on objectivity, study of a highly focused single reality, reductionism, control, and prediction. In contrast, *qualitative* research places value on subjectivity.

In contrast, *qualitative research* places value on subjectivity. Rather than focusing on one reality, qualitative methods emphasize the study of multiple realities. Discovery, description, and understanding a phenomenon are stressed, as opposed to reduction, control, and prediction. Rather than emphasizing measurement, qualitative research focuses on interpretation. In such interpretation, researchers may describe, account for, and make meaning of nuance and ambiguity in findings. While quantitative research requires that all parts must equal the whole, qualitative approaches view the whole as being much greater than the sum of individual parts. Rather than reporting numerical findings using statistical tests, qualitative methods report in-depth stories of participants' experiences. Finally, rather than being separate from the data collection process and context free, the researcher is part of a process that is considered context dependent. Finally, those who participate in the study are called "participants" rather than "subjects," again emphasizing their unique role in the study beyond simply providing answers to close-ended questions.[4]

APPROACHES

Qualitative research consists of six basic approaches: phenomenology, grounded theory, ethnography, historical research, discourse analysis, and triangulation.

Phenomenology

This approach is designed to describe a particular phenomenon or the appearance of things as a lived experience. Phenomenological methods focus on the contents of consciousness and provide ways of describing and analyzing those contents. Originally, phenomenology focused on describing researchers' own thoughts, feelings, and perceptions, such as the emotions experienced during anger or the cognitive processes involved in decision-making. Personal biases clearly influenced reports of this nature. Over time, other methods of examining phenomena were developed. Now this approach involves the researcher asking participants to write down or provide verbal descriptions of their experiences (such as the experience of visual hallucinations by a participant who is psychotic), with the goal of understanding participants' experiences as they experience them.

Grounded Theory

This is probably the most widely known and used qualitative method, and the most common one in R/S-health research. Developed in the 1960s, this method seeks to develop a theory about a phenomenon of interest that is grounded or rooted in observation.[5] Grounded theory involves an iterative process that goes from the general to the more specific. The researcher starts by asking some very general questions about a subject to identify core theoretical concepts. Loose linkages are then developed between these theoretical concepts and the responses provided by participants. The process starts out very open and can take literally months of interviewing before reaching its end. Strategies for analyzing the data collected from participants include coding (categorizing the data and describing the implications and details of these categories), memoing (recording the thoughts and ideas of the researcher as they evolve throughout the study), and creating integrative diagrams (used to pull the details together into a theory that makes sense of the data). As the research progresses, the researcher becomes more involved in verifying and summarizing the data. The initial core theories are revised over time, with the objective of identifying a well-considered explanation that is central to understanding the phenomenon—that is, the grounded theory. This process of refinement can go on indefinitely as the researcher approaches the true explanation.

Ethnography

This approach comes largely from the field of anthropology and involves the study of culture. Originally, "culture" was linked to a particular ethnicity or geographical location (inland tribes on Madagascar, for example). However, this has now broadened to include other defined groups and organizations as well (Buddhist herdsmen from Nepal, soldiers in Afghanistan, or even members of a local Lions Club). Participant observation is a key aspect of this form of qualitative research. In other words, researchers actually live in and immerse themselves into the culture as active participants and record their observations and experiences in field notes. The researcher seeks to have no limits on what may be observed. Again, as in grounded theory, there is an iterative process of acquiring information that goes on without any clear termination point as the truth is approximated.

Historical

Historical research involves systematic collection and objective evaluation of data in order to study interrelationships among ideas, events, institutions, or people in the past. The purpose is to test hypotheses concerning causes of, effects on, or trends in these events that may help to explain present events and anticipate future events. This method helps to answer questions such as, where have we come from, where are we now, and where are we going? Rather than interview participants, the researcher uses the techniques of library and information science[6] to identify primary sources of information (e.g., firsthand accounts, such as personal diaries, eyewitness accounts of events, or oral histories). Secondary sources may also be useful (e.g., reports or accounts by someone other than those who actually participated in or observed the event of interest), giving the researcher a better understanding of the topic and providing bibliographic information for further evidence-gathering.

Discourse Analysis

In this method, written language and spoken language are studied for their social significance. Researchers examine themes, patterns, sequences, and the use of particular words and phrases in recorded discourse. They then consider how these findings lend interpretive weight to their work.

Triangulation

Triangulation involves using a combination of the five methods above in a single study. The goal is to balance strategies so that each counterbalances the errors in the other, as exemplified by a group of blind people describing an elephant.

Triangulation also facilitates validation of data through cross-verification. This may involve the use of different sets of data, different types of analyses, different researchers, or different theoretical perspectives on a particular phenomenon. Techniques involve interviewing, observation, document analysis, or any other feasible approach, including combining qualitative and quantitative methods. Rather than seeing triangulation as a method for validation or verification, some qualitative researchers use this technique to ensure that an account is rich, robust, comprehensive, and well developed.

LITERATURE REVIEW

In quantitative research, the investigator must do an exhaustive review of the existing research literature before embarking on a study. In qualitative research, particularly when using the grounded theory approach, some researchers do only a limited literature review before the study. The purpose is to not bias the researcher with preconceived ideas that might limit vision and reduce openness to what study participants are saying. The literature review is not used to establish grounds for the study, and the aim is not to confirm existing findings. The purpose, often done after the data from the study is collected and analyzed, is to place the findings in the context of what is already known.

However, qualitative researchers have different views on this. Educational researchers in particular may do an extensive literature review and include this in their research proposals. This allows researchers to locate themselves within a body of work and to converse with it from the beginning. It also provides a basis for identifying and honing their own perspectives as they carry out their studies. Thus, while some qualitative researchers may steer away from initially familiarizing themselves with a body of literature to avoid bias, this is not true for all and may not even be true for the majority (depending on the discipline).

THE SAMPLE AND SETTING

Participants (or informants) take part in a study to help a researcher better understand their lives, experiences, and

> The participants in a qualitative study do not have to be randomly or systematically identified but instead can be selected purposefully, based on whether they have certain characteristics.

> Often only twenty to thirty subjects are needed to provide the kind of information that the qualitative researcher is seeking. The sample size is determined not by a power analysis as in quantitative studies, but rather by saturation.

social interactions. The participants in a qualitative study do not have to be randomly or systematically identified but instead can be selected purposefully, based on whether they have certain characteristics (e.g., have been severely traumatized during a natural disaster, have an illness such as cancer) or are located in certain contexts (e.g., a mental hospital, a hospice). The setting of the research is the field—the natural, unaltered circumstances where individuals of interest experience the phenomenon.

Because qualitative methods focus on the why and how of a phenomenon, smaller sample sizes are usually needed (compared to quantitative studies where sample size contributes to the likelihood of achieving statistical significance). Often only twenty to thirty subjects are needed to provide the kind of information that the qualitative researcher is seeking. The sample size is determined not by a power analysis as in quantitative studies (Chapter 21), but rather by saturation. *Saturation* occurs when the data being collected become repetitive so that additional data only confirm what has already been learned.

GENERATION OF DATA

Depending on the particular method, data are usually generated through open-ended and semi-structured interviews. This may involve narrative picturing, focus groups, written narratives, personal stories, participant observation, or extensive field notes. *Narrative picturing* combines private visualization with verbal narration in a process where informants are freed from the interactive dialogue of the interview to enter into their private thoughts, feelings, and experiences, allowing the images that describe their world, either lived or fantasized, to emerge spontaneously. In this way, the phenomenon is made more alive through participant engagement, improving the description and minimizing the influence of the researcher. A *focus group* consists of a group of six to ten participants who meet together and are asked to discuss their perceptions, opinions, beliefs, and attitudes toward a subject. In this interactive group setting, the researcher asks questions to members of the group who are free to talk with the researcher and other group members. Advantages of this method are that it is less expensive, can get results quickly, and can increase sample size and reduce time by talking with several participants at once.

Written narratives involve participants writing about their experiences. One benefit of this method is the provision of higher-quality information than verbal reports since it allows participants to think about what they wish to say. A second benefit is that it is less expensive because there are no transcription costs involved (as in verbal reports). The disadvantage of written narratives is that responses lack spontaneity, since they may be thought through and changed. *Personal stories* are descriptions of experiences reported verbally by participants, which are recorded and often analyzed line by line for content. These may involve full autobiographies or be focused more around a particular event or experience.

Participant observation involves researcher participation in a group or immersion in a culture in order to gain close and intimate familiarity with the group (religious, occupational, subculture, or community). It typically involves intense involvement with members of the group in their natural setting and may take place over long periods of time. Data are usually collected through informal interviews, direct observation, group discussions, examining personal documents, self-reflection, or collection of life histories. *Field notes* involve written documentation by the researcher of personal observations, feelings, or experiences while interviewing individual participants or interacting with group members in various natural settings.

> The qualitative researcher usually ends up with a lot of data that range from handwritten notes to transcripts from audiotapes to visual documents from pictures or videotapes. One of the biggest challenges is how to handle these data—that is, reducing, organizing, analyzing, and interpreting them.

ANALYZING THE DATA

The qualitative researcher usually ends up with a lot of data that range from handwritten notes to transcripts from audiotapes to visual documents from pictures or videotapes. One of the biggest challenges is how to handle these data—that is, reducing, organizing, analyzing, and interpreting them.[7] A variety of software packages are now available to analyze qualitative data (Atlas.ti, Ethnograph, HyperRESEARCH, nVivo, MaxQDA, C-I-Said, AnSWR, and so forth).[8] The objective of these software programs is to identify and categorize common data or themes, which can also be done by hand but with much more labor on the researcher's part.

> The greatest strength of these research methods is that they provide data that are rich, detailed, deep with meaning, salient, and relevant.

Whether using an analysis program or not, there are important steps in this process. The researcher should become familiar with the data by reading and rereading the text or listening to or watching taped recordings several times. The researcher must first determine the quality of the data. Sometimes the information does not add meaning or value, or may have been collected in a biased way. Next, the investigator should review the purpose of the study and identify key questions, and then organize the data by each of these questions, examining responses by all participants to identify consistencies and differences. Alternatively, the researcher may decide to group participant responses by case, individual, or group, depending on the goal of the research. Common themes are identified, and data are summarized into coherent categories (either preset categories determined beforehand or those emerging from the data). Next, patterns and connections between categories are identified. The software packages listed above can assist with this process. Using the categories/themes and connections between them, the researcher must then interpret the data by explaining what it all means and what is important.

PROBLEMS WITH QUALITATIVE RESEARCH

The greatest strength of these research methods is that they provide data that are rich, detailed, deep with meaning, salient, and relevant. Weaknesses include that it can be expensive and labor intensive, and the personality of the investigator may influence results. The most common criticisms of qualitative research include its "soft approach" that uses subjective procedures (i.e., lack of objectivity) and dependence on small samples that make the findings difficult to apply to anyone beyond the immediate participants in the study (i.e., problems with generalizability). Qualitative methods are viewed by some as too subjective and potentially influenced by the preexisting biases of the investigator, who can "read" into the data almost anything. As a result, qualitative research has become an unpopular method within the mainstream medical community, which has been trained to make decisions based on the results of quantitative studies and is largely unfamiliar with qualitative methods or how rigorous they have become. Rapid progress in the scientific development of qualitative methods is changing these common misconceptions, and there are now a number of highly credible qualitative research journals in the field. Furthermore, many of the concerns above are those used to critique quantitative studies; instead, researchers should apply standards to qualitative studies that are part of the paradigm of qualitative methods (e.g., credibility, trustworthiness). Otherwise, the result is a comparison of apples and oranges, using only one measuring stick that applies to one method and not the other.

> The most common criticisms of qualitative research include its "soft approach" that uses subjective procedures (i.e., lack of objectivity) and dependence on small samples that make the findings from such research difficult to apply to anyone beyond the immediate participants in the study.

In some cases, however, negative perceptions of qualitative research have a basis in reality, since qualitative methods are interpretive and implicit, rather than explicit and open to replication, making reliability and validity difficult to establish. Most open-ended interviews (the vast majority of qualitative research) involve the joint construction of an account between the researcher and the participant. When qualitative research occurs in health-care settings, the problem is that health-care researchers and the patients they interview both "have become highly practiced and defensive in the way they construct accounts."[9] Thus, given differences in perception that may be further magnified by the effects of cultural and political factors, it may be difficult to arrive at a complete and accurate picture. As a result, getting funding for qualitative research may be a real challenge, especially from government sources (NIH, NSF) and private foundations (Templeton). This frustration leads researchers away from qualitative methods, especially if they

> Quantitative research is not immune from problems either, and suffers from the fact that it often strips away the context and complexity of individual stories to arrive at an outcome that is objective and replicable but superficial and sometimes meaningless.

are in academia, because they have the added stress of trying to get tenure and so need to get grants.

While qualitative research does have problems, quantitative research is not immune from problems either, and suffers from the fact that it often strips away the context and complexity of individual stories to arrive at an outcome that is objective and replicable but superficial and sometimes meaningless. The truth is that qualitative and quantitative methods serve unique and different purposes, and the quality of each research method is determined by different criteria as well. Rigor in quantitative research is determined by its narrowness, conciseness, and objectivity, based on rigid adherence to research designs and precise statistical analyses. In contrast, rigor in qualitative research is determined by openness, scrupulous adherence to a philosophical perspective, thoroughness in collecting data, and consideration of all the data in the development of theory.

Summary and Conclusions

Qualitative methods are often ideal for R/S and health research, where relationships cannot be fully described by relying on quantitative methods alone. Qualitative research seeks to answer questions related to social experience, how it is created, and how it gives meaning to life. These methods are crucial early in a research program to obtain a deeper and richer understanding of a phenomenon, and are also important later on when the results of quantitative studies need interpretation and application to clinical practice. Qualitative processes leave room for addressing emergent and significant issues, problems and questions that were not part of the original research design. Qualitative methods of collecting information include phenomenology, grounded theory, ethnography, historical research, discourse analysis, and triangulation, each with inherent strengths for answering specific research questions. The data gathered from such approaches include narrative picturing, information from focus groups, written narratives, personal stories from verbal accounts, investigator observations from immersion within a group, and detailed field notes, depending on method.

Qualitative research has for many years been unpopular within the mainstream medical community, a group that is largely unfamiliar with this methodology and has been trained in a world where quantitative research rules. Common criticisms of qualitative research are that it is a soft approach that uses subjective procedures that provide weak explanations (lack of objectivity) and that the findings often reported from small samples are difficult to apply more generally (lack of generalizability). The reality is that quantitative and qualitative methods each serve unique and complementary purposes. The goal of quantitative research is to verify truth and predict outcomes, whereas the goal of qualitative research is to discover meaning and understanding. I strongly encourage that all research studies on R/S and health include a combination of quantitative and qualitative methods (mixed methods), since both are needed to arrive at a complete picture of what is really going on.

Observational Research

OBSERVATIONAL *QUANTITATIVE* STUDIES are the subject of this chapter, and include cross-sectional and longitudinal studies (retrospective and prospective). These are by far the most common research designs employed in R/S and health research. I discuss what kinds of research questions can be answered with these designs, describe the different kinds of observational studies, review their strengths and weaknesses, and provide examples of how to apply them in R/S and health research. Observational studies are distinct from experimental methods in that the role of the researcher is to observe and document what is naturally taking place, not intervene or change the system in any way. Indeed, some conditions or characteristics cannot be manipulated in experimental designs, leaving observational studies as the only possible scientific method. These types of observational studies also differ from observational

> Observational studies are distinct from experimental methods in that the role of the researcher is to observe and document what is naturally taking place, not intervene or change the system in any way.

qualitative research in that the goal is to quantify in terms of numbers the strength of relationships between characteristics/behaviors and health outcomes or to determine whether those characteristics/behaviors predict changes in an outcome, not to describe those relationships in detail.

PURPOSE

Observational studies (cross-sectional) can determine whether two variables (characteristics/behaviors) are associated and how strong that association is. They can also determine whether the association is independent of other factors that may explain the relationship (although there are limitations here since not all factors that affect the relationship are usually known or can be measured precisely). Observational designs (longitudinal studies) can also determine whether one variable at baseline predicts changes in another variable in the future. Adding the element of time to a relationship goes beyond simple cross-sectional association to the possibility that one variable actually affects or leads to changes in another variable, thereby providing evidence for a causal relationship (only partial evidence, though, since only a randomized clinical trial can demonstrate causality). I now examine in detail the two basic types of observational studies: cross-sectional and longitudinal. Some of the content of this chapter is a review and reinforcement of material presented in Chapter 5.

CROSS-SECTIONAL STUDIES

In this category I include case-control studies and the more classical cross-sectional studies involving survey research methodology.

Case-Control Studies

Case-control studies are optimal for studying conditions that are relatively rare or uncommon. The researcher collects a series of cases with "the condition" and then matches these cases to individuals without the condition to see what is uniquely different about cases that might help to explain the cause of the condition. Cases are matched to controls on as many relevant characteristics as possible, since the aim is to identify controls as similar as possible to cases except for the condition. This research design was often used in the early days prior to the development of more sophisticated statistical methods for examining associations.

> **Case-control studies are optimal for studying conditions that are relatively rare or uncommon.**

In R/S and health research, for example, an early study by Gallemore and colleagues[1] identified sixty-two patients with mood disturbances admitted to a psychiatric unit. Patients were matched to forty controls without psychiatric illness on age, gender, race, and socioeconomic status. Results indicated that patients were less likely than controls (15 percent vs. 35 percent) to come from religiously indifferent or antireligious backgrounds, and were more likely to report religious conversion or salvation experiences (52 percent vs. 20 percent). Investigators concluded that religious upbringing and religious experiences were more common among psychiatric patients with mood disturbance compared to controls, suggesting that this may have predisposed patients to mood disturbance.

In another example, consider a study by Friedlander and colleagues[2] who asked whether patients experiencing a myocardial infarction (MI) differed in level of religious involvement compared to healthy controls. Investigators identified 454 Jewish men and 85 Jewish women in Jerusalem who had experienced their first MI and matched these cases to 295 Jewish men and 391 Jewish women controls. Among the cases, 51 percent of men and 50 percent of women defined themselves as secular, compared to 21 percent of men and 16 percent of women in the control group. The difference was statistically significant, and remained significant after further controlling for age, ethnicity, education, smoking, physical exercise, and body mass index. The researchers concluded that religious involvement was less common among those experiencing their first MI compared to controls.

Hypothetically, another case-control study might be designed to determine what is uniquely different about individuals who report miraculous physical healings. Such a study might identify individuals who report a miraculous healing (cases) and match them to individuals with similar physical health conditions but without a healing. Besides having a similar physical condition, cases and controls might also be matched on age, gender, and socioeconomic status. The investigators would then administer a questionnaire both to cases and controls and gather information about characteristics that might be the cause for the miraculous healing (e.g., religious, social, mental, or physical health characteristics). Any significant differences between cases and controls on those characteristics might help explain miraculous physical healings.

Case-control studies can *only* determine whether a characteristic is more common among cases with a certain condition (i.e., establish an association). As in the next category of cross-sectional studies below, they cannot provide information about whether the characteristic preceded the condition or caused it.

Cross-Sectional Studies (Classical)

Cross-sectional studies used in survey research make up about 80 to 90 percent of studies in R/S and health. This design involves taking a snapshot of the association between two characteristics at one point in time. For example, a researcher develops a questionnaire that asks about age, gender, religious activities, social support, and well-being, and sends out the questionnaire through the mail to five hundred people. Of those who receive the questionnaire, one hundred fill it out (20 percent response rate, which is typical for a single mailed survey) and send it back to the researcher. The researcher enters the data into a data file and then analyzes the relationship between religious activity and well-being, controlling for age, gender, ethnicity, socioeconomic status, and social support. Since there is no follow-up and the questionnaire has only been administered once, this is a cross-sectional study.

Like a case-control study, a cross-sectional study is only

> Cross-sectional studies used in survey research make up about 80 to 90 percent of studies in R/S and health. This design involves taking a snapshot of the association between two characteristics at one point in time.

capable of determining whether one characteristic is associated with another, but cannot say anything about how that relationship came about (e.g., cannot isolate cause and effect). Since cross-sectional studies are conducted at one point in time, they provide no information about whether changes in one characteristic precede changes in another. By controlling for covariates, researchers can determine whether the relationship between one characteristic and another is an independent one and not confounded or explained by the covariates. If, after controlling for age, gender, ethnicity, socioeconomic status, and social support, it was determined (in the example above) that religious activity was associated with greater well-being, then the researcher could conclude that the relationship between religious activity and well-being is independent of these variables. In this example, age, gender, ethnicity, and socioeconomic status are called *confounders*, whereas social support would be considered a *mediator* or an *explanatory variable*. I discuss the differences between confounders and mediators in Chapter 16.

Strengths

Cross-sectional studies are relatively quick and inexpensive, and can involve large numbers of subjects. Compared to results from smaller longitudinal studies or experimental studies, results from cross-sectional studies can be more easily generalized to the population from which subjects come, especially if the sampling method is random, the response rate is high, and non-response bias is not a problem. Examples of cross-sectional studies in the United States are the General Social Survey (ninety-minute in-person interview of a random sample of three thousand to forty-five hundred people ages eighteen or older), the Gallup Poll (telephone survey of approximately one thousand adults ages eighteen or older), the National Health and Nutrition Examination Survey (NHANES) (in-person survey of five thousand adults ages eighteen or older), and the U.S. Census (in-person survey of approximately 2 million adults ages eighteen or older).

> Cross-sectional studies are relatively quick and inexpensive, and can involve large numbers of subjects.
>
> Results from cross-sectional studies can be more easily generalized to the population from which subjects come, especially if the sampling method is random, the response rate is high, and nonresponse bias is not a problem.

Weaknesses

As noted above, a downside of this method is that it provides no information on causality, direction of effect, or how the relationship came about. For example, many cross-sectional studies find that pain severity is positively correlated with frequency of prayer. What does such an association mean? Does prayer cause an increase in pain (i.e., perhaps prayer causes people to focus more on their pain thereby amplifying it)? Or, does pain cause an increase in prayer (i.e., perhaps people in severe pain turn to prayer to cope with the pain)? Furthermore, both pain and prayer may be related to another unmeasured factor that is common to both, in which case the relationship is completely spurious (i.e., there is actually no relationship between pain and prayer). Therefore, we know very little about what this correlation means.

Another weakness is that cross-sectional surveys usually collect relatively superficial information, especially if the survey was conducted for some other purpose. Researchers know that the longer the questionnaire, the less likely it is that subjects will fill it out, which reduces the response rate. Therefore, unless the study was being done specifically to study the R/S-health relationship (which is unlikely given the difficulty of getting funding in this area), the developers of the survey will probably not include detailed questions about R/S involvement. This is true for almost all of the large cross-sectional surveys of the U.S. population, which often include only one or two questions on R/S (typically, only frequency of religious attendance or religious affiliation). Finally, as noted above, cross-sectional studies cannot measure and control for all the characteristics or behaviors likely to influence the relationship between R/S and health, which means that an unmeasured factor may exist that accounts for the relationship.

> The sampling method and response rate are vital in cross-sectional studies and determine the quality of the study.

Sampling Method and Response Rate

As noted in previous chapters, the sampling method and response rate are vital in cross-sectional studies and determine the quality of the study (as does the use of reliable, valid measures). Today, random or systematic sampling and a relatively high response rate are needed for publication of a cross-sectional study in a respectable peer-reviewed journal. Interestingly, there has been debate about whether lower response rates actually yield less accurate results than high response rates. These debates have occurred mostly in the literature on public opinion polls related to predicting election results.[3] For example, one study compared two surveys of one thousand subjects, the first with a response rate of 25 percent and the other with a response rate of 50 percent. Researchers found that the results were similar in seventy-seven out of eighty-four comparisons.[4] Another study examined response rates to a marketing questionnaire that surveyed thousands of subjects, and found that excluding those who required two or more calls before responding (which reduced response rate by 50 percent) had little effect on the findings. Finally, a study examined the results of eighty-one national surveys with response rates varying from 5 percent to 54 percent, finding that surveys with low response rates were not that much less accurate than those with high response rates.[5] Nevertheless, in the social, behavioral, and medical sciences, I would strongly recommend aiming for the highest response rate possible to minimize nonresponse bias, since journal reviewers definitely consider the response rate when making decisions regarding publication. If, however, researchers end up with a low response rate, they may use the studies above to plead their case.

> For all cross-sectional studies, regardless of response rate, investigators should gather as much information as possible on nonparticipants. The researcher's job is to convince reviewers that nonparticipants are similar to those who participated in the study.

Nonparticipants

For all cross-sectional studies, regardless of response rate, investigators should gather as much information as possible on nonparticipants—that is, those who refuse to participate or otherwise do not respond (see Chapter 6). The researcher's job is to convince reviewers that nonparticipants are similar to those who participated in the study. One way to do this is to compare the characteristics of participants and nonparticipants to show that there are no significant differences. The most important characteristics involve exposure (R/S) and outcome (health) variables; however, since nonparticipants have either refused to answer or otherwise not answered those questions, that information is not available. Nevertheless, the investigator may have information on gender, age, race, or other demographic characteristics on nonrespondents that was recorded on the original contact list from which subjects were identified. If researchers can show that gender, age, race, and so on are similar between participants and nonparticipants, then this can be used to argue that other characteristics are similar as well. Whether researchers can use demographic characteristics on nonrespondents for this purpose depends on the Institutional Review Board (IRB) that approves the study. If nonrespondent information cannot be collected, researchers can always compare their final sample with known population parameters or previous studies of the same population (as noted in Chapter 5).

One method of reassuring reviewers that nonrespondents are similar to respondents is to compare the characteristics of those who initially responded to those who responded after multiple attempts to do so (i.e., multiple telephone calls or other methods of recruiting them). This requires keeping track of how often interviewers contacted subjects before they responded. The advantage here is that the researcher has complete information on exposure and outcome variables on all those who eventually decided to participate, so the characteristics of those who only agreed after much convincing can be compared with those who agreed right away. If no differences are found, then investigators can argue that there are no differences between participants and nonparticipants (based on the claim that "resistant" participants are similar to nonparticipants). Sometimes this logic convinces reviewers; other times it does not.

LONGITUDINAL STUDIES

In the category of longitudinal studies, I include retrospective and prospective cohort studies.

Retrospective Cohort Studies

As noted in Chapter 5, retrospective cohort studies involve looking back in time at data that others have collected for other purposes. This is possible when records exist that have measured the predictor variable (R/S) and the outcome variable (health), and there is evidence that the predictor variable preceded the outcome variable. For example, medical records may exist that have been collected over a period of time that contain information about R/S involvement (perhaps religious affiliation) or for some kind of R/S (such as a chaplain visit) as well as information about patients' health as it has changed over the years. These records document that the R/S "exposure" took place before changes in health occurred, so the longitudinal relationship between R/S and the health outcome can be examined. In this example, the information was collected solely for clinical purposes, but the researcher decided to take advantage of the already existing data to determine whether the earlier R/S exposure predicted future changes in health.

Strengths

The advantage of this method is that it adds the element of time, so that now investigators can determine if two variables are correlated and whether one variable (or changes in that variable) precedes changes in the other variable. This provides information about how the relationship may have come about over time, and contributes evidence toward a causal explanation (although, again, cannot demonstrate causality). Another advantage of retrospective cohort studies is that, because the data are already collected, the research is less expensive and time-consuming than prospective cohort studies.

Weaknesses

There are also disadvantages to this design. Records must exist that document that the exposure (R/S) happened before the outcome (change in health). The biggest problem is that the researcher cannot choose how R/S or the health outcome was measured, since the data have already been collected. Even more important, researchers have no control over what covariates were measured or how they were measured. Some may try to get around this by having chaplains or other clinicians use standard scales to measure R/S characteristics or document R/S interventions as part of their usual care of patients. These records will then be available at a later date for researchers to analyze. Unfortunately, if the data are collected for any reason other than exclusively for clinical purposes, researchers are obligated to get IRB approval and obtain consent from patients to allow their data to be used for this reason. Sometimes, however, things are not as clear-cut (e.g., the data could be used for clinical purposes, but might also be useful for research should someone at a later date wish to analyze these data). Whenever there is a possibility that clinical data may be used for research purposes, however, it is always best to check with the IRB on how to proceed.

Retrospective cohort studies are not common in R/S and health research. However, with the increasing use of electronic medical records that may contain patient information in a format that improves access, this method may become more popular (given its ease and low cost).

Prospective Cohort Studies

Prospective studies (also called longitudinal or cohort studies) collect data at one point in time and follow subjects forward in time. Although more expensive and time-consuming, prospective studies are almost always preferred over case-control, cross-sectional, or retrospective cohort studies.

> Although more expensive and time-consuming, prospective studies are almost always preferred over case-control, cross-sectional, or retrospective cohort studies.

> Prospective studies add the element of time, helping to explain how a relationship between two variables came about.

Strengths

Prospective studies add the element of time, helping to explain how a relationship between two variables came about (but cannot demonstrate causality). The biggest advantage over retrospective cohort studies is that investigators can measure whatever and however they want, having complete control over how to measure predictor variables (R/S) at baseline and health outcomes during follow-up. Using this research design, researchers can determine whether a certain characteristics at baseline (such as R/S) predicts changes in a health outcome measured between baseline and follow-up. Finally, results from prospective studies are easier to generalize than randomized clinical trials (RCT) because the strict inclusion and exclusion criteria of RCTs limit the population to which results apply. In addition, prospective studies can involve large numbers of persons who are more representative of the underlying populations from which they are sampled and are usually more heterogeneous than samples in highly focused RCTs.

Weaknesses

Prospective studies are more expensive, time-consuming, and complex than case-control, cross-sectional, or retrospective cohort studies. Subjects have to be located on follow-up and encouraged to participate two or more times (baseline and follow-ups). Prospective studies usually need interviewers to contact subjects and interview them, in contrast to other types of observational studies that don't usually require this. Having interviewers conduct the assessments increases the likelihood that subjects will agree to participate in both the baseline and follow-up evaluations, since refusing a live person is more difficult than tossing a questionnaire into a trashcan. This means that interviewers have to be hired and trained, and often retrained to avoid "drift"—that is, a change in the way that questions are presented to subjects that may influence their responses.

Another potential weakness is that dropouts can affect the ability to generalize the findings. Dropouts result from refusal, inability to locate subjects for follow-up, or worsening health of subjects, precluding their participation. There are several ways to minimize dropouts. First, collect information during the baseline interview on several contacts (family, friends, neighbors) so that subjects can always be located. Second, proxy interviews can be conducted with close family members or caretakers if subjects become too sick to complete follow-up assessments. Third, while researchers cannot do much with outright refusals, having friendly extraverted interviewers can make the interview experience a pleasant one and improve the chances that subjects will agree to follow-up interviews. Follow-up of at least 65 to 85 percent of those participating at baseline is usually needed for publication (depending on length of follow-up).[6] Thus, every effort should

> Follow-up of at least 65 to 85 percent of those participating at baseline is usually needed for publication (depending on length of follow-up).

be made to keep subjects in the study. Interviewers keep subjects interested and willing by offering small payments for study participation, being supportive during interviews, sending birthday and anniversary cards, and otherwise making subjects feel connected to the study.

When researchers interact with patients to keep them in the study, this can have unpredictable effects on health outcomes (a serious weakness of prospective studies). For example, in a study that examines the course of depression over time, repeated contact by caring supportive interviewers and other members of the research team can become an unintended intervention that improves symptoms and reduces the power of the study to detect the effects of baseline predictors (such as R/S). Interviewers face the difficult task of minimizing emotional support that may affect symptoms, yet providing sufficient support to keep subjects in the study.

Dropouts

As in cross-sectional studies, investigators must collect information on and compare the characteristics of nonparticipants with those of participants to ensure there are no significant selection effects that may bias results. Prospective studies require that researchers collect as much information on dropouts as possible so that they can show that dropouts do not differ significantly from participants. An advantage of prospective studies is that information on dropouts is collected during the baseline interview, so characteristics of completers and dropouts can be compared. Again, it is most important to compare dropouts and completers on the primary predictors, covariates, and health outcomes; if there are no differences on these characteristics, then investigators can claim that dropouts are similar to completers, and that the results from completers can be applied to everyone including the dropouts. Some IRBs require that investigators get permission from those who drop out to use their data collected earlier on in the study. We have dealt with this problem by providing a telephone number to dropouts to

> When researchers interact with patients to keep them in the study, this can have unpredictable effects on health outcomes (a serious weakness of prospective studies).

> Prospective studies require that researchers collect as much information on dropouts as possible so that they can show that dropouts do not differ significantly from participants.

call should they drop out they don't want their data to be used; if dropouts do not call, researchers can assume that it is permissible to use their data (subjects almost never call).

Prospective studies today are preferred in R/S-health research, since, as noted in Chapter 3, cross-sectional associations have already been established in many areas. What is most important now is to determine whether R/S characteristics can predict future changes in health outcomes.

Conducting an Observational Study

I now review from start to finish how researchers conduct a quantitative observational study (cross-sectional or prospective) (see Figure 8.1).

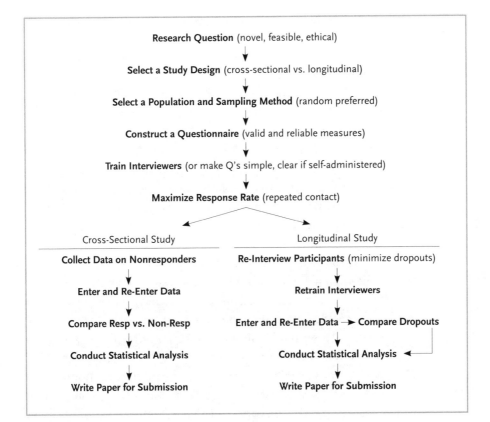

FIGURE 8.1. Conducting an Observational Study

First, investigators must decide on a research question that is novel, feasible, and ethical. Second, they must choose a sample in which to test their hypothesis (based on availability of subjects and funding support), and decide on a sampling method (systematic or random in most cases). Third, a study design needs to be selected based on the research question; if association only is desired, then a cross-sectional design may be sufficient; if information about order of effects is preferred, then a prospective design would be appropriate. Fourth, researchers must construct a questionnaire that asks about demographic information (confounders such as age, race, gender, education/income, living situation), R/S, mediating variables (such as social support, psychological traits, health behaviors), and health outcomes. Established measures of R/S, mediating variables, and health outcomes should almost always be used. By this, I mean measures whose psychometric characteristics (i.e., reliability and validity) are published in the research literature. The latter is particularly important for measures of R/S and the health outcome being studied.

Fifth, if the questionnaire is interviewer-administered (vs. self-administered), then interviewers need to be trained. Plans also need to be made to *retrain* interviewers on a regular basis throughout the study so that drift does not occur. Alternatively, if the questionnaire is self-administered, then subjects have to be healthy enough, motivated enough, and have adequate vision and reading ability to complete the questionnaire. Researchers also need to be sure that the questions and responses are written in a way that is clear and unambiguous and response options are simple. Subjects should also be provided with an easy way to return the questionnaire. If the questionnaire is sent out by mail, then include a self-addressed, stamped envelope; if questionnaires are distributed onsite, then a member of the research team should collect them directly from subjects.

Sixth, researchers should contact nonresponders repeatedly and in different ways to maximize the response rate. This might involve sending additional copies of the questionnaire to nonrespondents, postcards or e-mail to encourage completion, repeated phone calls, onsite visits, or communication through friends or relatives. The method used to contact and recontact nonresponders needs to be part of the study protocol, in the consent form, and approved by the IRB. A single mailing of a questionnaire is likely to result in a response rate of 20 to 30 percent; repeated contact can increase the rate by another 20 to 30 percent at most (a 50 percent response rate to a mailed questionnaire would be impressive). The researchers would then gather all the questionnaires and enter the data into an analysis program, and reenter the data to minimize errors (called "double-entry"). Finally, they would conduct the statistical analysis and write up the results for publication. If the design is cross-sectional, then the study is complete.

If the design is prospective, then subjects will have to be reinterviewed at established follow-up intervals (for example, at three, six, twelve, twenty-four, thirty-six, or sixty months). The baseline consent form needs to specify how often researchers will be contacting subjects so that subjects know what they are getting into when they sign up to participate. How often follow-up interviews take place and for how long depend on how rapidly the health condition changes over time (natural history) and how long it takes R/S to have an effect on the health outcome. Researchers also need to ensure that measures of the health outcome are sensitive enough to detect clinically significant changes during the follow-up period. Some measures are so insensitive to change over time that it may not be possible for R/S to predict significant changes even when they occur (Type II error). Thus, health outcome measures should have published information on how sensitive they are in detecting significant changes in the outcome over time.

Finally, researchers need to minimize dropouts throughout a prospective study, expecting to lose about 15 to 20 percent of participants on each follow-up evaluation. Information on dropouts needs to be carefully collected, including reasons for dropping out (could not locate, too sick to participate, no proxy available, outright refusal). Once all follow-up interviews are completed, researchers will enter and reenter the data from the questionnaires, conduct the statistical analysis, and write up the results for publication. At that point, the study is complete.

Example of a Specific Study

We recently completed a prospective study titled "Depression in Heart Failure Patients." The primary research question was, "Do changes in physical health affect the course of major depression in hospitalized patients over age 55 with heart failure (CHF) during the six months following hospital discharge?" A secondary research question was, "How do psychological, social, and spiritual factors mediate the relationship between changes in physical health and course of major depression over time?" We recruited patients with CHF at three regional hospitals located within about thirty miles of each other.

The sampling method was systematic and involved recruiting consecutive eligible patients admitted to the medical services of the three hospitals. Patients were identified using lists of daily hospital admissions that included age and primary medical diagnosis. Interviewers (trained research nurses with experience in psychiatry) were stationed at each of the three hospitals and screened patients at the bedside for major depression using the Structured Clinical Interview for Depression (SCID).[7] The SCID is a widely used, structured psychiatric interview that makes the diagnosis of major depression using established criteria. Changes in depression (the dependent or outcome variable) were measured at six, twelve, eighteen, and twenty-four weeks after discharge via telephone using the Longitudinal Interval Follow-up Evaluation (LIFE), a standard measure of depression outcome.[8] This measure also has established criteria for remission of depression that have been published.[9] Changes in physical health (the primary predictor) were measured using the Chronic Heart Failure Questionnaire, an established measure of CHF severity,[10] which also has published data on what constitutes a clinically meaningful change on the scale.[11] To maximize subject participation, the same interviewers who conducted the baseline evaluation in the hospital also did the follow-up interviews.

In order to address our secondary research question (regarding confounders and mediators), we measured a range of patient characteristics at baseline including demographics, social support, disability, global medical illness severity, religious involvement, comorbid psychiatric and medical diagnoses, history of depression, and treatments received for depression. Some but not all of these measures were reassessed at the follow-up evaluations (disability, medical illness severity, treatments for depression). Measures that were used to assess mediating variables were published in the literature with information on reliability and validity.

The baseline and follow-up interviews were computerized so that interviewers could directly enter subjects' responses into laptop computers, which helped to reduce data entry errors and prevent skipped questions. All research nurse–interviewers underwent intensive training together on how to recruit subjects, obtain consent, administer the questionnaires, and enter responses into the laptops. To avoid drift, this training was repeated every four to six months throughout the four years of subject enrollment and follow-up.

Identifying eligible subjects, diagnosing depression, and recruiting subjects into the study was difficult. Multiple consent forms were needed for baseline, follow-up, and proxy interviews at each of the three hospitals, which often led to confusion. Although the baseline interview was supposed to last only about 45 to 60 minutes, it actually took from 60 to 180 minutes, since patients wanted to talk. Each interviewer working full-time was only able to recruit only one new patient per day (and also complete follow-up evaluations of patients already in the study). This was anticipated in the grant proposal, so there were adequate resources to meet the study goals (i.e., to recruit and follow up with eight hundred patients).

Since this was a prospective study that focused on factors affecting the course of depression, the baseline response rate was less important than the follow-up response rate. Thus, once they were enrolled into the study, every effort was made to keep them in the study, including sending birthday and anniversary cards and making multiple attempts to contact subjects for follow-up interviews. Subjects were often difficult to locate, were too sick to complete the interview, died during follow-up, didn't have family members or caregivers to provide proxy interviews, were lost to follow-up (moved), or refused to continue. There were also numerous changes in study personnel, conflicts between study personnel, weather problems, and IRB issues that delayed subject recruitment. Despite these challenges, during the four years of recruitment, interviewers enrolled one thousand patients into the study (two hundred more than proposed), and 85 percent of enrolled patients completed at least one follow-up evaluation (60 percent completing all four follow-up interviews).

The first three months of this five-year NIH-funded study was spent hiring project personnel and training them, and the final nine months of the study were spent cleaning up the data, conducting the statistical analyses, and writing up the findings for publication. Nearly two dozen peer-reviewed scientific papers were published from the results.

SUMMARY AND CONCLUSIONS

The most common quantitative observational study designs are cross-sectional (case control and classical cross-sectional) and longitudinal (retrospective and prospective) studies. There are strengths and weaknesses of each research design and special considerations that need to be kept in mind. Cross-sectional and prospective cohort studies make up 90 percent of all R/S and health research. For cross-sectional designs, the easiest and cheapest studies to conduct, the emphasis should be on identifying a random (or at least systematic) sample from a population of interest, using reliable and valid measures to assess variables, maximizing the response rate, and accounting for all nonresponders. For prospective cohort designs, which are more expensive and time-consuming to conduct but almost always preferred over cross-sectional designs, the emphasis is on using reliable and valid measures of predictors, mediators, and outcomes; ensuring interviewer consistency through training and retraining; maximizing follow-up of all enrolled subjects; minimizing contact between interviewers and subjects that may affect health outcomes; and accounting for all dropouts. For cross-sectional and prospective studies, nonresponders and dropouts should be compared to participants to ensure that study results are not biased due to selective nonparticipation. In the latter part of the chapter, I reviewed how to conduct an observational study from start to finish, and then provided a specific example of a prospective study, discussing the challenges that such studies often present.

Clinical Trials

OUTLINE

A RANDOMIZED CLINICAL TRIAL (RCT) is a prospective study that compares the effect and value of an intervention against a control in human subjects, where subjects are randomly assigned to either the intervention or the control group. The first RCT was in 1931 and tested the efficacy of gold in the treatment of tuberculosis.[1] Subjects were randomized to intervention or control groups by the flip of a coin. The gold treatment turned out ineffective, and it was abandoned.

Importance

Given the uncertain knowledge about factors that affect the course of illness and the large variations in the natural history of illness, it is usually impossible to say whether a predictor (such as religion/spirituality) has made a difference in an illness except by conducting an RCT. In the hierarchy of strength of scientific evidence for treatment decisions, the randomized clinical trial is at the top, followed by prospective cohort studies, retrospective cohort studies, case-control studies, cross-sectional studies, case series (series of in-depth case descriptions, such as reported in qualitative studies), and unsystematic clinical observations.[2]

> In the hierarchy of strength of scientific evidence for treatment decisions, the randomized clinical trial is at the top.

Unlike observational studies that can only establish whether two characteristics are associated and the strength and timing of that association, a clinical trial can determine whether a risk factor actually leads to or causes changes in a health outcome. Observational studies use designs with stronger *external validity* by studying relationships as they occur in real-world settings. Clinical trials, in turn, validate findings from observational studies by using designs with *internal validity* by examining effects using random assignment.

Limitations

While there is no doubt that the RCT is a powerful scientific design, one that health-care professionals are most familiar with and give the greatest value to, this method also has many limitations.

Feasibility

RCTs are simply not feasible in many circumstances, particularly when investigating causes that may produce considerable harm. For example, randomizing subjects to either cigarette smoking or a control group is ethically unacceptable. Likewise, there might be ethical concerns about randomizing atheists to an intervention that makes them more religious or to a control condition where atheistic beliefs are affirmed. Finally, there are many research questions that RCTs simply cannot answer. As noted in Chapter 3, no RCT can establish whether R/S can affect health through supernatural pathways, since the RCT is a scientific method designed to study forces that exist within, not outside of, nature.

Translation into Real World

RCTs are "staged." Interventions are administered to a highly select group of subjects in ways that maximize the likelihood of detecting benefit and so may not translate easily into real-life situations.

Volunteer Bias

Subjects usually hear about a trial through advertisements or by referral from health professionals, and then volunteer to participate. In general, volunteers tend to have less severe disease, are younger, are better educated, and are more likely to be women. Can the results of a trial conducted in volunteers be generalized to those who are not volunteer-minded? Sometimes they can't. Although the problem of volunteer bias is present for all studies regardless of design, this is particularly concerning for clinical trials. Those who participate in observational studies are usually approached by researchers first and then make a decision to participate, which is the reverse of what happens with RCTs, where subjects make a decision to participate and then approach the researchers.

Volunteer bias may be particularly problematic in studies testing the efficacy of R/S interventions. Those who volunteer for such studies are often quite religious and want the religious intervention. Because they expect to receive benefit from the religious intervention, they often do—whether the treatment is effective or not. An even bigger problem occurs when religious volunteers are randomized to the control condition where they get something other than the R/S intervention. Expecting the religious intervention, they learn that they aren't getting it and may be quite

> Interventions are administered to a highly select group of subjects in ways that maximize the likelihood of detecting benefit and so may not translate easily into real-life situations.

disappointed. Consequently, just as the religious volunteer who received the religious intervention may do better due to positive expectations, the religious volunteer who gets the "other treatment" may do worse. Again, none of this has anything to do with the effectiveness or lack of effectiveness of the intervention.

Inclusion-Exclusion Criteria

As noted in Chapter 6, stringent inclusion and exclusion criteria (i.e., restrictive enrollment criteria) usually limit participants in a clinical trial to a very specific group of individuals who may be quite different from the general population. Results of a clinical trial, then, may apply only to this small select group and not to others. The inability to generalize is particularly evident in psychopharmacology studies that examine the effects of antidepressant medication on depressive symptoms. Subjects participating in such studies often have milder depressions (those with severe depression are usually too sick to sign up for such studies). Furthermore, those with suicidal thoughts, comorbid medical problems, or alcohol or substance abuse issues are typically excluded. The result is that the findings from antidepressant drug studies usually apply to patients whom clinicians seldom see and may not be relevant to the vast majority of patients who are more seriously depressed and often have problems with substance abuse, other chronic medical conditions, or suicidal thoughts. Similar concerns apply to all intervention studies, including those examining R/S interventions.

Expensive and Time-Consuming

Because of their complexity, the costs and time involved in conducting a RCT can quickly add up. While this is a concern even for drug studies that compare an active pill with an identical-looking inactive placebo, the challenge is magnified many times for RCTs that involve psychosocial interventions that are difficult to administer and require a lot more monitoring.

Consider the many components to an RCT involving an R/S intervention. First, the intervention must

> Because of their complexity, the costs and time involved in conducting a RCT can quickly add up.

be carefully documented in a manual that describes every aspect, including the minutest details of the R/S intervention. Second, the intervention needs to be tape recorded or video recorded so that outside experts can evaluate a random sample of sessions in order to establish treatment fidelity (i.e., how closely those who administer the intervention are following the study protocol). Third, an independent monitoring group is needed that randomizes subjects and ensures that all recruitment and intervention procedures are followed and that no harm occurs to subjects. Fourth, interviewers doing the baseline and follow-up assessments need to be blinded to treatment group, requiring that those assessing the outcomes are different from those administering the intervention. Fifth, RCTs usually require a large, multitalented research team of specialists and consultants (including experts in clinical trial design, experts in the condition being treated or health outcome being measured, and experts in the intervention). Sixth, subjects themselves may need to be paid in order to retain them in the study, as might those referring subjects to the study to ensure adequate recruitment. Finally, if biological outcomes are being studied, then the researchers must consider the costs of collecting, packaging, transporting, and analyzing the specimens, which can add up quickly.

Given the many components of a well-done RCT, conducting such a trial and managing the large research team involved in it can be extremely time-consuming. This means that directing a clinical trial may not be feasible for researchers with heavy administrative, clinical, or teaching responsibilities. Multicenter trials, which allow for greater generalization of results, are even more difficult to manage and coordinate. Failure to appreciate the complexity, cost, and time involved in an RCT can easily result in findings that are misleading. In other words, failure to identify an intervention's effect may not be due to lack of efficacy, but rather because the study was not properly conducted due to inadequate resources or investigator time. Sometimes the opposite is true as well; ineffective or useless interventions may end up appearing beneficial for the same reason.

Basic Features of Clinical Trials

The objective in many clinical trials is to see if an intervention plus standard care is better or worse than a control condition plus standard care, for example, an R/S intervention plus standard care vs. social attention (control) plus standard care. Alternatively, an R/S "version" of a standard treatment may be compared against the standard treatment to see if the former is superior to the latter in affecting the disease outcome.

I now describe seven basic features involved in conducting clinical trials, and then go on to discuss intervention standardization, types of controls, subject selection, randomization, outcome measurement, types of blinding, and ways of analyzing results.

> The objective in many clinical trials is to see if an intervention plus standard care is better or worse than a control condition plus standard care.

1. All subjects recruited into a clinical trial must be followed forward in time. They need not all be followed from an identical calendar date, although each subject must be followed from a well-defined point (time zero) and for a similar time period.
2. The intervention must be defined, documented, and applied in a standard fashion directed at changing some aspect of the subject's health.
3. An RCT must contain a control group that does not receive the intervention being tested and to which the intervention is compared; alternatively, the intervention may be compared to another intervention, which basically serves as the control group.
4. At baseline the control group must be similar to the intervention group on all characteristics affecting the outcome so that any differences in outcome can be attributed to the intervention. Random assignment usually accomplishes this, but not always (if not, then this needs to be adjusted for in the analysis phase).
5. Subjects in both intervention and control groups can and usually are receiving other interventions, either self-administered, from family/friends, or from other health professionals. This should be considered in the

design, limited to the extent ethically permissible, and at least measured during the study and controlled for in the analysis.

6. Investigators cannot force subjects to comply with the intervention. Thus, researchers must consider the degree to which subjects will fail to strictly comply with the protocol, measure this, and control for it in the analysis.

7. Random assignment is necessary in an RCT, since this removes bias in assignment, produces comparable groups, and guarantees the validity of statistical tests.[3]

Standardization of the Intervention

Every aspect of the intervention must be documented in detail from start to finish. A manual should be developed that lays out step by step the sequence of activities taken by the person administering the intervention (and the qualifications of that person). This assures that (1) the intervention will be administered the same way each time during the trial, and (2) when investigators at other institutions seek to replicate the study's findings, they can administer the intervention in the same way that the original investigators did. Audiotaping or videotaping all sessions helps to document that the intervention is being administered each time in a standardized manner according to protocol.

> **Every aspect of the intervention must be documented in detail from start to finish.**

Types of Control Group

There are five basic types of control group: randomized control, nonrandomized concurrent control, historical control, wait-list control, and withdrawal control.

Randomized Control

This is the usual control. A central coordinating body (preferably not involving the researchers) randomizes subjects to either the intervention or the control group using a standard randomization protocol.

Nonrandomized Concurrent Control[4]

This control group consists of subjects treated without the intervention at approximately the same time as those receiving the intervention. For example, researchers wish to examine whether admission to a faith-based hospital (A) increases the likelihood of survival compared to admission to a secular hospital (B). The intervention in hospital A is treatment that emphasizes spirituality in the care of patients. The control hospital B does not emphasize spirituality. Outcome is length of survival of patients admitted from January 1 to March 31 at each of the hospitals. Subjects in this study are not randomized, but they are being treated at the same time, and presumably the only difference is the inclusion of spirituality in the treatment of patients in hospital A. In this example, using a nonrandomized concurrent control is a much weaker design than randomizing subjects to either hospital A or B, since there could be differences in the types of patients admitted to each of these hospitals (due to self-selection, socioeconomic class, disease severity, etc.) and differences in the kinds of treatments available to patients (one hospital may offer a risky surgery for a disease with a poor prognosis, whereas the other hospital may not). For such a study to produce meaningful results, everything needs to be the same in both hospitals except the spiritual aspects in hospital A. In fact, without random assignment there is no way to ensure that hospitals A and B are equivalent, even if there appears to be no difference in the two hospitals (since there may be unknown factors that differentiate the two hospitals and could affect patient outcomes).

Historical Control

Here the control group is previously treated patients. The intervention is applied to a series of subjects, and the outcomes are compared to those of a previous series of comparable subjects (control group). For example, researchers wish to examine the effects of four twenty-minute chaplain visits on surgical complications and length of hospital stay among one hundred consecutive patients admitted for coronary artery bypass graft surgery (CABG). The control group against which the intervention is compared consists of the one hundred consecutive patients admitted for CABG immediately prior to the one hundred patients receiving the intervention. Again, this is a weaker design because subjects are not randomized, so the characteristics of subjects in each group may be different, which could affect the outcome. Furthermore, changes in surgical technique or quality of patient care between the two time periods may also impact the outcome, favoring one group over another.

A difference between using historical controls and the previous example concurrent controls (where patient outcomes are compared between hospital A and hospital B) is one of individual comparison versus group comparison, with the latter comparing patients in two different hospitals and the former comparing patients given treatments at different time periods within the same hospital.

Wait-List Control

A wait-list control group is commonly used in RCTs that test R/S interventions. In this design everyone eventually gets the intervention, but those in the control group have to wait until after the test group gets it. In other words, subjects are randomized to a control group that eventually gets the intervention, but only after the effects of the intervention in the test group have been compared to the control group that has not yet received the intervention. This allows the intervention to be administered to all subjects, and may be particularly relevant for situations where researchers are reluctant to deprive any subject of the intervention. The wait-list control group is equally credible to the randomized control group. The one major downside is that it truncates the follow-up period for assessing outcomes in the intervention group. The comparison ends (as well as the study) as soon as the control group starts getting the intervention. For example, investigators wish to know whether an R/S intervention is effective in treating anxiety disorders. Subjects in the intervention group receive a three-month intervention and are then compared to subjects randomized to a wait-list control group. If the wait-list control group then receives the intervention, researchers can no longer assess the effectiveness

> A wait-list control group is commonly used in RCTs that test R/S interventions. In this design everyone eventually gets the intervention, but those in the control group have to wait until after the test group gets it.

of the intervention beyond the time when the control group starts the intervention. Consequently, investigators will not be able to determine if the response in the test group is maintained beyond the actual three-month treatment period since there is no longer a control group that has not received the intervention.

To get around this problem, the researchers may decide to wait an additional three months before administering the intervention to the wait-list control group in order to determine if the treatment response persists for three months beyond the actual treatment. There are problems, however, with doing this. One is that the wait-listed controls now need to "wait" for six months with active symptoms before getting the intervention. They may get tired of waiting and drop out of the study (or seek other treatments). A second concern is an ethical one. Based on how severe and distressing the underlying condition is, investigators must judge how long it is ethical to allow subjects to remain untreated.

Withdrawal Control

Although not commonly used in R/S-health research for obvious reasons, this method involves withdrawing a treatment or intervention from those who have been receiving it in order to determine whether a relapse in symptoms occurs with the discontinuation of treatment. For example, researchers may wonder whether weekly attendance at religious services improves the well-being of individuals experiencing recent foreclosure on their homes. One way to answer this question would be to identify one hundred weekly attendees who have undergone foreclosures in the last six months and then ask them to participate in a clinical trial. Fifty of the one hundred subjects would be randomly assigned to the control group and would be instructed to discontinue attending religious services for the next six months. Well-being would be assessed in both groups at three and six months and compared. Although such a study would not likely be done, nor would it likely be approved by the local IRB, this illustrates a withdrawal control group (see Chapter 10 for a study that examined outcomes after withdrawing chaplain services from a hospital).

Related to withdrawal controls is another type of experimental design sometimes used in psychology, communication, and education research. In this design, a group of subjects is selected and then randomly assigned to either a control group or an intervention group. After a period of treatment, subjects in the intervention group have the treatment withdrawn (e.g., become controls) whereas those in the control group begin receiving the treatment (e.g., become the intervention group). There are potential pitfalls with this design, however, such as carryover effects and order effects.

Subject Selection

The inclusion and exclusion (I/E) criteria define the study population and determine the population to whom the results can be applied. As indicated in Chapter 5, investigators need to achieve a balance between having a homogeneous vs. a heterogeneous group of subjects. The more homogeneous the group is (i.e., extensive I/E criteria that narrow the sample to subjects with very specific characteristics), the easier to detect the effect of the intervention (increases "power"). Therefore, having a homogeneous group of subjects is critical for a successful clinical trial. On the other hand, strict I/E criteria make it more difficult to enroll patients and also limit the ability to generalize the results.

> The inclusion and exclusion (I/E) criteria define the study population and determine the population to whom the results can be applied.

The opposite applies when I/E criteria are less stringent and the result is a heterogeneous group of subjects. A benefit of having a heterogeneous sample is that if an effect of the intervention is detected, then the results can be generalized to a broader population of individuals. However, heterogeneity adds to the variance in the outcome, reducing investigators' ability to detect the impact of the intervention (i.e., decreasing power). The reason is that the factors that contribute to heterogeneity may influence the outcome and add "noise" that may drown out the effects of the intervention. However, loosening I/E criteria makes it easier to enroll subjects and achieve the sample size that researchers are targeting. Investigators are under tremendous pressure to reach the target sample size, both in terms of meeting their obligations to the organization that funded the study and in terms of achieving sufficient power to detect the effects of the intervention. Therefore, both homogeneity and heterogeneity of samples affect study power, although for different reasons. A clinical trial is always a compromise between the ideal and the doable. Ability to identify a truly efficacious intervention increases in proportion to how well investigators can approximate the ideal balance between homogeneity and heterogeneity.

Outcomes

A single, well-defined outcome needs to be identified that addresses the primary research question. In medical research, outcomes are categorized as "hard" vs. "soft." *Hard outcomes* include death and other events (recurrence of a myocardial infarction, occurrence of a stroke, complications after surgery, length of hospital stay, etc.). Hard outcomes are usually well defined, easily measured, and often determined by a central organization, laboratory, or independent group. *Soft outcomes* include well-being, depression, quality of life, and other psychosocial measures that are largely subjective and harder to measure precisely. Identifying accurate and reliable measures of the outcome is important for both hard and soft outcomes, although it is especially important for soft outcomes. Evidence for the psychometric rigor of the outcome measure needs to be available in the published scientific literature. Finally, those administering the baseline and follow-up outcome measures need to be "blind" to treatment group (even if outcome measures are completed by subjects themselves).

One can also distinguish intermediate outcomes that precede the primary outcome that may give clues as to the process by which a treatment has its effects on the primary outcome. In addition, one should always use fidelity/implementation measures that assess the extent to which the treatment was actually implemented and therefore has a chance of affecting the primary outcome.

Types of Consent

Once the intervention has been carefully documented, the control group selected, I/E criteria established, and valid/reliable measures of the outcome determined, then subjects can be enrolled into the study. Before enrollment can occur, however, subjects must be fully informed about the nature of the study, i.e., they need details about what they are agreeing to participate in, and then must sign a document that indicates they are informed. Consent forms describe the expectations that researchers have of subjects, as well as any compensation or special benefits that subjects receive for participating. The risks of the intervention must be clearly spelled out, alternative proven treatments described, and potential benefits of participating in the study discussed. Subjects must be assured that their health care will not be influenced by participation or failure to participate in the study. Subjects must be informed that they can drop out of the study at any time without influencing their health care. Consent forms are usually four to six pages even for simple studies, and need to be signed and witnessed before research can begin. All research of any kind requires informed consent. No research data may be collected from subjects until after they have formally given written consent (with some exceptions—e.g., low-risk mailed questionnaires where completion and return of the questionnaire is evidence of consent). For an RCT, consent may be obtained either before or after randomization.

> **Subjects must be fully informed about the nature of the study, i.e., they need details about what they are agreeing to participate in, and then must sign a document that indicates they are informed.**

Consent before Randomization
The usual procedure is to obtain informed consent before subjects are randomized to the intervention and control groups. A single consent form is used for both intervention and control subjects.

Consent after Randomization
Although much less frequent and often not allowed by the IRB unless there is strong scientific justification, consent after

randomization involves obtaining consent from subjects after they have been randomized to one group or the other. In this case there would be two consent forms, one for those randomized to the intervention group and one for those randomized to the control group. The primary reason for this approach is to conceal from control subjects the type of intervention that those in the intervention group are receiving. Why would researchers want to do this? As noted earlier, clinical trials involving R/S interventions usually attract subjects who are religious themselves and interested in receiving an R/S intervention. Subjects who are assigned to the control group without an R/S intervention may be disappointed, which could affect the outcomes being studied. Therefore, the scientific integrity of the study may be influenced by whether those in the control group "know what they are missing." When researchers obtain consent after randomization with the use of two consent forms, this problem is avoided.

How might this work? A centralized body randomizes the next potential participant to either the intervention or the control group. This information is then communicated to the research personnel *before* they see the next potential subject, which allows them to determine which consent form to use with that subject. One drawback of this method is that research personnel enrolling subjects in this manner must be different from research personnel who do the baseline and follow-up assessments, since blinding would otherwise be compromised.

The result of consenting subjects after randomization is that those randomized to the intervention group simply have to decide if they want to participate in the intervention. The consent form they sign only provides details regarding the intervention. Subjects know what they would be getting and can decide on whether they want to participate in the intervention. Subjects randomized to the control group receive a different consent form at the time of enrollment. This consent form describes exactly what is expected of control subjects, the benefits and risks of being a control subject, and the consequences of choosing to participate as a control. The consent form describes in a general way what the overall research study is about, although specifics about what the intervention group gets is not provided since it is not relevant to what the controls are signing up for.

For example, in an R/S intervention study, the consent form for controls may indicate that a new psychosocial intervention is being tested, and this study will provide information about the effectiveness of the new treatment for the condition the subject has. The consent will make clear that although no intervention will be provided, the subject's participation in the study will help investigators determine whether the new treatment is effective. The subject can then decide whether to participate in the control group. The consent form for controls would indicate that involvement in the control group will involve periodic assessments of the subject's condition (if a no-treatment control) or may involve participating in a health education class or other type of social activity (an "attention" control). Subjects might be paid for being in the control group, increasing their willingness to participate without getting an intervention.

Unfortunately, IRBs may not allow consent after randomization with two separate consent forms as just described. Researchers will not know this, however, unless they discuss the situation with their IRB. If investigators can provide a good enough argument that consent after randomization with two separate consent forms could avoid compromising the scientific integrity of the study, then the IRB may allow this method. For the reasons described above, I think there is good rationale for doing so in clinical trials testing R/S interventions.

Randomization

As noted earlier, randomization eliminates selection bias,[5] balances both known and unknown characteristics influencing the outcome across treatment groups, and forms the basis for statistical tests used to compare the outcome between groups. An independent central coordinating group should be responsible for randomizing subjects to intervention vs. control groups. This will help to maintain the blind for research personnel who are interacting with subjects by coordinating schedules, conducting

> Randomization eliminates selection bias, balances both known and unknown characteristics influencing the outcome across treatment groups, and forms the basis for statistical tests used to compare the outcome between groups.

assessments, or collecting specimens. Software programs (such as SAS or SPSS) are widely available to generate random numbers to guide assignments.[6] I now describe several common methods of randomizing subjects: simple, block, stratified, and unequal randomization.

Simple

Simple randomization involves a method similar to tossing an unbiased or fair coin (heads = intervention group A, tails = control group B). In reality, there is no difference between this and other methods of random assignment. This method can be considered a true experiment. A coin toss, however, is sometimes discouraged because it "looks bad." A random numbers generator using a software programs described above is usually preferred and produces group assignments that are totally unpredictable (the same result as the flip of a fair coin). With both methods, however, imbalances in assignment between intervention and control groups can result and cause a reduction in statistical power, especially when small sample sizes are involved. Bear in mind that alternate assignment (i.e., ABABAB) is not considered random.

Blocked

Blocked randomization is a method to ensure that the number of subjects assigned to intervention and control groups are roughly equal. This is accomplished by dividing subjects into z blocks of size 2x, creating all possible combinations for each block where x subjects are allocated to intervention group A and x subjects to control group B, and then choosing the blocks randomly to determine assignments. For example, let's say investigators wish to randomly assign one hundred subjects to intervention and control groups. They decide to divide up their sample into twenty-five blocks of block size $2 \times 2 = 4$, where z = 25 and x = 2. This will result in six possible treatment allocations: AABB, BBAA, ABAB, BABA, ABBA, and BAAB. Twenty-five different blocks of these six types would then be chosen randomly to guide assignments. This would result in roughly fifty subjects in each group. Investigators should be kept blind to block size, since otherwise they may be able to guess to which group subjects are assigned, resulting in selection bias.

Stratified

While imbalances in intervention vs. control group size can reduce statistical power, imbalances in subject characteristics that affect the study outcome can likewise increase variability in the outcome that reduces the power of the study to detect intervention effects (Chapter 21). Intervention and control groups, then, should be balanced on significant prognostic factors (e.g., race, gender, age, or religiosity in R/S-health research). For example, if race (B/C) and gender (M/F) have a strong influence on the primary outcome, then this would require randomization by 2 × 2 = 4 strata (BM, BF, CM, CF). Block randomization (see previous paragraph), then, would be performed separately for each of these four strata. Block size should be kept relatively small to maintain balance between groups. More stratification variables result in fewer subjects per stratum, so stratified randomization on two characteristics (producing four strata) is probably the most that investigators would be able to do in small clinical trials (e.g., < 100 subjects). Large RCTs usually don't stratify since subject characteristics tend to balance out during the randomization process; this is not the case, however, for small trials. Other sorts of biases, however, may occur with stratified randomization, mostly having to do with the order in which participants are recruited. As the number of blocks increases, the less likely are these biases.

Unequal

Although most clinical trials seek to have equal numbers of subjects assigned to intervention and control groups to maximize statistical power, there may be other reasons to assign more subjects to the intervention than the control group. For example, in R/S interventions that involve terminal oncology patients, investigators may wish to assign subjects to the intervention arm using a 2:1 ratio that minimizes subjects in the control group. Although this results in a modest loss of statistical power, ethical reasons may argue for choosing this method.

Randomization ratios of 3:1 result in a considerable loss of statistical power, and ratios greater than 3:1 are not useful unless sample sizes are huge.

Types of Blinding

Blinding study investigators and subjects helps to remove bias in the application of the intervention, in outcome assessments, and in subjects' preconceived notions regarding the benefits of the intervention. For most purposes, there are three types of blinding in clinical trials: unblinded, single-blind, and double-blind.

> Blinding study investigators and subjects helps to remove bias in the application of the intervention, in outcome assessments, and in subjects' preconceived notions regarding the benefits of the intervention.

Unblinded

In unblinded clinical trials, also called "open-label" trials, everyone is aware of subjects' group assignments—including study investigators, subjects, and those assessing subject outcomes. This method is typically used in feasibility trials to work out the details of study protocols. Not much can be said about treatment effects using this method since the delivery of the intervention and outcome assessments may be biased. This is also the method used in experimental studies that do not involve a control or comparison group (and so would not be considered clinical trials, strictly speaking).

Single-Blind

This is where either research team's members or subjects in the trial are not aware of the subjects' treatment groups. A single-blind would be indicated in a clinical trial where researchers must know who is and isn't getting the intervention in order to conduct the trial (e.g., when conducting a sham intervention vs. a real intervention) or the nature of the intervention makes it impossible to blind the subjects in the trial. A single-blind is appropriate if bias will not be introduced by researchers or subjects knowing which treatment group subjects are in. The worry is that knowledge of who gets the treatment could influence how researchers interact with subjects or affect subjects' expectations of the treatment, influencing subjects' responses to the intervention. With R/S-health interventions, subjects and investigators are usually not blinded, although research team members assessing the outcomes of the trial or otherwise interacting with subjects (besides those actually administering the intervention and control treatments) must be blinded so that this does not affect assessments or subjects' responses.

Double-Blind

In this instance, neither the subjects nor the investigators know who is receiving the intervention. This removes bias in application of the intervention (experimenter bias), removes bias in assessments of outcome (experimenter bias), and removes bias by subject's preconceived ideas about the effectiveness of treatment (subject bias). Double-blinded studies have the highest standard of scientific rigor. For this reason, many early studies of distant intercessory prayer involved "double-blinded" experiments. This was the kind of design that most health-care professionals were familiar with, and so investigators thought that this would provide credible evidence that "prayer works." Unfortunately, as indicated in Chapter 3, these efforts were misguided. Usually it is not possible to conduct a double-blinded clinical trial when testing an R/S intervention, since this is a psychosocial intervention that is delivered by researchers to subjects who know what they are getting. In some instances, it may be possible to blind patients to what treatment group they are in (as in sham R/S interventions) and blind most investigators on the research team (if a group separate from the research team is administering the intervention and control treatments).

Triple-Blind

An extension of the double-blind, a triple-blind study is conducted in a way such that not only are investigators and subjects blinded to who is getting the intervention, but so is the clinical trial monitoring group keeping track of results. Thus, no one knows who is receiving the active treatment. This design also is not possible in R/S-health research and is not being used

> With R/S-health interventions, subjects and investigators are usually not blinded, although research team members assessing the outcomes of the trial or otherwise interacting with subjects (besides those actually administering the intervention and control treatments) must be blinded so that this does not affect assessments or subjects' responses.

much in any other type of research either. The reason is that it is important to have a monitoring board that has access to the data for periodic determination of safety or extraordinary benefit that might lead to a premature stopping of the trial.

Analysis of Results

Analysis of results in clinical trials involving R/S intervention would typically involve a mixed model repeated measures analysis of variance (ANOVA), which allows examination of differences both within subjects and between subjects in the two treatment groups (intervention vs. control) when more than one outcome assessment is involved.[7] For example, consider a clinical trial that examines the effects of religious psychotherapy vs. conventional psychotherapy in depression, where depression is measured as a continuous variable involving a count of symptoms assessed at four time points. Subjects in both groups are assessed at baseline, at the end of treatment, and at three and six months later. This analysis would consist of one "within subject" factor (scores on the four assessments) and one between subjects or treatment factor, with two levels (religious psychotherapy and conventional psychotherapy). In the mixed model approach, the treatment factor is considered as a fixed effect and the subject factor a random effect. The mixed model approach (also known as a general linear mixed model or GLMM) is considered a further refinement of repeated measures ANOVA. Growth curve models, in particular, are used in such situations since they allow the modeling of trajectories of response to the interventions for each subject and predictors of between-subject variation in those responses. The aim of these approaches is to determine whether subjects receiving the religious psychotherapy (1) significantly improved from the beginning to the end of the trial, and (2) did significantly better or worse than those receiving conventional psychotherapy.

> Analysis of results in clinical trials involving R/S intervention would typically involve a mixed model repeated measures analysis of variance (ANOVA), which allows examination of differences both within subjects and between subjects in the two groups (intervention vs. control or other treatment) when more than one outcome assessment is involved.

Intent-to-Treat vs. Per-Protocol Analysis

In a clinical trial there will be those subjects who complete the trial and those who drop out of the study before it is completed. This applies to both intervention and control groups. If the analysis includes only those who completed the entire study, then this is called "per-protocol analysis." If the analysis includes all those who were randomized (including the dropouts), then this is called an "intention-to-treat analysis." From a scientific standpoint, and for grants in particular, researchers should always plan to conduct an intention-to-treat analysis since this is considered more rigorous. When reporting results of the clinical trial it is also permissible to conduct a per-protocol analysis along with an intention-to-treat analysis, since it is important to know whether those subjects who were in the study from start to end and received the full course of treatment did better than controls. However, the issue of attrition (study dropouts) is one of the most serious threats to the validity of RCTs since subjects who are not invested in the intervention or less healthy may be more likely to drop out.

Inaccurate Findings

For a number of reasons, clinical trials may not find significant differences even if the intervention is effective. These include low statistical power (sample too small), poor or incomplete implementation of the intervention, unreliable measures of outcomes and weak potency of the treatment. There are fewer reasons for finding significant differences when the treatment is actually ineffective, although there may be confounding factors associated with the implementation of the treatment (e.g., Hawthorne effect).

> For a number of reasons, clinical trials may not find significant differences even if the intervention is effective.

SUMMARY AND CONCLUSIONS

A randomized clinical trial is a powerful design that is capable of determining whether a religious or spiritual intervention causes changes (improvement or worsening) in a health outcome. In terms of the hierarchy of evidence, the RCT is at the top of the pyramid and is the most convincing design capable of showing that R/S actually affects health. Despite some strengths, however, RCTs also have a lot of weaknesses and limitations. Among those limitations are (1) RCTs are only feasible for certain research questions, (2) results often do not translate easily into real-world situations (since clinical trials are "staged"), and (3) they are expensive, time-consuming, and require expertise in RCT design and management. Failure to consider any of the above limitations is likely to produce misleading results.

In addition to discussing the strengths and limitations of clinical trials, I also described the basic features of RCTs that include standardization of the intervention, choosing a control group, selecting subjects, measuring outcomes, types of informed consent, types of randomization, types of blinding, and methods of analyzing results. In the next chapter I review a number of clinical trials that have examined the effects of R/S interventions on health outcomes.

CHAPTER 10

Clinical Trials with Religious Interventions

H AVING EXAMINED the strengths and weaknesses of clinical trials and described how to go about conducting a randomized clinical trial (RCT) in the last chapter, I now review clinical trials that have tested the effectiveness of religious/spiritual (R/S) interventions. By examining closely the trials that have been done (and some that have not yet been done), my hope is that we can learn lessons about how to conduct an RCT to examine the effects of R/S interventions on health. The studies presented in this chapter are categorized into those examining effects on mental health outcomes, those examining effects on physical health, and those involving the effects of various kinds of R/S interventions on a variety of outcomes.

MENTAL HEALTH

Many more clinical trials have examined the effects of R/S interventions on mental health than physical health. I review some of these studies below, focusing on clinical trials of religious psychotherapy in patients with depression, bereavement, and anxiety.

Depression

In one of the first studies of this kind (1980), Rebecca Propst randomized mildly depressed religious college students to either cognitive behavioral therapy (CBT) with Christian religious imagery or CBT without it.[1] A total of forty-four subjects received one-hour sessions twice weekly for four weeks. Outcomes were assessed immediately following the treatment and six weeks later. Subjects receiving the religious imagery experienced a significantly greater reduction in depressive symptoms (measured by Beck Depression Inventory, BDI) compared to standard cognitive therapy (14 percent vs. 60 percent, respectively, had elevated BDI scores at the end of the trial).

In 1992 Propst and colleagues conducted a larger RCT comparing religious CBT with conventional CBT in fifty-nine religious Christian patients with depression.[2] Depression was diagnosed using standard research diagnostic criteria. Both religious CBT and conventional CBT were carefully documented in manuals was used by therapists in the study. Subjects were randomized to religious CBT (n = 19), conventional CBT (n = 19), or two control groups (n = 21) (pastoral counseling or a wait-list control group [WLC]). Eighteen to twenty one-hour sessions were delivered over twelve weeks, and outcomes were assessed at completion of treatment and at three months and two years later. Results indicated that only subjects receiving the religious CBT reported significantly lower posttreatment BDI scores than did the WLC group (p < 0.001), whereas the conventional CBT showed only a nonsignificant trend in that direction. Likewise, only religious CBT showed a clinically meaningful change on BDI score compared to WLC group (68 percent vs. 27 percent). In both studies above, a Christian form of religious CBT was utilized. Interestingly, the effects were greatest in subjects who received the religious CBT from nonreligious therapists.

In 1995 Azhar and Varma examined the effects of religious psychotherapy based within the Islamic faith tradition in sixty-four depressed Malaysian Muslims with strong religious beliefs.[3] All subjects received fifteen to twenty sessions of weekly supportive psychotherapy plus low doses of antidepressant medication. Half of the sample (n = 32) was randomized to a group that received additional religious psychotherapy that involved discussions of religious issues specific to patients and the prescription of religious practices (such as reading verses from the Holy Qur'an and prayer). Depressive symptoms were assessed using the observer-rated Hamilton Depression Scale that was administered by a psychiatrist blind to treatment group. Patients receiving the additional psychotherapy with a religious perspective experienced more rapid improvement of depression during the first three months of treatment, but after six months the difference between treatment groups became nonsignificant. What is not clear in this study is whether the initial benefits were due to the religious aspects of the therapy or to the additional psychotherapy time spent with therapists.

In both studies above, a Christian form of religious CBT was utilized. Interestingly, the effects were greatest in subjects who received the religious CBT from nonreligious therapists.

What is not clear in this study is whether the initial benefits were due to the religious aspects of the therapy or to the additional psychotherapy time spent with therapists.

Bereavement

In the same year (1995), Azhar and Varma examined the effects of Muslim psychotherapy on bereavement in thirty highly religious Muslims in Malaysia.[4] Subjects were randomized to either supportive therapy plus low-dose antidepressant medication (n = 15) or to supportive therapy plus medication plus twelve to twenty additional sessions of religious psychotherapy (n = 15). Religious psychotherapy again involved discussions of religious issues specific to patients and prescription of religious practices such as reading from the Qur'an and prayer. After six months of treatment, subjects receiving the additional religious psychotherapy experienced significantly greater improvements on the Hamilton Depression Scale than did subjects receiving supportive psychotherapy plus medication alone. Again, as in the previous study of depression, it is not clear whether improvement was due to the effects of the religious psychotherapy or to the additional time spent with therapists.

Anxiety

In their third study of Muslim psychotherapy in Malaysia, Azhar and colleagues randomized sixty-two religious Muslims with generalized anxiety disorder (GAD) to religious psychotherapy plus standard treatment or standard treatment alone.[5] The standard treatment involved antianxiety drugs (benzodiazepines) and twelve to sixteen weekly forty-five-minute sessions of psychotherapy. Those randomized to religious psychotherapy (n = 31) received the standard treatment plus additional religious psychotherapy involving the discussion of religious issues specific to patients (and reading verses of the Holy Qur'an and praying to help with relaxation). Subjects were assessed at baseline, three months, and six months on the Hamilton Anxiety Scale, administered by a psychiatrist blind to treatment group. Subjects receiving the additional religious psychotherapy did significantly better at the three-month evaluation compared to subjects receiving only the standard regimen, although no differences were observed between the two groups at six months.

More recently, Razali and colleagues randomized 165 Malaysian Muslim patients with GAD to either religious CBT (n = 87) or to standard treatment (n = 78).[6] The unique aspect about this study is that 85 subjects were religious and 80 subjects were nonreligious, allowing investigators to examine whether religious CBT might be effective in nonreligious patients. The religious CBT used cognitive-behavioral techniques guided by the Qur'an and Hadith (sayings and customs of the Prophet) to correct negative thinking, discussed religious issues related to GAD with subjects, and taught them effective coping skills from an Islamic perspective. All subjects in both study groups received standard treatment for GAD including benzodiazepines (for up to six weeks), supportive psychotherapy (reassurance, improving coping, reinforcing adaptive behaviors), and/or simple relaxation exercises. Duration of treatment was not specified. Subjects were evaluated at baseline, four, twelve, and twenty-six weeks. Among religious subjects, those receiving the additional religious CBT improved significantly more than those receiving standard treatment at the four-week and twelve-week evaluations (i.e., symptoms improved faster), although by twenty-six weeks, differences between groups had disappeared. No additional benefit from adding the religious CBT to standard treatment was seen in nonreligious subjects at any time.

Finally, Zhang and colleagues examined the effects of Chinese Taoist cognitive psychotherapy for treatment of GAD.[7] Investigators randomized 143 Chinese outpatients seen in clinics in south central China to Chinese Taoist cognitive psychotherapy (CTCP) (n = 46), benzodiazepines (BDZ) only (n = 48), or combined CTCP and BDZ (n = 49). The religious "therapeutic core" of CTCP (besides standard cognitive therapy) involved explaining the complementary roles of Taoism and Confucianism and interpreting the thirty-two-character Taoist formula word for word to assimilate its spirit into the patient's psychological conflicts and coping styles (based on the Lao-zi, the sacred text followed by 20 million Taoists worldwide). Subjects in the CTCP and combined CTCP and BDZ groups received one-hour sessions of CTCP weekly for four weeks and then twice monthly for the remaining five months. Subjects receiving only BDZ remained on the same dose for the last five months of the study. Results indicated that subjects receiving BDZ treatment alone experienced a rapid reduction in GAD symptoms by one month, but beneficial effects were no longer present by six months. CTCP alone had little effect on symptoms at one month (compared to BDZ group), but showed significant symptom reduction at six months. Those receiving combined CTCP and BDZ did the best, with significant symptom reduction observed at one and six months. However, we don't know whether it was the CBT or the religious aspects of the CBT that was responsible for these benefits.

Summary

With the possible exception of the Propst studies above, each of the studies reviewed above has serious weaknesses. We don't know whether the initial faster improvement in the Islamic psychotherapy studies was due to the religious nature of the psychotherapy or to the additional time spent with therapists. We also don't know whether the beneficial effects of Taoist cognitive therapy in the Zhang study were due simply to cognitive therapy alone or anything unique to the Taoist aspects of the treatment. What seems clear, however, based on the Razali study, is that using religious psychotherapy to treat nonreligious patients is not particularly useful, even when therapists spend additional time with patients. The ideal and most rigorous study of religious vs. conventional psychotherapy for treating emotional disorders would be a head-to-head clinical trial of religious vs. conventional CBT in religious subjects, keeping everything the same in both groups except the religious nature of the therapy. This would be a high standard to meet, however, since most clinical trials that compare different types of psychotherapy have not found one therapy superior to another. Our research team is now carrying out such a study.[8]

> Using religious psychotherapy to treat nonreligious patients is not particularly useful, even when additional time is spent with therapists.

PHYSICAL HEALTH

Compared to clinical trials in mental health, much less research exists on the effects of R/S interventions on physical health.[9] Most of the research thus far has examined the effects of Eastern meditation (Transcendental Meditation from the Hindu religious tradition or mindfulness meditation from the Buddhist tradition). I begin by describing completed, attempted, or proposed clinical trials assessing R/S interventions from a Western religious perspective.

Breast Cancer

Dr. Diane Becker at Johns Hopkins University[10] and our team at Duke collaborated on an R/S intervention that was to be administered to African American women with stage I breast cancer one to two months after undergoing radiation therapy. The proposal was submitted to NCCAM in February 2000 and was funded in August 2000 as part of the Hopkins CAM

Center. To my knowledge, this was the first rigorous prospective trial of a prayer intervention supported by NIH. The study was initiated in March 2001. Eighty women were to be randomized to four months of either a prayer intervention or to a wait-list control group. The prayer intervention, called centering prayer[11] or contemplative prayer, consisted of twice daily practice for thirty minutes. Subjects were asked to read a book on centering prayer and participated in five one-hour sessions with research personnel on a one-on-one basis in participants' homes. Study outcomes were (1) neuroendocrine markers (plasma adreno-corticotropic hormone, responses to corticotropin-releasing hormone stimulation, twenty-four-hour urinary cortisol, and cortisol circadian rhythm using salivary cortisol), (2) immune markers (peripheral blood CD4/CD8 T-cell subsets, monocytes, natural killer cell activity, lymphocyte proliferation and cytokine release in response to breast-cancer-specific antigens), and (3) psychosocial outcomes (perceived stress, psychosocial functioning, and quality of life) to be assessed at baseline, one month, and six months.

By May 2003, however, we had fallen behind in recruitment, enrolling only twenty of the eighty subjects planned. After an NCCAM site visit, they decided to halt the study after it became clear that we could not recruit the necessary number of subjects during the time remaining in the grant to complete the study. The reason for lack of recruitment was notable. Once the women completed radiation therapy, they felt "cured," wanted to distance themselves from their long-term link with the medical care system, and so did not wish to participate in the four-month prayer study. We proposed to the NCCAM committee that we change the time of recruitment, and enroll the remaining sixty women during the six weeks when they were actually receiving radiation therapy (a time when there was much more motivation to participate). However, the NIH site reviewers were afraid to take any risks with the study due to the fact that it involved prayer. Throughout the development of the project, the NIH review process, and the study implementation, there appeared to be bias against this type of research study (received much closer scrutiny than other CAM studies because of fear of criticisms from the government). Thus, many lessons were learned.

Congestive Heart Failure

Dr. Becker also developed a similar protocol for the treatment of patients with congestive heart failure. The plan was to randomize eighty subjects with class III-IV CHF and dilated cardiomyopathy to either four months of centering prayer or to an attention-matched control group. The intervention proposed in this study was the same one used in the breast cancer prayer study described above. Outcomes to be assessed at baseline, one months, and six months were (1) catecholamines (epinephrine and norepinephrine) and heart rate variability (as an indicator of sympathetic nervous system activity), (2) circulating neurohormones and cytokines reflective of CHF progression (endothelin-1, atrial natriuretic peptide, brain natriuretic peptide, tumor necrosis factor-α), (3) functional status (six-minute walk test), (4) left ventricular function (rest gated cardiac blood pool imaging), and (5) psychosocial measures (perceived distress, psychosocial functioning, quality of life). The study was submitted to NIH and received an excellent priority score in the first round indicating that it would be funded. However, Dr. Becker's circumstances changed, so she had to get a colleague to replace her as principal investigator on the project. As a result, NIH required that the proposal be resubmitted for an entirely new review. The NIH committee that first reviewed the proposal, however, changed composition between the initial submission and the resubmission. This new review group expressed many more criticisms of the proposal and eventually turned it down.

Malignant Melanoma

Dr. Brenda Cole, then at the University of Pittsburgh Cancer Institute, developed an R/S intervention titled "spiritual focused therapy" (SFT) for adults diagnosed with stage IV unresectable metastatic melanoma. The plan was to randomize subjects to SFT, to a cognitive behavioral therapy (CBT) condition, or to a usual care control condition, with fifty participants in each group. Assuming a refusal rate of 50 percent and an attrition rate of 40 percent, investigators estimated that they needed to identify approximately five hundred eligible participants for the study (budget was $300,000 in direct costs). Primary outcomes in the study were survival and quality of life. Both SFT and CBT were to be administered following structured treatment manuals. Both interventions included equivalent amounts of time spent on the structured interventions, semistructured discussion, and meditative practices. The only difference was that the SFT condition integrated spiritual material into the treatment. That spiritual material involved strengthening one's relationship or connection to the Sacred (i.e., God) to enhance coping support, meaning, and insight, meditation with explicit spiritual content, and discussion of spiritually related concerns and resources. The treatment manual was constructed to incorporate the beliefs of the participants and included discussion time to help therapists identify the participant's language and symbols for the Sacred. This well-designed, carefully thought-through study was submitted to and funded by National Cancer Institute on the *fourth* submission. Results of the study are now pending.

Summary

Notice how focused and specific the patient populations selected for these studies were, and also the rigorous evaluation of biological outcomes, especially in the Becker studies above. Also, consider the challenges that these highly qualified investigators faced as they sought funding support for their proposals.

Other Clinical Trials

Clinical trials that involve chaplain interventions, in-person intercessory prayer, and Eastern meditation are reviewed in this section.

Chaplain Interventions

The most common R/S interventions currently taking place in the health-care system involve interventions by chaplains. Several studies have now examined the health benefits of chaplain visits.

Orthopedic Surgery

In 1973 Florell divided 150 orthopedic surgery patients into three groups: (1) those who received support by a chaplain (regular visits where patients talked about their feelings and anxieties, with reassurance that feelings were acceptable and the chaplain would be available if needed) (n = 30), (2) those who received support plus information (the support above was augmented by information about the hospital routine, expectations of patients, practical information about how to get relief from pain, recovery procedures, etc.) (n = 70), and (3) control patients receiving normal hospital care without support or information (n = 50).[12] Outcomes were length of stay, use of pain medication, anxiety and stress level, pain level, and number of lines of nursing notes written on patients (the latter served as a proxy for the amount of nurse's time needed for help and assistance). No information was given on who assessed outcomes, whether this was done blinded to treatment group, or whether subjects were randomized to treatment group. However, groups did not differ on any of the outcomes at baseline.

When health outcomes were compared after the hospitalization, the investigator reported that those in the control group stayed over a day longer than those in the support group and two days longer than those in the support plus information group. Likewise, anxiety levels, use of pain medication, lines of nursing notes, and number of calls for pain medication, bedpan, service, nurses and physicians were all significantly higher in control patients, especially when compared to those in the support plus information group.

Elimination of Chaplain Services

In an example of a clinical trial that used a "withdrawal" control group, Gartner and colleagues measured effects on source of chaplain referrals before and after chaplain staff was substantially reduced at Northwestern Memorial Hospital in Chicago.[13] Elimination of the clinical pastoral education program in 1985 reduced pastoral care staff from five and a half full-time chaplains plus nine students to four and a half full-time chaplains and no students. Before chaplain services were reduced, chaplains initiated forty-two referrals per week whereas staff initiated only ten referrals per week. After chaplain services were cut, chaplain-initiated referrals dropped from forty-two per week to only seventeen per week, whereas staff-initiated referrals increased from ten referrals per week to twenty-one referrals per week ($p < 0.01$). Researchers concluded that when pastoral care was less available, the demand for pastoral services from nursing and medical staff increased substantially.

Chronic Obstructive Pulmonary Disease

Iler and colleagues at the Lewis-Gale Medical Center in Salem, Virginia, alternately assigned (not random) fifty hospitalized patients with COPD to either a chaplain-visited intervention group or to a non-chaplain-visited control group.[14] The chaplain intervention (conducted by Iler) involved an average of four visits, approximately twenty minutes each. During the visit, the chaplain prayed with patients and allowed them to vent their emotions. Nonvisited controls received only brief visits on admission and discharge for purposes of collecting information. Controlling for baseline anxiety on admission, chaplain-visited patients on discharge had significantly less anxiety (measured by Beck Anxiety Inventory), significantly shorter hospital stays (5.7 days vs. 9.0 days, $p = 0.002$), significantly greater satisfaction with care ($p < 0.05$), and tended to be more likely to say they would recommend the hospital to others ($p = 0.056$). The only weaknesses of this study were that assignment was alternate (vs. random) and that it was not clear whether outcomes were assessed blinded to treatment group.

Coronary Artery Bypass Graft Surgery

Bay and associates at Clarian Health Partners in Indianapolis, Indiana, randomized 170 patients undergoing CABG surgery to either a chaplain-visited intervention group (n = 85) or a control group that did not receive chaplain visits (n = 85).[15] Of 485 patients screened, 311 met inclusion and exclusion criteria; 107 of those declined, leaving 204 patients who were randomized to treatment or control groups. Of randomized patients, 38 patients did not complete the study and 34 of those had no follow-up data, resulting in 170 randomized subjects on whom data were available for analysis. The chaplain intervention (administered by Chaplain Bay, primarily) consisted of four visits with the patient and one visit with the patient's family (average forty-four minutes of contact total). The visit involved listening, support, identification of a single general coping question, and discussion of hopes, positive future, and grief related to limitations of disease. The description of the intervention sounds like the chaplain focused primarily on psychological rather than religious concerns. Patients assigned to the control group received no chaplain visits, although may have been visited by their own clergy.

Outcomes assessed at baseline, one month, and six months after surgery were anxiety, depression, hope, religious coping, and religious problem-solving styles and the use of health services. A research assistant enrolled patients and conducted baseline and outcome assessments. Results indicated no difference between groups on anxiety, depression, hope, number of hospital readmissions, unscheduled physician office visits, postsurgery length of stay, or cost of hospitalization. The only benefits documented in chaplain-visited patients were an increase in positive religious coping and decrease in negative religious coping at six months. The major weaknesses of this study are (1) chaplains spent less

> Chaplain-visited patients on discharge had significantly less anxiety, significantly shorter hospital stays, significantly greater satisfaction with care, and tended to be more likely to say they would recommend the hospital to others.

> The only benefits documented in chaplain-visited patients were an increase in positive religious coping and decrease in negative religious coping at six months.

than ten minutes per visit with patients and families, which may not have been sufficient to affect the health outcomes in this study; (2) the focus was largely on psychological rather than religious issues (i.e., the unique role of chaplains); and (3) since enrollment and assessments were both conducted by the same research assistant, assessments did not appear to be blind to treatment group.

Intercessory Prayer Studies (In-Person)

In contrast to double-blinded distant intercessory prayer studies, which as noted above have little theological or scientific rationale, proximal person-to-person prayer and proximal intercessory prayer studies have clear theological relevance and scientific rationale (acting via plausible mind-body mechanisms).

Depression and Anxiety

Boelens and colleagues examined the effects of proximal person-to-person prayer on depression, anxiety, positive emotions, and salivary cortisol levels in sixty-three depressed/anxious adults (95 percent women) being seen in primary care medical clinics.[16] Subjects were randomized to either the prayer intervention (n = 27) or a wait-list control (n = 36). Those in the intervention group received one ninety-minute and five sixty-minute prayer sessions over six weeks conducted by a nondenominational college graduate in her late sixties (trained at Christian Healing Ministries). Those in the wait-list control group received no prayer or any other intervention during the six-week intervention (although they did receive the six-week prayer intervention after that time).

Salivary cortisol (8 a.m., noon, 5 p.m., 9 p.m.) and measures of depression and anxiety were assessed at baseline and six-week follow-up in both groups. The depression and anxiety measures (Hamilton Depression Scale and Hamilton Anxiety Scale) were observer-rated and performed by the senior author, a physician, who was not blinded to treatment group. Results indicated a significant reduction in both depressive symptoms

> In contrast to double-blinded distant intercessory prayer studies, proximal person-to-person prayer and proximal intercessory prayer studies have clear theological relevance and scientific rationale (acting via plausible mind-body mechanisms).

and anxiety symptoms in the intervention group compared to controls, although no difference was found on cortisol measures. The primary weakness of this study is that the physician assessing outcomes was not blinded to treatment group.

Hearing and Vision

In a remarkable and highly controversial experimental study (without a control group, so it is technically not a clinical trial), Brown and colleagues examined the effects of a single session of proximal intercessory prayer (PIP) on hearing sensitivity and visual acuity during charismatic Protestant meetings in twenty-four rural Mozambican subjects with auditory or visual impairments.[17] Consecutive subjects who received prayer for vision or hearing loss and agreed to diagnostic tests (all subjects assented) were included in the study. PIP involves direct-contact prayer to God for healing. This frequently involved touch by one or more persons, usually lasting between one and fifteen minutes, although sometimes lasting an hour or more. Those administering the intervention were in direct contact with subjects, and subjects knew they were receiving the intervention. Approximately half of the subjects ($n = 13$) received the intervention from a single individual, whereas the remaining participants received PIP from others trained in this method. Researchers who conducted the assessments of hearing and vision were not blinded to treatment group since all subjects received the intervention. However, the measurements were objective: a handheld audiometer (Earscan ES3) for hearing thresholds and standard visual acuity charts (Precision vision) for vision assessment. Results indicated significant improvements in both hearing ($p < 0.003$) and visual acuity ($p < 0.02$) following PIP (before vs. after assessments).

The major weaknesses here are (1) the absence of a control group and (2) researchers assessing outcomes in an unblinded fashion (although the objectivity of the assessment methods helped to minimize bias, the possibility of investigator bias remains). One way to improve on this study would be to randomize subjects to PIP or sham PIP (someone pretending to pray, but not actually praying) and ensure that those assessing outcomes were blind to the treatment group.

Eastern Meditation

Many studies have examined the effects of Hindu-based Transcendental Meditation (TM) or Buddhist-based mindfulness meditation (MM) on mental and physical health outcomes using an RCT design. These studies have examined effects on blood pressure, cerebrovascular disease, immune function, endocrine function, and pain level, besides many studies on depression and anxiety. Here are some recent examples of clinical trials examining physical health outcomes.

Blood Pressure (BP)

Paul-Labrador from Cedar-Sinai Medical Center in Los Angeles and associates from Maharishi University examined the effects of TM on BP and components of the metabolic syndrome in 103 subjects with stable coronary heart disease.[18] Subjects were randomized to sixteen weeks of TM or health education. The TM group received three hours of introductory lectures, a fifteen-minute personal interview, one and a half hours of personal instructions, four and a half hours of group meetings, and three hours per week of maintenance meetings during the first four weeks and one and a half hours per week during the remaining twelve weeks. In addition, subjects practiced TM twice daily throughout the sixteen weeks. Controls in the health education (HE) group attended the same number and frequency of group meetings as the TM group, and home assignments were given to match the time practiced at home by the TM group. Before-after results following sixteen weeks of the intervention revealed that the TM group dropped their systolic BP by 2.9 mmHg, compared to an increase of 3.1 mmHg in the control group ($p = 0.03$, comparison between TM and HE groups at study end, adjusted for baseline differences); there was no difference between groups on diastolic BP. Note the time and intensity of the intervention necessary to achieve these small differences.

Barnes and colleagues from the Georgia Prevention Institute examined the effects of TM on BP in a sixteen-week clinical trial involving 156 African American adolescents.[19] Randomization was not done at the student level but rather at the school level (five schools involved). Students in the TM group received personal instruction on the technique, engaged in fifteen-minute sessions at school and at home each day, and practiced twice daily at home on weekends. Those in the control group received fifteen-minute lifestyle education lectures twice daily. Outcome was measured using an ambulatory BP monitor. Subjects were reassessed at two months, four months, and eight months following the start of the study. Since there were 56 dropouts, outcome analysis was conducted only on subjects in TM and control groups who completed the clinical trial (per-protocol analysis). Daytime systolic BP in the TM group decreased significantly greater than in the control group (4 mmHg vs. 1 mmHg, $p < 0.04$); there was also a trend toward greater daytime diastolic BP decrease in the TM group compared to controls (2.4 mmHg vs. 0.1 mmHg, $p < 0.06$). There was no difference in nighttime BP. The randomization by school rather than individual student, high number of study dropouts, and the per-protocol analysis were all study weaknesses.

In the largest study of TM and BP to date, Schneider and colleagues from Maharishi University randomized 234 African Americans with hypertension to one of three groups: TM, progressive muscle relaxation (PMR), or health education (HE).[20] Over one-third of subjects (36 percent) dropped out, leaving 150 who completed the protocol and assessments at baseline and twelve-month follow-up. The TM intervention consisted of several hours of introductory lectures, a personal interview, one and a half hours of personal instruction, and four and a half hours of maintenance instruction and practice in a group format, and subjects were required to practice TM for twenty minutes twice daily for twelve months (a massive intervention!). Members of the PMR control group practiced twenty minutes twice daily, and those in the HE control group received written materials, lectures, and group support for modifying cardiovascular risk factors, and were encouraged to exercise and become involved in restful activities at home for twenty minutes twice daily. According to researchers, the TM and control groups all had a similar number of follow-up meetings and attention from instructors. Results indicated that members of the TM group decreased diastolic BP significantly more than PMR and HE control groups (−4.8 vs. −2.6 and −2.6 mmHg, respectively, p < 0.05 for intent to treat analysis), and there was a similar but nonsignificant trend for systolic BP (−3.1 vs. −0.5 and −0.9 mmHg, respectively, p = ns). Despite the high number of dropouts, this was a well-done study, although the effects seem small given the intensity of the intervention.

Cerebrovascular Disease

Castillo-Richmond and colleagues, again from Maharishi University, examined the effects of TM on carotid artery atherosclerosis, a precursor of cerebrovascular disease and stroke.[21] African Americans over age twenty with high blood pressure were randomized to either TM or a health education control group. Those receiving TM underwent a week of initial instruction followed by meetings held every two weeks for two months and then every month for three months, and were instructed to practice TM for twenty minutes twice daily for seven months. Those in the HE control group received similar amounts of instruction and home practice. B-mode carotid ultrasound was used to measure carotid intima-media thickness (IMT) at baseline and six to nine months later. Of the 138 initial participants, only 60 subjects completed the pretest and posttest assessments (31 in TM group and 29 in the health education control group). Members of the TM group who completed the protocol experienced a significant decrease of −0.098 mm in IMT compared to the control group's increase of +0.054 mm in IMT (p = 0.04). Of course, the major weakness of this study is that only 43 percent of subjects completed the study, requiring a per-protocol analysis. As in the Paul-Labrador and Schneider studies, note the intensity of the intervention.

Immune Function

Davidson and colleagues from the University of Wisconsin in Madison randomized forty-eight subjects using a 3:2 ratio to either Buddhist-based mindfulness meditation (MM) or a wait-list control group; of these, forty-one subjects completed the baseline and at least some follow-up assessments.[22] The MM intervention (n = 25) consisted of a three-hour class that met once per week for eight weeks, attendance at a seven-hour silent retreat during week six, and one hour of daily meditative practices at home throughout the study. Following the intervention, subjects in the MM and control group were vaccinated for influenza, and antibody titers were assessed four and eight weeks later. Results indicated that those receiving the MM intervention had a significantly greater rise in antibody titer from week four to week eight, compared to members of the control group ($t = 2.05$, $p < 0.05$). The per-protocol analysis is the primary weakness of this study.

Endocrine Function

Granath and associates examined the effect of a Hindu-based Kundalini Yoga program on salivary cortisol in adults in Sweden.[23] Researchers randomized thirty-seven subjects to either a cognitive-behavioral therapy (CBT) stress management program (n = 17) or to the Hindu yoga program (n = 16). Both interventions were administered during ten group sessions that were delivered over four months. The yoga program consisted of physical exercise, Hindu meditation, emphasis on mantra knowledge, and intuition. Both interventions were guided by and documented using treatment manuals. Outcomes were based on single samples of salivary cortisol and urinary catecholamines (norepinephrine and epinephrine) obtained at baseline and follow-up after the interventions. Results indicated no significant change in salivary cortisol either within each group or between groups. Norepinephrine levels decreased significantly from baseline to postintervention in the yoga group ($t = 3.15$, $p = 0.007$), but not in the CBT group, whereas there was a near significant decrease in epinephrine in the CBT group ($t = 2.07$, $p = 0.06$), but no change in the yoga group. When compared across intervention arms (rather than within), no significant difference was found. Technically, this was a fairly well-done study (with the exception of a weak measure of salivary cortisol).

Chronic Pain

In a well-designed clinical trial that examined the effects of short-term intensive residential Hindu yoga on chronic low back pain, Tekur and colleagues from the Swami Vivekananda yoga Research Foundation in Bangalore, India, randomized eighty Indian subjects with back pain to either the yoga intervention or a physical exercise control group.[24] The yoga intervention involved a weeklong intensive residential program consisting of asanas (physical postures) designed for back pain, *pranayamas* (breathing practices), meditation, and didactic and interactive sessions on the spiritual concepts involved in yoga. The physical exercise control group practiced physical exercises and had didactic and interactive sessions on lifestyle change. Both groups received the same amount of intervention time and attention. A member of the research team blinded to treatment group assessed pain level before and after the interventions using a standard scale (Oswestry Disability Index). Results indicated a reduction in pain scores in the yoga group that was significantly greater compared to the exercise group (p = 0.01).

Summary and Conclusions

Randomized clinical trials can be done (and must be done) to assess the effects of R/S interventions on mental and physical health outcomes. With the exception of studies on Eastern spiritual meditation, most studies that tested explicitly religious interventions have focused on mental health outcomes (depression or anxiety). There is great need for clinical trials in the Americas, Australia, Africa, and Europe that examine the effects of Western religious interventions on physical health outcomes. Several such interventions show substantial promise, and a number of those have been reviewed in this chapter.

> There is great need for clinical trials in the Americas, Australia, Africa, and Europe that examine the effects of Western religious interventions on physical health outcomes.

Many lessons can be learned from the experiences of investigators who have attempted studies of this kind and have not been able to complete them due to lack of funding support, difficulty recruiting subjects, or inadequacies in design. We can also learn much from studies of Eastern meditation—those of Hindu Transcendental Meditation done by the research group at Maharishi University and those of Buddhist mindfulness meditation developed by Kabat-Zinn at the University of Massachusetts and others. These interventions typically last from two to twelve months, with intensive instruction, preparation, and twice-daily practice.

Despite this, the effects (at least when conducted in Western nations) are often quite small given the size and intensity of the intervention. In contrast, the designs of clinical trials testing Western religious interventions are often quite weak, with investigators expecting positive results from short, brief, anemic attempts to alter health outcomes. Is it surprising that a chaplain intervention consisting of a few visits each lasting less than ten minutes finds that such an intervention has no effect? Not surprising at all.

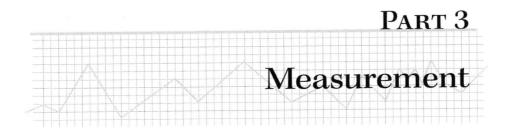

PART 3

Measurement

Definitions

D EFINITION OF TERMS is essential for clear communication and precise understanding of what is being discussed. Yet definitions can be a thorny issue, especially in the area of religion, spirituality, and health. Since there are no clear gold standards, everyone has their own definitions of terms such as "religion" and "spirituality." These definitions are often viewed as sacred, held passionately, and defended fervently. I propose my own definitions here and provide rationale for them. I argue that the definitions chosen for terms such as "religion" and "spirituality" depend on the setting and purpose for which they are used. The two settings relevant for our purposes here are research settings and clinical practice settings. Each has different criteria for defining constructs such as religion and spirituality that are specific to the setting's unique needs.

Research vs. Clinical Practice

The following are criteria for defining constructs used in quantitative research settings:

1. A construct must be clear and unambiguous. Quantitative research involves reducing an entity to its basic elements so that it can be measured and quantified in terms of numbers.
2. A construct must be distinct and unique, and must not overlap with similar constructs to which researchers may wish to relate it.
3. A construct must not be confused with its outcome (health) or with other constructs (psychological and social factors) that lie along the path that leads from that construct to the outcome.
4. A construct must be measurable and quantifiable. Quantitative research seeks to measure constructs numerically and precisely, so that the construct can be correlated with other constructs (health outcomes) that are likewise measured numerically and precisely.
5. Measures of a construct must be able to identify those with the construct, and separating them from those without it, since the goal is *comparison*.

For clinical settings, the criteria for defining constructs are different than for research, since the goals of clinical practice are different. In clinical practice, the definitions of constructs we are interested in must be applied to a wide range of patients and be capable of comprehensively addressing topics that are personal and sensitive.

1. A construct need not always be clear. In fact, ambiguity may be an advantage, especially when health professionals do not wish to force their own definitions of sensitive topics onto patients.
2. A construct may have some overlap with similar constructs, including the outcomes of the construct.
3. A construct need not be precisely measured or quantified.

4. Since there is no gold standard or "correct" view applicable to everyone, definitions can be broader, applying to patients with many different views and perspectives.

5. Definitions should promote conversation and focus on similarities, not differences, since the goal is *dialogue* and *engagement* (not comparison).

While having a common definition of terms such as "religion" and "spirituality" is important when talking with patients, that need is magnified many times in the world of research because research seeks to determine whether religion/spirituality (R/S) is related to health and how this relationship comes about. Clear definitions in research settings are important because they will determine the content of measures used to assess and quantify R/S in observational studies. The results from observational studies, in turn, will inform the design of effective interventions that will be used to change health outcomes.

Constructs in R/S-health research that need clear, unambiguous definitions include *predictors* such as religion or spirituality; *control* and *moderating variables* such as demographics and genetic influences; *explanatory variables* such as psychological, social, and behavioral factors; and *outcome variables* having to do with mental and physical health (see Chapter 16 for an explanation of these variable classes). Many constructs used in R/S-health research already have standard definitions within the social, behavioral, psychological, and medical sciences and relatively precise measures to assess them. I focus here then on the three predictor variables used in R/S-health research and define them for research purposes: religion, spirituality, and secular. The definitions I present here come with a disclaimer. None are universally accepted. They are based on my understanding of quantitative research, reading of the literature, and, admittedly, personal biases.

> While having a common definition of terms such as "religion" and "spirituality" is important when talking with patients, that need is magnified many times in the world of research because research seeks to determine whether religion/spirituality (R/S) is related to health and how this relationship comes about.

> The definitions I present here come with a disclaimer. None are universally accepted. They are based on my understanding of quantitative research, reading of the literature, and, admittedly, personal biases.

Religion

I define "religion" as beliefs, practices, and rituals related to the Transcendent or the Divine. These beliefs and practices are often held with considerable emotional intensity and thus are considered sacred (set apart as holy). In Western religious traditions, the Transcendent is also called God, Allah, HaShem, or a Higher Power, and in Eastern traditions, the Transcendent is variously called Vishnu, Krishna, Buddha, or closely related to concepts such as Ultimate Truth or Reality. Religion may also involve beliefs about spirits, angels, demons, or other supernatural forces that exist outside the natural world, yet are thought to interact with it. Religions usually have doctrines about life after death and rules to guide behavior during the present life to prepare for the life to come. Religions also provide guidance on how to live within a social group in order to maximize harmony and cooperation, and minimize conflict and harm to self or others. Religion is usually organized and practiced within a community made up of those who seek to adhere to the doctrines of a particular faith tradition, and is often organized and maintained as an institution. Religion, however, can also exist outside of an institution and may be practiced alone and involve private expressions of devotion to the Transcendent. At its core, religion involves an established tradition that arises out of a group of people with common beliefs about and rituals concerning the Transcendent.[1]

> I define "religion" as beliefs, practices, and rituals related to the Transcendent or the Divine.

Although some may disagree with this definition, particularly the strong emphasis I place on the Transcendent (certain Jewish and Buddhist traditions may not require belief in the existence of God or Divinities), there is general agreement on what the term "religion" means. Certain parts or components of religion, however, may sometimes be used to signify the entire construct. As described in Chapter 12, there are at least sixteen different aspects of religion. However, some individuals see "institutional" religion as synonymous with the entire construct or may contrast institutional religion with personal forms of sacred involvement that are viewed as more valid. For others, the word "religion" has negative connotations, reflecting divisions, political views, war, or indoctrination. Nevertheless, most persons at least recognize religion as distinct and separate from states of mental or physical health.

SPIRITUALITY

In contrast to religion, "spirituality" is often viewed positively and personally. It is perceived as a more inclusive term that individuals can define for themselves and which carries little of the baggage (rules, authority, responsibility, divisions) associated with religion.[2] Because of this focus on individuality, however, it is challenging to come up with a common definition for "spirituality," especially one that fulfills the criteria necessary for research purposes.

To address this challenge, I prefer a more traditional definition of "spirituality" that is described in the work of theologian Philip Sheldrake at the Cambridge Theological Federation (United Kingdom).[3] The word "spirituality" has distinctly religious and Christian origins, deriving from the Latin *spiritualitas* and *spiritualis*, and the Greek versions of those terms contained in St. Paul's epistles in the Bible. According to this traditional definition of "spirituality," those considered "spiritual" are a subgroup of religious persons whose lives are rooted in and directed by their religious beliefs (i.e., the deeply religious). These individuals, then, would be distinguished from those who are either not religious or who are religious but not deeply so (see Figure 11.1).[4] This traditional definition of spirituality contrasts with the more contemporary and popular view of spirituality as much broader than religion, even including those who are not religious at all ("spiritual but not religious").

According to the historical definition of "spirituality," being religious is a *necessary but not sufficient criterion* for being spiritual. Individuals described as spiritual were those who dedicated their lives to religion, such as the clergy or committed religious leaders (e.g., Gandhi, Buddha, Confucius, Jesus, Mother Teresa). Spiritual persons, however, were not limited to the clergy but also included individuals who were deeply involved in religious

> According to the historical definition of "spirituality," being religious is a *necessary but not sufficient criterion* for being spiritual.

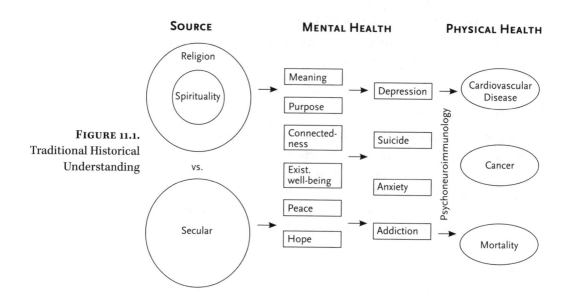

FIGURE 11.1.
Traditional Historical
Understanding

SOURCE   **MENTAL HEALTH**   **PHYSICAL HEALTH**

activity or were sincerely seeking to develop a religious view and way of life reflected in their relationships with others, themselves, and the world around them.

Such a definition, while not perfect, is more easily measured for research purposes than the contemporary definition of spirituality, which is so diffuse and broad (see below). For example, identifying those who are spiritual using the traditional definition is accomplished by developing a measure of religiosity that assesses a person's degree of commitment and level of practice, and then assigning the term "spiritual" to individuals who score in the top 10 or 20 percent on this measure—that is, the deeply religious. The health status of these individuals identified as spiritual, then, could be compared to the less devoutly religious or the nonreligious (secular). Spirituality defined in this way is a clear, nonoverlapping construct, and its association with health outcomes can be easily interpreted.[5]

SECULAR

The secular, distinct from both religion and spirituality, is a philosophical approach that understands human existence and behavior without reference to the Transcendent. The secular focuses on the rational self and human community as the ultimate source of meaning and hope. This definition of the secular is generally agreed upon, is clear, and does not overlap with other constructs. I do not include here, as many others do, a category of "secular spirituality"—at least not for research purposes. Such a term is a confusing combination of opposites. The language for research purposes must be crystal clear in terms of description and measurement so that its relationship with health can be examined.

> The secular focuses on the rational self and human community as the ultimate source of meaning and hope.

CONCERNS ABOUT SPIRITUALITY

As noted above, "spirituality" as used today is a popular term for describing a wide range of people and experiences, almost always referring to something good or positive. While this use of the word "spirituality" may be fine for public discourse and for discussing the topic with patients in clinical practice, it is not appropriate for the kinds of precise language necessary for research. Many researchers, however, are now defining spirituality in exactly this way. Unfortunately, attempts to measure spirituality as a broad, overarching, inclusive construct have resulted in scientifically unacceptable construct overlap.[6] This situation came about quite gradually, and the driving force has been a legitimate desire to include both the religious and the nonreligious among those defined as spiritual (see Figure 11.2).

> Attempts to measure spirituality as a broad, overarching, inclusive construct have resulted in scientifically unacceptable construct overlap.

What exactly qualifies a person who is not religious to describe himself or herself using religious language (i.e., spiritual)? How does one identify such a person? What are the unique criteria that mark persons who consider themselves spiritual but not religious as spiritual (other than by simply asking individuals to categorize themselves as religious, spiritual, both, or neither)? This has created a vacuum that researchers have filled with all sorts of indicators, resulting in a further expansion of the term "spirituality" (see Figure 11.3). The problem is that some of those indicators include positive character traits (forgiveness, moral values, altruism), positive emotional states (meaning, purpose, peacefulness, harmony,

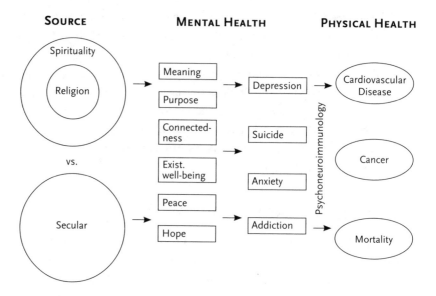

FIGURE 11.2. Modern Understanding

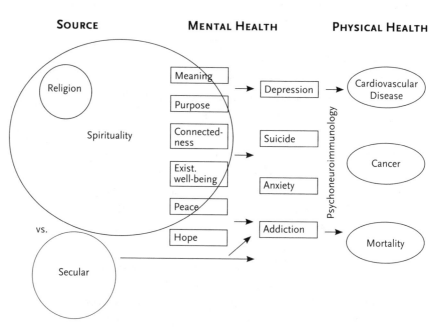

FIGURE 11.3. Modern Understanding—Tautological Version

sense of wholeness), and positive social characteristics (social connectedness).

By defining spirituality a priori as a positive psychosocial state and measuring spirituality using indicators of positive psychological and social health, this contaminates measures of spirituality with the very outcome that researchers are trying to predict (i.e., good mental health). There is a word for this circular type of reasoning: "tautology," that is, process of correlating something with itself. Investigators using measures of spirituality contaminated with such mental health indicators will of course find positive correlations between spirituality and mental health (and often with physical health as well, since good mental health positively influences physical health via psycho-physiological processes). The resulting positive correlations between spirituality and mental health, however, have been set up a priori by defining spirituality as good mental health in the first place. Hence, the findings from such research are meaningless.

Not only is this scientifically unacceptable, but there are other problems as well with this tautological version of spirituality. First, atheists and agnostics may deny any association with spirituality and yet rightly claim that they are forgiving, have meaning and purpose in life, have strong social connections, and live by high moral values. Second, those with mental illness—the depressed, anxious, or those struggling with terrifying delusions and hallucinations—now can no longer be called spiritual. Indeed, a lack of purpose or meaning in life, absence of peace and harmony, and a desire to withdraw from social contact and disconnect from others are exactly the criteria used to define many mental, emotional, and behavioral disorders. Finally, research that defines spirituality as a positive mental health state and measures it using indicators of good mental and social health can no longer examine the negative effects of spirituality. Spirituality cannot possibly be expected to have positive effects in all people, in all settings, and under all circumstances. Thus, there are many problems with defining and measuring spirituality in this manner.

Measurement Contamination

Let's now examine some widely used spirituality scales that illustrate the problem of measurement contamination discussed above.

Functional Assessment of Chronic Illness Therapy–Spiritual Well-Being (FACIT-Sp)[7]

This measure is the most commonly used (and almost required) for assessing spirituality in patients with cancer. Indeed, it is a recommended measure on the website of the National Cancer Institute.[8] The rapid rise to fame for the FACIT-Sp is likely because of its close relationship to the Functional Assessment of Cancer Therapy–General (FACT-G), the standard measure of quality of life in field of oncology today.[9] Thus, it would seem natural that a spirituality measure connected to that tool would gain the acceptance that it has. Here is an example of the statements contained in the twelve-item version of the FACIT-Sp:

- I feel peaceful.
- I have a reason for living.
- I have trouble feeling peace of mind (score in reverse).
- I feel a sense of purpose in my life.
- I am able to reach down deep into myself for comfort.
- I feel a sense of harmony within myself.
- I feel comfort in my faith or spiritual beliefs.
- I know whatever happens with my illness, things will be okay.

These items—peacefulness, purpose and reason for living, sense of harmony, feeling comforted or strengthened—are the *results* of living a spiritual life, not spirituality itself.

Daily Spiritual Experiences Scale (DSE)[10]

The DSE seeks to measure daily spiritual experiences that people have. Several of its items, however, stray away from anything distinctly spiritual to instead measure some of the positive mental or social health states that genuine spirituality may produce.

Below are examples of items in the sixteen-item version of the scale.

- I experience a connection to all life.
- I feel deep inner peace or harmony.
- I feel a self-less caring for others.
- I accept others even when they do things I think are wrong.

Although the items above reflect measurement contamination, the DSE also has many valid items that tap experiences that are distinctly spiritual. Unfortunately, the inclusion of contaminating items helps to weight scores in favor of positive psychological or social health.

Spiritual Transcendence Scale (STS)[11]

This scale is often used when a broad measure of spirituality is desired, and has even been described as a separate dimension of personality. Consider the following items included in the nine-item brief version of the scale:

- In the quiet of my prayers and/or meditations, I find a sense of wholeness.
- I find inner strength and/or peace from my prayers and/or meditations.
- Although individual people may be difficult, I feel an emotional bond with all of humanity.
- My prayers and/or meditations provide me with a sense of emotional support.

Descriptors such as finding a sense of wholeness, inner strength or peace, an emotional bond with all of humanity, or a sense of emotional comfort—all reflect a positive state of emotional health, and so would be expected (and guaranteed) to correlate with good mental health.

Spiritual Well-Being Scale (SWB)[12]

The last example of a scale that illustrates measurement contamination is the SWB scale—a measure that has been around for almost 30 years and has been used in hundreds of studies. In fact, it is among the most cited of all R/S scales by Google Scholar (437 citations as of November 2010). The SWB scale consists of two subscales, a ten-item religious well-being subscale and a ten-item existential well-being subscale. The existential well-being subscale is sometimes described as the spiritual aspects of the scale, whereas the religious well-being subscale is said to reflect the religious aspects. Actually, the existential well-being subscale is a measure of well-being (not spirituality). Consider the following items:

- I don't know who I am, where I came from or where I'm going (scored in reverse).
- I feel that life is a positive experience.
- I feel very fulfilled and satisfied with life.
- I feel a sense of well-being about the direction my life is headed in.
- I don't enjoy much about life (scored in reverse).
- I feel good about my future.
- I feel that life is full of conflict and unhappiness (score in reverse).

Clearly, this is measuring mental health and positive emotions. How can one automatically equate this with spirituality?

Summary

When spirituality is measured using scales like those described above, especially when examining relationships between spirituality and mental health (well-being, happiness, depression, anxiety, psychosis, substance abuse, etc.) or social health (social support, social connections, etc.), the results of such research should be suspect and are likely influenced by measurement contamination. If these measures are used, however, there is a way of handling measurement contamination in the analysis phase, and that is to examine relationships between these spirituality measures and health outcomes in two ways: with and without the contaminating items. If results come out the same, then there is no problem; if not, then only the results from the uncontaminated measure should be emphasized. Likewise, investigators can separate contaminating items into a separate subscale and then model relationships between the measure of spirituality made up of noncontaminated items and health outcomes by using the subscale composed of contaminating items as a mediator (see Chapter 18).

RECOMMENDATIONS

For the reasons presented above, when I conduct research on R/S and health, I usually measure religion, since this is the language that is clearest, most distinctive, and most separate from health outcomes. When measuring spirituality for research purposes, especially when examining relationships with mental or social health, I strongly recommend not using measures that are contaminated with items tapping positive character traits, positive psychological states, or positive social qualities. This will help to avoid defining "spirituality" a priori as good health (and prevent the tautological relationships that would otherwise result). In fact, I recommend the traditional way of defining and measuring spirituality, which identifies those who are spiritual as the deeply religious (eliminating entirely the category of spiritual but not religious). In contrast, when *applying* the research results to clinical settings (i.e., identifying spiritual needs, taking a spiritual history, learning about spiritual background), I would use "spirituality" in the broadest and most inclusive sense possible, preferably defined by patients themselves, so that social connection, engagement, and conversation are maximized.

For the reasons presented above, when I conduct research on R/S and health, I usually measure religion, since this is the language that is clearest, most distinctive, and most separate from health outcomes.

SUMMARY AND CONCLUSIONS

In this chapter I provide definitions for the terms "religion," "spirituality," and "secular." I describe criteria for definitions of these constructs when used in research settings and in clinical settings, criteria that I argue are quite different. I define "religion" as beliefs and practices (public and private) regarding the Transcendent and use a historical definition of spirituality that views the spiritual person as someone who is deeply religious.

I take issue with the now popular and widely used definition of spirituality, especially dominant in academic settings, that views spirituality as much broader than religion and even include those who are completely secular under this term.

I take issue with the now-popular and widely used definition of spirituality, especially dominant in academic settings, that views spirituality as much broader than religion and even includes those who are completely secular under this term. I provide examples here of spirituality scales that suffer from measurement contamination and increase the risk of tautological and meaningless results when examining relationships with health outcomes. I acknowledge the harshness of this approach, but argue the necessity of doing so on practical and scientific grounds.

Measurement I

MEASUREMENT LIES AT the heart of research on religion/spirituality (R/S) and health. Clear definitions enable the development of measures that accurately operationalize those definitions. In this first chapter on measurement, I begin with a general discussion of approaches to measurement, and then spend the remainder of the chapter examining the major dimensions of religion and describing measures that have been developed for use in specific religious groups.

Approaches to Measurement

The overall approach to measurement that this chapter focuses on is quantitative, seeking to assess the degree of R/S involvement in terms of numbers (vs. qualitative measurements). Quantitative measurement usually involves subjects filling out scales contained in a questionnaire, interviewers reading scale items and recording subjects' response, or interviewers filling out scales based on their observations and then making judgments regarding how much of a belief, attitude, or behavior is present. Self-administration and interviewer-administration, then, are the two most common methods of administering R/S scales. I now discuss these methods along with more novel assessment procedures.

> **Measurement lies at the heart of research on religion, spirituality, and health.**

Self-Administration

> **Self-administration by subjects themselves is the easiest, most prevalent, and least expensive way of collecting information.**

Self-administration by subjects themselves is the easiest, most prevalent, and least expensive way of collecting information. Many scales were meant to be self-administered (called "self-report scales"), and this is how the reliability and validity of the scales are often established. However, this method does not work as well in subjects who are elderly or sick, those with reading or language barriers, or persons who are less cooperative. In those populations it is better to have interviewers administer the scales (even if the reliability and validity of those scales are based on self-administration). For self-administered scales, it is important to make it as easy as possible for subjects to respond—that is, for example, use scales that are made up of questions that are easy to read and understand (clear, simple sentences), easy to respond to (clear, unambiguous response options), and make it easy to return the questionnaire (self-addressed stamped envelope or collected in person). Examples of scales designed to be self-administered include the Center for Epidemiological Studies-Depression (CES-D) scale, the Symptom Check List-90 (SCL-90), the Duke Religion Index (DUREL), and Hoge's Intrinsic Religiosity Scale (IR).

Interviewer Administration

Interviewer administration of scales is more expensive since an interviewer needs to be hired and trained, and also needs to be retrained periodically to ensure that the questions are being asked in the same way (to avoid drift). The way the interviewer asks the question—that is, the tone of voice and emphasis placed on different words—can influence subjects' responses. This is especially true since subjects may wish to please the interviewer or provide the answers they think the interviewer wants. Hence, training and retraining are essential. Interviewer-administered scales can be self-reported (i.e., interviewer reads the scale questions that were designed to be read and answered by subjects, such as the CES-D, DUREL, and IR) or interviewer-rated (i.e., interviewer makes judgments and fills out responses based on their observations, such as the Hamilton Depression Scale, or Hamilton Anxiety Rating Scale, Structured Clinical Interview for Depression, and Hall's fluent vs. nonfluent religiosity scale).

Combination

Some scales may have components that are self-reported and other components that are interviewer-rated, although all the questions are usually interviewer-administered since at least one of the questions requires interviewer administration. The Religious Coping Index (RCI) is an example of such a scale. This measure consists of three items: two self-reported and one observer-rated. The first question (self-reported) asks subjects how they usually deal with problems—that is, what beliefs, behaviors, or resources they use to cope with stressors; if the subject gives a religious response, then a score of 10 is given, and if a nonreligious response, then a score of 0 is given. The second question (self-reported) asks subjects to rate the extent to which they use religion to cope with stress, using visual analog scale that ranges from 0 (not at all) to 10 (most important factor that keeps me going). The third question (observer-rated) asks subjects to describe exactly what they mean by "using religion to cope" and to give examples of how they did so recently; the interviewer then writes down verbatim what the subject says and rates the response on a 0 to 10 scale on how much the interviewer thinks the subject really uses religion to cope (based on the details and specificity of the subject's responses).

Novel Methods

There are also novel methods of assessment that seek to get away from the subjectivity of self-reporting and make measurements more objectively. These include continuous monitoring, tests of application, computer algorithms, and collection of data from informants. Continuous monitoring may involve subjects wearing pagers and being paged randomly throughout the day to ask them whether they had any R/S thoughts or engaged in any R/S activity in the past fifteen minutes (recall is better, and lying is more difficult for recent events). Tests of application may involve manipulating a situation and observing subjects' responses. For example, an opportunity to attend chapel services may be offered to a group of students unaware of their being assessed and then those attending the services noted. Computer algorithms may involve a computer game that requires choices to be made regarding preferences to spend time or other resources on religious vs. secular activities. Finally, informants (spouse, children, friends, coworkers) may be asked about the degree of the subject's religious devotion or activities. As noted above, these novel methods all seek to enhance the objectivity, accuracy, and reliability of assessments.

> There are many other aspects of religion besides affiliation with a particular denomination or frequency of attendance at religious services

DIMENSIONS OF RELIGION AND RELIGIOUSNESS

As noted in the last chapter, many people tend to equate religion with institutionalized religion. There are many other aspects of religion, however, besides affiliation with a particular denomination or frequency of attendance at religious services. I describe sixteen of these dimensions below.

Denomination/Affiliation

In order to get a sense of subjects' religious background, religious denomination or affiliation should always be obtained (Protestant, Catholic, nontraditional Christian, Jewish [Orthodox, Conservative, Reform], Islam [Shiite, Sunni], Buddhist, Hindu, and so forth).

Belief/Orthodoxy

Type of religious belief or religious orthodoxy assesses the degree to which subjects' beliefs correspond to liberal, mainstream, conservative, or fundamentalist doctrines. For example, Glock and Stark—sociologists at the University of California at Berkeley in the 1960s—developed a Christian orthodoxy scale that asked about subjects' beliefs about a personal God, the divinity of Jesus, authenticity of biblical miracles, and existence of the devil.[1]

Public Religious Practices

Religious activities that occur in social groups include attending religious services, participating in prayer or Bible study groups, altruistic group religious activity, and other religious activities that include participation with others.

Private Religious Practices

This would include religious activities performed in private or alone. Private prayer, reading religious scriptures, watching religious television, and listening to religious radio are among these activities.

Subjective Religiousness

A single self-reported question about religiousness, religious salience, or importance of religion is commonly used to assess this subjective dimension of religiousness.

Religious Motivation

One of the most important measures of religious commitment is religious motivation. Gordon Allport, a psychologist at Harvard who studied religious prejudice, developed notions of intrinsic vs. extrinsic religious commitment in the 1960s.[2] Those described as intrinsically religious were persons whose master motive lay in religion as an end in itself. Intrinsically religious persons pursued religion as the object of ultimate concern, building and living their lives around their religious beliefs. This was contrasted with the extrinsically religious who used religion as a means to some other, more important end (i.e., social or economic gain). Religious attendance per se is not considered extrinsic religiosity.

Religious Well-Being

Religious well-being involves the sense of well-being and satisfaction in one's relationship with God. This dimension of religiousness is one of the two subscales of Paloutzian and Ellison's Spiritual Well-Being Scale (the other subscale, as discussed in the last chapter, is existential well-being).

Religious Coping (RC)

Religious coping consists of religious beliefs and behaviors used to cope with and make sense of negative life experiences (and sometimes positive ones, too). This might involve behaviors such as praying to derive comfort and hope during trying emotional times; reading religious writings for inspiration and guidance; attending religious services to be uplifted by singing and worshiping together with others; and seeking support from members of one's congregation, or giving support to others for religious reasons. RC may also involve cognitive processes, including beliefs about a better life after death when pain and suffering will be no more, or belief in a loving, caring God who is in control, has a purpose for every person in every situation, and has the power to transform difficult circumstances so that good outcomes are possible. RC can be measured in global, general terms (overall degree to which a person uses religion to cope, for example, as measured by RCI) and specific ways of using religion to cope (Pargament's RC scales).

Religious History

Measures of religious history seek to determine "exposure" to religion over the lifetime of a person, rather than only currently. This includes major religious transitions in life, number of years of religious belief and activity, and the intensity of religious belief and behavior over the years. A religious history scale has been developed, although it needs further work to adequately capture lifetime exposure.[3]

Religious Support

Social support is often obtained from involvement in religious community activities, and this dimension of religiosity seeks to determine the positive and negative aspects of religion-related support. Krause has developed both long and short versions of a church-related support scale that I discuss later.[4]

Religious Experience

Religious experiences include conversion experiences, mystical experiences, and less intense but common spiritual experiences that some may be had on a daily basis. The Hood mysticism scale[5] assesses experiences in areas of ego quality, unifying quality, inner subjective quality, and temporal/spatial quality, and is more oriented toward Eastern spirituality. The Daily Spiritual Experiences scale assesses religious and spiritual experiences from a Western spiritual perspective, and includes experiences that are more common than the more rare conversion or mystical experience.[6] While this particular measure is at risk for measurement contamination (as discussed in Chapter 11), it does include many items that are valid measures of religious experience and so may be useful for this purpose.

Religious Attachment

In many Western religions, an important dimension of religious involvement is having a warm, positive, intimate relationship with God. Indeed, this may be the core dimension of religion that drives all others. While research in this area is still very early, investigators have developed scales assessing love from God,[7] or more specifically, the quality of one's relationship with or attachment to God.[8]

Religious Giving

Religious giving (i.e., giving for religious reasons) may involve donations of money, possessions, time, or other resources. This may be measured by percent of gross income given to religious organizations or religious causes, or by number of hours spent per week volunteering for religious reasons. Giving of money and time, then, are frequently used to measure this dimension.

Religious Knowledge

Individuals vary widely in their knowledge about their faith tradition and the sacred writings on which that faith is based. One might assume that those who are more knowledgeable about religion are more religious, since time and effort have presumably been taken to acquire that knowledge. Besides an individual's motivation and desire to learn about one's religion, education level and rearing environment are also major determinants. After discovering that two-thirds of American Christians did not know who delivered the Sermon on the Mount, Stark and Glock developed a measure of religious knowledge.[9] Examples of questions testing religious knowledge from their scale are, "If you were asked, do you think you could recite the Ten Commandments?" "Do Jews believe in the Ten Commandments?" Other questions ask about whether certain statements come from the Bible (e.g., "God helps those who help themselves"), or whether subjects can correctly choose Old Testament prophets from a list (e.g., David, Isaiah, Elijah, Jesus, Paul).

Religious Growth

Finally, religious growth is a dimension of religiosity that involves growing deeper in experience of and commitment to one's religious faith. Among the dimensions of religious involvement developed by Morton King is a five-item subscale assessing "openness to religious growth" that numerous investigators have used and which involves questions asking about interest in moral growth and the degree to which a person is engaged in a continuous struggle to understand religion better.[10]

Religious Quest

Daniel Batson developed a dimension of religiosity that is similar to religious growth that he called religious "quest." Batson claimed that there are individuals who "view religion as an endless process of probing and questioning generated by the tensions, contradictions, and tragedies in their own lives and in society,"[11] and argues that this form of religious expression should also be acknowledged and measured.

Three-Dimensional Categorization

A simpler and more condensed summary of the major dimensions of religion (besides the sixteen categories above) involves only three dimensions: organizational religiosity, nonorganizational religiosity, and religious importance or salience. These were the three major dimensions of religiosity that members of an interdisciplinary consensus panel came up with after studying and discussing this topic.[12] Organizational religiosity is equivalent to public religious practices and is often measured by questions asking about frequency of religious attendance or other group religious activity. Nonorganizational religiosity is equivalent to private religious practices such as personal prayer, scripture reading, or viewing or listening to religious media. Religious importance or salience is an indicator of an individual's commitment

> A simpler and more condensed summary of the major dimensions of religion involves only three dimensions: organizational religiosity, nonorganizational religiosity, and religious importance or salience.

to religious beliefs and may be measured by subjective religiousness, religious importance, or intrinsic religious motivation.

Religion-Specific Scales

I now present several scales that were developed for use in specific religious groups. Most religiosity scales used today were developed for Protestant or Catholic Christians. No scales currently exist for assessing religiosity in nontraditional Christian groups such as Mormons, Jehovah's Witnesses, or Unitarians, or for assessing religiosity in American Indians or other indigenous religions. Scales have been developed for Jews, Muslims, Hindus, Buddhists, and New Age groups, and I review them here.

> No scales currently exist for assessing religiosity in non-traditional Christian groups such as Mormons, Jehovah's Witnesses, or Unitarians, or for assessing religiosity in American Indians or other indigenous religions. Scales have been developed for Jews, Muslims, Hindus, Buddhists, and New Age groups.

Jews

There are no specific measures for use in each of the primary subdivisions of Judaism (Reform, Conservative, Orthodox), although there is a measure assessing traditional Jewish beliefs and practices based on a random survey of the population of Israel in the 1970s. This measure was developed by Ben-Meir and Kedem, and consists of six statements about belief and twenty statements about religious practice.[13] Statements about Jewish belief have to do with belief in God, the continued existence of the soul after death, the coming of the Messiah, something supernatural that directs the history of the Jewish people, and the Jewish people being a chosen people. Statements concerning religious practice include activities such as attending synagogue, wearing a yarmulke, praying with phylacteries, refraining from travel on the Sabbath, praying on the Sabbath, lighting and blessing Sabbath candles, and so forth. Some may view this scale as a measure of Jewish orthodoxy, although Reform and Conservative Jews (and perhaps even some secular Jews) may also have some of these beliefs and engage in traditional Jewish practices. David Rosmarin and colleagues have also developed a Jewish religious coping scale.[14]

Muslims

The *Journal of Muslim Mental Health* devoted two special issues in 2007 and 2008 to measures of Islamic religiosity.[15] Included there are measures of Muslim religious commitment, Islamic religiousness, Islamic fundamentalism, Muslim religious reflection, Muslim intrinsic religiosity, Islamic moral values, attitudes toward Islam, Islamic knowledge and practice, and Arabic religious coping. This represents the most extensive information on measures of Islamic religiosity ever assembled in a single place. It is interesting, though, that many religious measures developed in Christian populations work very well in Muslim populations (with a few adaptations in wording).[16]

Hindus

At least two measures of religiosity have been developed for use in Hindu populations, the Bhushan religiosity scale[17] and the Hassan and Khalique scale.[18] These measures assess adherence to traditional Hindu beliefs and practices. In addition, at least one measure of religious coping has been tested and found reliable and valid for Hindus living in the United States.[19] The coping strategies in this measure were based in Hindu theology and consist of three factors: "God-focused" religious coping, "spirituality-focused" religious coping, and religious guilt, anger, and passivity.

Buddhists

At least one measure of Buddhist beliefs and practices exists. Emavardhana and Tori developed the Buddhist beliefs and practices scale, an eleven-item instrument that inquires about agreement to statements such as "I believe in the doctrine of no-soul," "The teachings of the Buddha are very important in my life," "I observe the Five Precepts," "I believe in the theory of karma and rebirth," "I practice meditation," and so forth.[20] Based on a large sample of Buddhists in Thailand, the internal consistency coefficient for this scale is high (alpha = 0.69).

New Age

Granqvist and Hagekull have developed a twenty-two-item New Age Orientation Scale to assess New Age beliefs and practices.[21] Examples of scale statements, each rated on a 1 to 6 scale from strongly disagree to strongly agree, are as follows: "The position of the stars at birth affects how one will live one's life or how one's personality will develop," "I am convinced that thought transference and/or the ability to move things by mere thinking actually do work," "There are some objects or places that have a special spiritual meaning, for instance by being surrounded by a certain type of energy," "With the assistance of a 'medium' it is possible to get in touch with dead people or with life on other planets," "Tarot cards, horoscopes, or fortune telling can be a good starting points from which to develop oneself and one's possibilities," "Spirituality to me is above all about realizing my true nature or becoming one with cosmos," and so forth.

SUMMARY AND CONCLUSIONS

In this chapter I discussed approaches to quantitative measurement that involve self-administered and interviewer-administered scales. I also explored novel methods of measurement to increase objectivity and accuracy. I then examined sixteen dimensions of religion or religiousness, including religious affiliation, belief, public religious practices, private religious practices, subjective religiousness, religious motivation, religious well-being, religious coping, religious history, religious support, religious experience, religious attachment, religious giving, religious knowledge, religious growth, and religious quest. I indicated that these dimensions could also be summarized into three basic categories: organizational, nonorganizational, and religious importance/salience. I then examined religion-specific scales that have been developed for studying religious groups such as Jews, Muslims, Hindus, Buddhists, and members of New Age religions. In the next chapter on measurement, I describe the most commonly used scales today and make recommendations on the best scales to use depending on the researcher's purpose.

CHAPTER 13

Measurement II

I N THIS SECOND chapter on measurement, I describe and discuss the strengths and weaknesses of commonly used scales, make specific recommendations on the best scales to use depending on circumstances, and discuss how to develop a scale from scratch if no scale exists that meets the researcher's needs.

COMMONLY USED SCALES

In this section I examine the most commonly used scales today for studying relationships between religion/spirituality (R/S) and health, and also something about their strengths and weaknesses.

Multidimensional Measure of Religiousness/ Spirituality (MMRS)

This is a commonly used measure when investigators have space in surveys for many questions on R/S. A short version of this measure consists of thirty-eight items, the Brief MMRS (BMMRS) was developed by a consensus panel of the Fetzer Institute and the National Institute on Aging.[1] National norms were established for the U.S. population by including the BMMRS in the 1997–1998 General Social Survey. To obtain a copy of both the long and brief versions of this scale, contact the Fetzer Institute.[2] I would use the thirty-eight-item BMMRS, but not include the BMMRS's forgiveness, values, and meaning subscales as measures of R/S itself. Instead, I would model those subscales as mediators along the path that leads from R/S to health outcomes (see Chapter 18). Another way to employ the scale is to select individual subscales of various R/S dimensions and use those subscales separately; long and short versions of each of the subscales are provided in the MMRS booklet.

Religious Orientation Scale

Allport and Ross in 1967 developed a measure of intrinsic and extrinsic religious motivation that consisted of two subscales, a nine-item intrinsic and an eleven-item extrinsic subscale.[3] Statements are responded to on a five-point scale (1–5) from strongly disagree to strongly agree. This scale has become one of the most widely used, most widely criticized, and most widely modified of all religiosity scales.[4]

Intrinsic Religiosity Scale

Dean Hoge shortened the Allport-Ross scale from twenty items to ten (seven intrinsic and three extrinsic), and the resulting scale is the most widely used intrinsic religious measure today. It is my personal favorite of all religiosity scales and has been my favorite for more than twenty-five years. Like the Religious Orientation Scale, each item is assessed on a 1 to 5 scale from strongly disagree to strongly agree, producing a score range from 10 to 50. Unlike many other R/S scales, researchers have actually established the validity of this IR scale based on judgments of religious professionals (ministers, priests, rabbis).[5] A weakness of this scale (as with the Allport I/E scales) is that it does not assess organizational religiosity or public religious involvement, which is one reason that we developed the DUREL.

Duke University Religion Index (DUREL)

The DUREL is a five-item scale that measures the three major dimensions of religiousness described earlier: organizational, nonorganizational, and religious commitment / intrinsic religiosity.[6] The first two items of the scale (frequency of religious attendance and frequency of private religious activities) were taken from several large community and clinical studies conducted in North Carolina, so there are normative data on response rates for these populations. These serve as one-item measures of organizational and nonorganizational religiosity. The final three items of the index form a subscale that assesses intrinsic religiosity and were extracted from Hoge's ten-item intrinsic religiosity scale based on their relationship to health outcomes. The psychometric characteristics of the DUREL have been established, and the index has been used widely to examine relationships with physical, mental, and social health.[7] Although collecting only superficial information on religion, this short scale is ideal for use in large epidemiological studies where investigators can include only a few questions and yet desire to cover the major dimensions of religiosity.

> The researcher needs to know the most commonly used scales today for studying relationships between religion/spirituality (R/S) and health, and also something about their strengths and weaknesses.

Francis Scale of Attitude toward Christianity

Widely employed in Europe, this scale has been used in many different populations and consists of several different versions. The scale assesses how positively people feel about God, Jesus, the Bible, prayer, and church. The most commonly used versions are the twenty-four-item[8] and seven-item[9] scales. There are even junior versions of this scale available that have been tested in nine- to eleven-year-old English schoolchildren.[10]

Quest Scale

Batson developed a nine-item scale that assesses the "interactional" or quest dimension of religiosity that includes statements such as, "It might be said that I value my religious doubts and uncertainties," "I find my everyday experiences severely test my religious convictions," and "Questions are far more central to my religious experience than are answers."[11] The Quest Scale (nine-item and twelve-item versions) has been used in relatively few studies (compared to those assessing religiosity using the IE scales of Allport and Hoge). The Quest Scale is not a particular favorite of mine and doesn't predict outcome very well.

Spiritual Well-Being Scale (SWB)[12]

As discussed in Chapter 11, the SWB scale is used a great deal, although depending on how its two subscales are analyzed and reported, it can provide misleading results. The ten-item religious well-being subscale is a fine measure of a person's satisfaction with his or her relationship with God. The ten-item existential well-being subscale is simply a measure of psychological well-being and so should be viewed as a mediator of the effects of religious well-being on health outcomes. Results from the two subscale scores should always be reported separately and not combined into a total SWB score.

Functional Assessment of Chronic Illness Therapy—Spiritual Well-Being (FACIT-Sp)[13]

As noted in Chapter 11, the twelve-item FACIT-Sp consists of two subscales, an eight-item "meaning and peace" subscale and a four-item "faith" subscale. This measure is widely used in patients with cancer, congestive heart failure, and other serious or chronic medical illnesses. The meaning and peace subscale is a measure of positive mental health, and while the faith subscale comes closer to something distinctively spiritual, it includes two items that are phrased in a way that indicate a feeling of comfort or strength that could favorably bias associations with good mental health. A third item on this subscale is simply a measure of optimism ("I know that whatever happens with my illness, things will be okay") and so is a marker of good mental health (i.e., successful coping). I would avoid using the FACIT-Sp.

Self-Transcendence Scale (STS)

Two different STS scales have appeared in the literature. The first STS is a thirty-three-item subscale of Robert Cloninger's Temperament and Character Inventory,[14] and consists of three subscales (self-forgetfulness, transpersonal identification, and spiritual acceptance). The second STS scale was developed by a nurse, Pamela Reed, and consists of fifteen items that assess intrapersonal, interpersonal, and transpersonal experiences (have hobbies and interests, social involvement, adjusting well to present life, finding meaning, helping others, enjoying life, etc.).[15] These scales are only marginally related to anything distinctively spiritual, are contaminated by positive psychological and social indicators, and are not recommended.

Mysticism Scale

Developed by psychologist Ralph Hood, this thirty-two-item scale assesses four dimensions of mystical experiences: ego quality (loss of sense of self while conscious, absorption into something greater than ego), unifying quality (extent to which everything is experienced as One), inner subjective quality (perception of an inner subjectivity to all), and temporal or spatial quality (modification of time and space so that experience is perceived as timeless and spaceless).[16] As noted earlier, this measure of mysticism most accurately captures Eastern forms of spiritual experience, is expressed largely in psychological terms, and is recommended only for assessing Eastern spiritual mysticism.

Spiritual Transcendence Scale (SpTS)[17]

The SpTS, developed by psychologist Ralph Piedmont, is a twenty-four-item scale with three subscales (universality, prayer fulfillment, connectedness). There is also a nine-item version[18] of the scale available (see Chapter 11 for commentary on this version). Items on the prayer fulfillment subscale focus on fulfillment, strength, peace, and bliss experienced during prayer or meditation; those on the universality subscale focus on the interconnectedness of all of life and meaning in life; and the items on the connectedness subscale focus on images of dead relatives influencing life, emotional bonds with the dead, and the importance of giving back to the community.

Daily Spiritual Experiences Scale (DSES)[19]

Lynn Underwood, former vice president of the Fetzer Institute, developed the DSES in order to assess common daily spiritual experiences (feeling God's presence, God's love, God's guidance, closeness to God, and so forth). There are two versions of the scale: a long version (sixteen items) and a shortened version (six items). As noted in Chapter 11, there is some concern regarding items on this scale that indicate good mental health (peace, harmony, joy, connection). Nevertheless, among the spirituality scales currently being used, I like this one and have used it myself to assess daily spiritual experiences. As noted in Chapter 11, if investigators choose to use the scale, I suggest that they analyze results with and without the items that may be contaminating the measure (items 2, 3, 5, 6, 11–14), and then report the findings both ways.

Love from God Scales

Developed by epidemiologist Jeff Levin at Baylor, this four-item "religious love" subscale of the Sorokin Multidimensional Inventory of Love Experience (SMILE)[20] assesses a key dimension of religiousness with the following statements that respondents agree to on a 1–5 scale: "I feel loved by God (or a higher power)," "God loves all living beings," "God's love is eternal," and "God's love never fails." Scores on this scale have been strongly related to self-rated health in primary care patients.

Similar to the Levin scale, psychologist David Rosmarin has developed a sixteen-item "Trust/Mistrust in God" scale that assesses perceptions of God's love for a person.[21] There also exists a shorter six-item version in which subjects indicate their strength of belief on a five-point scale; three statements are stated in a positive manner and three statements are stated in a negative manner.[22] Positive statements include, "God loves me immensely," "God cares about my deepest concerns," "No matter how bad things may seem, God's kindness to me never ceases"; negative statements are "God ignores me," "God doesn't care about me," and "God hates me." Responses to this short scale relate to levels of anxiety and depression.

Attachment/Relationship to God Scales

Psychologists Wade Rowatt and Lee Kirkpatrick have developed a nine-item Attachment to God scale, with each item rated 1 to 7 from not characteristic to very characteristic of the responder.[23] Two subscales make up this measure, a six-item subscale and a three-item subscale. The first subscale items include negatively worded statements ("God seems impersonal to me," "God seems to have little or no interest in my personal problems," "God seems to have little or no interest in my personal affairs") and positively worded statements ("I have a warm relationship with God," "God knows when I need support," "I feel that God is generally responsive to me"). The second subscale includes the statements, "God sometimes seems responsive to my needs, but sometimes not," "God's reactions to me seem to be inconsistent," "God sometimes seems very warm and other times very cold to me." The advantages of this scale are its brevity and strong face validity.

Similarly, psychologists Richard Beck and Angie McDonald developed a twenty-eight-item Attachment to God Inventory, also divided into two subscales; items are rated 1 to 7 from strongly disagree to strongly agree.[24] The fourteen-item subscale includes statements such as "I just don't feel a deep need to be close to God (reverse scored)," "I am totally dependent upon God for everything in my life," "My experiences with God are very intimate and emotional," "Daily I discuss all of my problems and concerns with God," and so forth. The second fourteen-item subscale includes statements such as "I worry a lot about my relationship with God," "I often worry about whether God is pleased with me," "I crave reassurance from God that God loves me," and so forth. For a comprehensive measure of attachment to God, this seems like a pretty good measure, and in my estimation, has solid face validity. The length of the scale, though, makes it a bit unwieldy.

Religious Coping (RCOPE)

Developed by psychologist Ken Pargament, the RCOPE assesses specific ways that persons may use religion or spirituality to cope with stress. A 105-item long form and a 14-item abbreviated RCOPE have been developed. The 105-item RCOPE consists of 21 subscales (3 items per subscale rated on a 0–3 scale) indicating five ways in which religion is used to cope: (1) find meaning, (2) gain control, (3) gain comfort and closeness to God, (4) gain intimacy with others and closeness to God, and (5) achieve a life transformation.[25] The 14-item Brief RCOPE is a shorter version of the RCOPE that consists of two 7-item subscales, for positive and one for negative religious coping.[26] Positive religious coping items include "looked for a stronger connection with God," "sought God's love and care," "tried to put my plans into action with God," "asked forgiveness for my sins," and so forth. Negative religious coping items include "wonder whether God had abandoned me," "felt punished by God for my lack of devotion," "questioned God's love for me," "wondered whether my church had abandoned me," and so forth. The Brief RCOPE, especially the 7-item negative religious coping subscale (which is almost always related to health outcomes), is strongly recommended for research related to religious coping.

Religious Coping Index (RCI)

The RCI is a short, three-item, interviewer-administered measure of overall religious coping.[27] The first item is an indirect way of assessing religious coping, where the interviewer does not mention religion but instead asks an open-ended question about what the person does in order to cope with stress. If a religious response is offered spontaneously, then the interviewer gives the subject a score of 10; if religion is not included in the response, then a score of 0 is given. The second item involves directly asking the subject to rate on a 0 to 10 visual analog scale to what extent he or she uses religion to cope, where 0 means not at all and 10 means religion is the most important factor that keeps the person going. In the third and final item, the interviewer rates the subject's degree of religious coping based on an in-depth discussion, recorded verbatim, about how specifically the subject uses religion to cope, when the subject did so last, how frequently this is done, and so on (with responses recorded verbatim). The interviewer than rates the subject's response on a 0–10 scale, where 0 indicates that religion is not being used to cope and 10 signifies specific and frequent use of religion. Summing the three items results in a score that ranges from 0 to 30. The RCI has a test-retest reliability of 0.81 (when administered on separate occasions by different interviewers with different religious backgrounds), and predicts lower rates of depression both in cross-sectional and longitudinal analyses.[28] For a short, global measure of religious coping, the RCI is hard to beat, but again it must be interviewer-administered.

Religious Support Scale

Developed by sociologist Neal Krause at the University of Michigan, this scale measures the kinds of support received and given within religious settings (also called church-based support).[29] Two versions of this scale exist, a twelve-item scale and an abbreviated eight-item version, each with items that are self-rated from 1 to 4. Both versions of the scale are made up of four subscales: emotional support received from others, emotional support provided to others, negative interaction, and anticipated support. This is an excellent scale and recommended for research that seeks to understand whether and how involvement in a religious community affects health.

Religious History Scale

Developed by nurse Judy Hays and colleagues at Duke University Medical Center, this twenty-three-item scale seeks to measure individuals' religious involvement across the lifespan.[30] Each statement is self-rated from 0 to 4 based on agreement or disagreement. Examples include "When I was a child, religion was a natural part of my life," "When I was a child, I was very involved in the church," "When I was about 60, I looked for God's guidance in my daily life," and "When I was 50, I was very involved in the church." The Fetzer Institute's Multidimensional Measure of Religiousness/Spirituality also has a twenty-item measure of religious/spiritual history, developed by sociologist Linda George.[31] Unfortunately, the Hays and colleagues' scale applies only to persons over age sixty, and the items are not stated in a way that would allow calculation of lifetime exposure to religion (which is what is really needed). George's scale is not limited to those over age sixty and goes a long way toward meeting this goal of quantitatively assessing lifetime exposure, so in my opinion that scale would be a better place to start (vs. the Hays scale).

Religious Preference

In order to determine the religious background of participants in a study, it is important to measure religious preference or affiliation. An excellent, easily available measure of religious preference is in the Fetzer Institute's MMRS, which provides seventy-two religious affiliations grouped along theological lines.[32]

Other Measures

Many other measures of religiousness/spirituality are contained in the book *Measures of Religiosity* by Peter Hill and Ralph Hood.[33] The value of this source is that it also contains the measure's psychometric characteristics when available. A new, updated version of this book is forthcoming.

RECOMMENDED MEASURES

One of the most common reasons that R/S-health researchers contact me is to obtain a recommendation on what measure of R/S to use. The R/S measure chosen depends on the research question, the population being studied, and especially, the amount of space in the questionnaire available for questions on R/S. I now make recommendations on the "best" scales to use depending on the researcher's situation.

Best Measure Overall

In my opinion, the best measure of R/S is the ten-item intrinsic religiosity (IR) measure developed by Hoge.[34] Although it does have its weaknesses (e.g., it does not assess religious practices or involvement in the faith community), this is the most accurate measure of what I think is at the heart of religious devotion—relationship with and commitment to God (the object of ultimate concern). I have used this measure for nearly three decades and have included it in virtually every study I've designed. I am convinced that this is the best measure to use when studying Western religiosity. Finally, it is the only measure that I am aware of that has established validity based on at least two studies that have subjected the scale to multidenominational ministers' judgments (priests, pastors, rabbis).

> In my opinion, the best measure of R/S is the ten-item intrinsic religiosity (IR) measure developed by Hoge.

Shortest Measure

The Duke Religion Index (DUREL) is hard to beat in terms of both brevity and comprehensiveness.[35] In order to include the strengths and compensate for the weaknesses of the Hoge IR measure, we developed this five-item scale for use in epidemiological studies that examine relationships between R/S and health. It contains three items from the Hoge scale that most centrally capture IR and have been shown to relate to health outcomes. It also makes up for the Hoge scale's failure to assess religious practices or faith community involvement by including single items on private and public religious practices. The DUREL's brevity allows it to be included in large studies focused on health outcomes that do not have room for lots of questions on R/S, and yet still meets investigators' need to comprehensively measure religiosity. The established psychometric properties and availability in nearly a dozen languages also increases its value and usefulness.[36]

Most Comprehensive Measure

If investigators want a comprehensive measure of R/S and there is no limitation on the space available in a questionnaire, then I would choose the Fetzer Institute's Brief Multidimensional Measure of Religiousness/Spirituality (BMMRS),[37] which includes subscales on daily spiritual experiences, meaning, values, beliefs, forgiveness, private religious activities, religious and spiritual coping, religious support, religious/spiritual history, religious commitment, organizational religiosity, self-rated religiosity and spirituality, and religious preference. As noted above, national norms exist for responses to the questions on this measure since it was included in the 1997–1998 General Social Survey of the U.S. population; thus, investigators can compare the responses by participants in their research with the responses obtained from a national U.S. sample. Furthermore, psychometric properties of this measure (at least for college students) have now been published.[38] I would not, however, include the items for the forgiveness, values, or meaning subscales, since these are outcomes of R/S, not R/S itself (as discussed previously). Specifically, I would not include the three items on forgiveness, the one item on values, and the two items on meaning. I would also probably eliminate questions 2, 3, and 6 from the Daily Spiritual Experiences subscale, since there is risk that these items are measuring mental health and may introduce bias into the measure. If all of these recommendations are followed, then the number of items on the BMMRS is reduced to thirty-one. An alternative is to include these eliminated items but to model them as mediators (see Chapter 18).

Many researchers, however, do not have room in their questionnaires for thirty-one items on R/S, or would prefer to choose specific R/S measures to address the particular needs of their study. Thus, an alternative to the BMMRS is to identify specific scales in the literature that measure what the investigator wishes and then use those scales from their original sources. A concern with some of the subscales of the BMMRS is that they do not always include the same items as published in the original source, where psychometric properties of the scale were established.

Best Combination of Measures

The best combination of measures that is still relatively brief and yet captures the three major dimensions of R/S (organizational, nonorganizational, and subjective or intrinsic religiosity) would be to use the first two items on the DUREL, covering public and private religious involvement, and then add the full ten-item Hoge IR scale. This involves a total of twelve questions.

The best combination of measures that is still relatively brief and yet captures the three major dimensions of R/S (organizational, nonorganizational, and subjective or intrinsic religiosity) would be to use the first two items on the DUREL, covering public and private religious involvement, and then add the full ten-item Hoge IR scale.

Other Recommended Measures

If researchers have room in their questionnaire, I would next include the seven-item negative religious coping subscale from the Brief RCOPE, the eight-item version of the Krause religious support scale, and one of the love from God or attachment to God scales (depending on space available).

Including negative religious coping ensures that investigators have at least some significant findings, since this subscale is almost always related to poor mental and physical health (from greater depression to higher levels of interleukin-6 in the blood). Furthermore, findings on negative religious coping have immediate practical significance in that interventions are now being developed to specifically address this, which could possibly result in a reversal of the poor health outcomes associated with negative religious coping.[39]

The Krause measure on religious support is important because it helps to dig deeper into the relationship between religious community involvement and health outcomes. In all the research on R/S and health, the most consistent predictor of physical health and longevity is attendance at religious services. Currently, this remains somewhat of a mystery. Why attendance at religious services? While investigators have already attempted to address this important question,[40] the Krause scale allows future research to unpack the association further in order to better understand it.

Finally, more research needs to examine what role having a strong, secure relationship with God has on health outcomes. In trying to understand the mechanisms by which R/S affects health, in Chapter 16 I emphasize the importance of identifying the primary source for the health effects of R/S (i.e., the engine that runs the whole process), and I'm willing to bet that this primary source has something to do with an individual's attachment to God.

> The Krause measure on religious support is important because it helps to dig deeper into the relationship between religious community involvement and health outcomes. In all the research on R/S and health, the most consistent predictor of physical health and longevity is attendance at religious services.

> More research needs to examine what role having a strong, secure relationship with God has on health outcomes.

SCALE DEVELOPMENT

Although researchers can choose from many scales, certain aspects of R/S may not have yet been measured or at least not measured in the way that investigators want. In that case, a researcher may need to develop a scale from scratch. How does one go about doing this? Neal Krause, one of the top R/S research methodologists in the world, has published an article that identifies the step-by-step process of scale development.[41] Although that article focuses on development of surveys for older adults, its principles apply to scale development for all populations in survey research. Although I briefly summarize the steps for scale development here, researchers who are seriously considering developing their own scale need to consult that article.

A researcher may have an idea about a certain aspect of R/S that relates to a particular health outcome in a particular population of interest. For example, the researcher wants to measure closeness to God in Muslims with terminal cancer, and assess this as people get nearer and nearer to death. None of the existing R/S measures captures exactly what this researcher wants to assess, so she decides to develop a new measure of closeness to God. The first step would be to assemble a group of eight to ten Muslims with terminal cancer and hold an open discussion about the topic. This is called a focus group, where the focus is on the subject of interest (i.e., closeness to God as death approaches). Based on this discussion, a list of maybe one hundred items would be generated that could be used to measure closeness to God. The researcher would then group the one hundred items in plausible categories that might ultimately make up four or five subscales for a closeness-to-God scale.

Although some investigators might recommend coming up with these subscales based on administering the one hundred items to a group of Muslims with terminal cancer and then factor analyzing the responses, I would recommend against this approach. While the researcher wants the items on each subscale to hold together (i.e., have high internal reliability), I think it is too risky to allow statistics to drive what items end up on what subscale; otherwise, strange items may end up together that make no common sense and lack face validity. Instead, I would recommend first grouping the one hundred items into plausible categories (potential subscales) based on their face validity (i.e., be sure it makes good sense that certain items should be grouped together), and only then do factor analysis within each of these categories to identify items that hold strongly together (high internal reliability).

Once these groups of items are identified for potential subscales, then the researcher should take the items back to the focus group and get feedback from the group. Do the closeness-to-God subscales and the items that constitute them make sense to persons in the group—that is, Muslims with terminal cancer? Are the items stated clearly and easy to respond to? Which items on the subscales or entire subscales should be eliminated because they are too vague or don't relate to the group members' experiences? The scale would then be modified accordingly and again readministered to another small group of Muslims with terminal cancer, and the process repeated until a final, relatively short scale of, say, twenty items is developed consisting of two or three subscales with high internal reliability. This scale would then be administered to a large random sample of Muslims with terminal illness, and norms developed for the scale, subscales, and items composing the subscales. The scale would then be ready for use in a prospective study that examines how closeness to God changes as Muslims with terminal illness get closer to death (the investigator's primary research question).

SUMMARY AND CONCLUSIONS

In this second chapter on measurement, I described and commented on nineteen scales used commonly in R/S and health research, noting their strengths and weaknesses. I then made recommendations on which scales to use, depending on whether investigators want the best overall measure, the briefest measure, the most comprehensive measure, or the best combination of measures, and recommended other scales that should be included if researchers have space in their questionnaire. Finally, I rounded out this chapter with a discussion of scale development, describing how to develop a new scale from scratch. Measurement is at the heart of research on R/S and health. Choosing the right scales to assess the aspect of R/S that a researcher is interested in will likely have a significant impact on a study's findings. Knowing about the various measures that currently exist, their strengths and weaknesses, and the best scales to use depending on circumstances can help researchers choose the right measures for their study that will increase their likelihood of success.

> Measurement is at the heart of research on R/S and health. Choosing the right scales to assess the aspect of R/S that a researcher is interested in will likely have a significant impact on a study's findings.

PART 4

Statistical Analyses and Modeling

Statistics I: General Considerations

THOSE WHO CONDUCT research on religion/spirituality (R/S) and health need statistical skills to correctly analyze their data and interpret the findings. In this chapter I describe ways of handling data and cover a broad range of practical information that I think R/S-health researchers will find useful. I discuss fundamental rules to follow when conducting statistical analyses, make recommendations on how to prepare data for analysis, discuss general approaches to analyzing religious variables, and address the issue of multiple statistical comparisons. While R/S-health researchers can perform many statistical procedures without expert advice, it is always a good idea to involve a statistician early in study design. Recently, national attention was focused on a cancer researcher at Duke whose findings could not be validated by a number of top institutions. As a result, some journals (big and small) have started coming down pretty hard on manuscripts where a statistician did not analyze the data. Unfortunately, many R/S-health researchers may not have access to a statistician, and so must learn to do the analyses themselves.

Fundamental Rules

1. Learn about statistics—including how to write and run analysis programs. Waiting for a statistician to donate time to analyze an unfunded researcher's data can be frustrating and discouraging. Even when a researcher has the funds to pay a statistician, other priorities often come up and the researcher may end up at the bottom of the statistician's task list. Finally, because a statistical consultant will not likely be as interested in or as exact about the data analysis as the researcher, the consultant will require monitoring. Life is much easier when researchers have some basic knowledge about statistics, can analyze their own data when the need arises (e.g., analyze original data or reanalyze data in response to reviewers' comments), and can check over the analyses conducted by others to ensure that those analyses have been done properly. Knowing about what statistical tests are appropriate for which questions (Chapter 15) gives the researcher important tools for formulating research questions and planning research.

> Those who conduct research on religion/spirituality (R/S) and health need statistical skills to correctly analyze their data and interpret the findings.

2. Learn about statistics by taking a course on the topic (either online or attend classes at a local college). There are also a number of excellent books on statistics that are easy to read and that will help enhance the researcher's knowledge. I list several such books in Table 14.1.

> Learn about statistics—including how to write and run analysis programs.

3. Find an easy-to-use statistical software package to analyze data. Several such packages exist. One that is completely free and can be downloaded to any computer is Epi Info. Epi Info is a public-domain statistical package available from the Centers for Disease Control website.[1] Data can be entered directly into this software program and statistical analyses performed.

One should also not overlook Excel, which most people already have and know how to use. Excel's data validation tools prevent out-of-range entries, and the data can be exported to all major statistical packages, including Epi Info. Besides its use for data entry, Excel has a free add-in called Analysis ToolPak that performs nineteen statistical tests. Type "ToolPak" in Excel Help, and it will give directions for installing it. After ToolPak is installed, Excel has a new drop-down menu offering statistical tests that include three forms of ANOVA, three t-tests, correlation (can create a correlation matrix), covariance, regression, and others. If more sophisticated analyses are needed, packs of statistical macros can be installed that give Excel the power of the more traditional analysis programs, such as SAS and SPSS. While many of these packs are free, the better ones do require a purchase. For example, StatistiXL, designed and written by Alan Roberts and Philip Withers, both university professors, costs $75.

While the Excel program has been useful to many, there are problems with it. Some nationally renowned statisticians are now telling researchers to stop using Excel.[2] The claim is that Excel may not always produce reproducible results (the Duke cancer researcher whose results were disputed used Excel). Furthermore, if problems develop, it is more difficult to determine exactly what went wrong with the analysis if using Excel. Not much has been published on this, however, so it may be too early to draw any firm conclusions—but be aware.

If advanced analyses are planned, then it may be wise to take a course to learn SAS or SPSS. These statistical software programs can be run either on a PC or on a university mainframe computer (for university researchers, the cost is minimal or free). If the researcher is a registered student, it is possible to rent SPSS very reasonably through companies offering academic discounts, such as http://www.studentdiscounts.com/. This company offers a basic version of SPSS for $63.99 and an advanced version for $93.99 for a one-year rental (as of 2011). Taking only one class qualifies one as a student.

An intermediate approach might involve purchasing a good but somewhat costly statistical package[3] called STATA11, which is used widely by researchers. In 2010, STATA11 cost $1,395 for a perpetual license, and students and faculty could obtain a license for as low as $425. Training courses on how to use STATA11 are readily available online, costing $95 to $295 per course in 2010.

> When analyzing data, always follow an analysis plan, technically known as a statistical analysis plan (SAP).

4. When analyzing data, always follow an analysis plan, technically known as a statistical analysis plan (SAP). Before analyzing data (and preferably before

TABLE 14.1.

Recommended Introductory Books on Statistics

J. H. Abramson and Z. H. Abramson, *Making Sense of Data*, 3rd edition (Oxford University Press, 2001).

S. A. Glantz, *Primer of Biostatistics*, 5th edition (McGraw-Hill, 2002).

Leon Gordis, *Epidemiology*, 3rd edition (W. B. Saunders Company, 2004).

T. A. Lang and M. Secic, *How to Report Statistics in Medicine*, 2nd edition (American College of Physicians, 2006). Available at https://www.acponline .org/atpro/timssnet/products/tnt_products.cfm?action=long&primary_id =330351060.

Harvey Motulsky, *Intuitive Biostatistics* (Oxford University Press, 2010). Describes things verbally, rather than numerically.

J. T. Newsom, R. N. Jones, and S. M. Hofer, *Longitudinal Data Analysis: A Practical Guide for Researchers in Aging, Health, and Social Sciences* (Routledge, 2011).

Geoffrey Norman and David Streiner, *Biostatistics: The Bare Essentials*, 2nd edition (PMPA USA, 2000). Excellent, easy to read, humorous, lots of examples.

collecting the data), develop a written plan for the sequence of statistical tests that will be performed in order to answer the primary research question and related secondary research questions. If a researcher does not obtain significant results following this planned procedure, looking at other variables to try to achieve significance is called "post-hoc analyses." Although it is possible to statistically correct for post-hoc analyses, any study doing so loses credibility in the eyes of reviewers. Remember that for every statistical test done beyond the one necessary to test the primary research question, researchers need to lower their p-values accordingly (see below). Therefore it pays to run only those statistical tests that are carefully thought through and absolutely essential.

5. Don't dredge the data. "Dredging data" (also called going on a fishing expedition) means that the researcher is not following an analysis plan but instead running as many statistical tests as necessary until a significant correlation comes up. The researcher then reports only the significant correlation, devel-

oping a hypothesis retrospectively to fit the finding. For a single statistical test, the scientific convention for statistical significance is a p-value less than 0.05, meaning that such a correlation would occur in a population by chance alone in fewer than one in twenty tests. Following this convention, if the researcher conducts one hundred statistical tests, five of those tests could be statistically significant based on chance alone, even if there is no true correlation between variables (called a Type I error).[4]

Honest researchers, then, should avoid dredging their data, and when reporting the results of their analyses, should state how many statistical tests were done and report the results of each test. Do all researchers report the results of every test they perform? Believe me, they do not. But R/S-health researchers should.

Preparing to Analyze Data

Several preliminary steps are necessary before analyzing data to reduce errors and to increase the accuracy of results.

1. Be sure that the data are entered correctly from paper questionnaires into the analysis program. Data entry errors are common; they add unnecessary variability to the data and reduce the chances of significant findings. If data are entered directly into a computer during the interview, then entry errors are less of a problem (assuming that the computer program has checks on score ranges so that unusual scores cannot be entered). Double entry of data from paper questionnaires—entering the data twice into two separate programs and then comparing the results for differences—is a good way to minimize such errors.

> "Dredging data" (also called going on a fishing expedition) means that the researcher is not following an analysis plan but instead running as many statistical tests as necessary until a significant correlation comes up.

> Be sure that the data are entered correctly from paper questionnaires into the analysis program.

2. Clean the data. In this step, descriptive statistics on all variables are carefully examined, looking for potential errors. Out-of-range responses and outlier responses (those that are much higher or much lower than others) can be detected in this way, and researchers can then go back to the questionnaires to help sort this out.

3. Learn how to handle missing data statistically. Computer programs have been written that estimate missing values using algorithms based on answered responses to questionnaire items. These algorithms can fill in missing data to prevent subjects from dropping out of multivariate regression analyses because one or more covariates are missing. These methods, also called "imputation," include model-based techniques that are able to handle all sorts of missing data. Most large epidemiological studies now address missing values this way, which is especially important when constructing scale scores from multiple items. Although not all statisticians agree, my experience is that at least 60 percent of scale items need to be answered before inserting the average scores of answered items into the missing values.

4. Be sure to recode reverse-scored items. This step includes those items that make up either single-item scales (e.g., self-rated religiosity) or multi-item scales (e.g., intrinsic religiosity). A researcher who fails to recode may find the exact opposite of the true result. For example, some versions of the Duke Religion Index have all items reverse-scored and thus require recoding before analysis. I'm aware of one study in which investigators forgot to recode the reverse-scored items and reported a positive relationship between religiosity and blood pressure. The real finding, however, was the exact opposite—an inverse relationship. Another example where recoding is necessary is the ten-item Hoge intrinsic religiosity scale. This scale has three reverse-scored items that require recoding, and failure to do so can change the total score by up to twelve points (24 percent of the total score range). Other sorts of recoding may also be necessary, including recoding contingent questions (if yes, how often) into single variables or handling "don't know" or "not applicable" responses.

5. Check computer-calculated scores with scores calculated by hand from the actual paper questionnaires. Statisticians write analysis programs that automatically calculate multi-item scale scores by adding up the scores on individual items. However, sometimes the programming is written incorrectly, resulting in systematic errors. The researcher can

check scores by hand-calculating the scale scores, then comparing the hand-calculated scores with the computer-calculated scores. There is no problem if they are the same. If not the same, then an error in the programming needs correcting. The researcher should do this since the statistician may not.

6. Keep a record of what is done with the data. For example, in SPSS, menus can be used to recode data, but unless there is a record of this being done, the researcher may not remember that it was done or how it was done. In SPSS, if syntax is not used in the original program (a good way to keep the records), it can be pasted into the output or otherwise saved for record keeping. Failure to keep such records can result in re-recoding errors that leads to the opposite of the findings expected.

> Keep a record of what is done with the data.

7. Leave variables in their original state rather than collapse scores into categories and lose data (and precision). For example, if education is assessed by years of schooling, then researchers should not collapse the response categories into grammar school, high school, and college, but instead leave them as number of years (a continuous variable). Likewise, depressive symptoms assessed using a count of symptoms from a depression scale should be left as

> Leave variables in their original state rather than collapse scores into categories and lose data (and precision).

a continuous count of symptoms, rather than collapsing them into depressed vs. nondepressed categories. Collapsing scores almost always results in a cruder measure of the variable than leaving responses as originally given by participants.[5] Dichotomizing (collapsing scores into two categories) can also lead to incorrect results, sometimes showing relationships that don't exist with the continuous scale.[6]

There are occasional exceptions, however. Religious attendance, for example, is best examined after collapsing responses into categories of weekly attendance or more vs. less than weekly, or alternatively, any attendance vs. no attendance. Similarly, frequency of daily prayer is best examined after collapsing responses into once-daily prayer or more vs. less than daily, or alternatively, any prayer vs. no prayer. In general, measures should be coded based on theory, clinical standards, or the distribution of the variable. If no clear theory or standard exists or

Translate research
questions into analytic
methods.

distributional issues are present, the measure should
be left as continuous.

8. Translate research questions into analytic methods; for example, comparing groups requires analysis
of variance (ANOVA), whereas looking at continuous
variables probably requires some form of regression. Be
sure to know what the different analytic methods are designed
to do (see below).

ANALYZING RELIGIOUS VARIABLES

Chapter 15 describes many different statistical tests and when
to use them. However, I think it is important for R/S-health
researchers to follow a certain procedure for analyzing R/S
variables that cuts across the particular statistical test chosen.
When analyzing R/S variables as predictors of a health outcome, it is important to consider the following. I focus here on
the order of entry of R/S variables into regression models, the
need to analyze R/S dimensions in separate models, concerns
about combining R/S variables into total scores, and the need to
check for interactions. What follows may be more easily understood after reading the next four chapters, so it may be fruitful
to return to this section later.

Order of Entry

When building a regression model that includes an R/S predictor, confounders, mediators (or suppressors), and interactions,
and the primary research question is whether R/S predicts a
health outcome in an observational study, researchers should
pay attention to the order of entering variables into the model.
I recommend the following procedure.

Main Finding

Using multistep hierarchical multiple regression, first enter
the R/S variable into the model; this step provides a parameter coefficient for the bivariate relationship between the R/S
variable and the health outcome. Next, enter the confounders
into the model (age, race, gender, education, etc.). This step, as

noted in Chapter 16, determines the study's primary finding—that is, whether there is a significant relationship between the R/S variable and the outcome.[7] If there is a significant positive (or negative) relationship with the health outcome, then test for moderation and mediation in separate models.

Moderation

Often the association between R/S and health is stronger at one level of a variable than at another level, indicating that an interaction is present. In that case, the variable is said to moderate the relationship between R/S and health. Moderators determine under what conditions R/S affects a health outcome (i.e., the "when"). Moderators may be either confounders (e.g., age, race, gender, education, socioeconomic status, or physical illness severity) or mediators (e.g., stress level or social support). To test whether a moderator influences the strength of the relationship between R/S and the health outcome, enter in the model the R/S variable, the moderator, and the interaction term (the product of R/S and the moderator variable). If the parameter coefficient for the interaction term is statistically significant, then this indicates a moderator effect. Several moderators can be tested in a single statistical model.

Mediation

Next, test for mediation in a separate model containing the R/S variable and confounders by entering mediators (e.g., social support, health behaviors, mental health) that might help to explain "how" and "why" R/S affects the health outcome.[8] If the parameter coefficient for the R/S variable weakens or disappears with the mediator(s) in the model, then this provides evidence for mediation and helps to explain the mechanism by which R/S might affect the health outcome.

Mediation of Moderation

Finally, to determine how the moderator effect is mediated or explained, in a separate model (containing the R/S variable and confounders), add the moderator, the interaction term (product of moderator and predictor), *and* potential mediators to determine if the strength of the moderator effect (parameter coefficient of the interaction term) weakens or disappears with the addition of mediators to the model. For example, stress level moderates the effects of religious attendance on a health outcome such as depression (i.e., the parameter coefficient for the interaction term represented by the product of religious attendance and stress level is statistically significant). A researcher might then wish to examine social support as a mediator of this moderator effect. The researcher would do so by entering social support to a model that contains religious attendance and confounders, the moderator (stress level), and the interaction term (attendance by stress level). If the parameter coefficient for the interaction term weakens or loses significance, then this indicates that social support mediated or helped to explain the interaction (e.g., individuals who attend religious services frequently and are under high levels of job stress are less likely to be depressed because they have greater access to social support).

To complicate matters even further, a variable such as social support can be *both* a mediator and a moderator of the relationship between R/S and health. In other words, social support could both help to explain why R/S affects health and under what circumstances it does so (i.e., in those with high or low social support). The researcher's hypothesis always guides such analyses.

Analyze Religious Variables Separately

Because many R/S variables are closely linked, each d*imension* of R/S should be examined in a separate statistical model (see below for definition of "dimension"). In other words, don't lump denomination, religious attendance, prayer, daily spiritual experiences, religious well-being, religious coping, and so on, all into the same model. Instead, examine each religious dimension in separate regression models.[9] A reason for doing so is that many R/S dimensions are highly correlated with each other, increasing the chances of multicollinearity. Multicollinearity is when two or more predictors in a multiple regression model are highly correlated with one another

> **Because many R/S variables are closely linked, each *dimension* of R/S should be examined in a separate statistical model.**

and do not provide unique or independent information to the regression. As a general rule, correlations need to be above 0.40 before there is increased risk (some experts say correlations need to be above 0.60 or 0.70). Since multicollinearity can occur within a combination of more than two predictors, bivarate correlations may not provide sufficient information to rule this out. Specific indices of multicollinearity do exist, such as tolerance and variance inflation factor (VIF).

The result of multicollinearity is that the parameter coefficients may change erratically in response to small changes in the model or in the data. The size of the effect of each predictor may be influenced adversely and precision lost. Using uncorrelated or weakly correlated predictor variables gives the greatest power in regression techniques. Thus, it is better to avoid this issue entirely by examining each dimension of R/S individually in separate models. This approach requires that the researcher identify and combine all R/S variables assessing a particular dimension (e.g., organizational religious activity, nonorganizational religious activity, subjective religiosity) into a total score for each dimension and then analyze each of those total scores in its relationship to health in separate models.

There are also exceptions to this general rule. For example, if a researcher wants to know whether "religious commitment" (subjective religiosity) adds anything over "religious attendance" (organizational religiosity) in predicting depression, then one would want to include both of these R/S dimensions together in a single statistical model.

Combining Religious Variables

Investigators should only combine R/S variables into "total scores" when creating scales to assess a specific "dimension" of R/S. The major R/S dimensions as noted in Chapter 12 are organizational religiosity, nonorganizational religiosity, and subjective religiosity. For example, it is fine to combine responses to questions such as frequency of religious attendance, participation in prayer groups, participation in Bible study groups, or attendance at other group church functions

> **Investigators should only combine R/S variables into "total scores" when creating scales to assess a specific "dimension" of R/S.**

into an overall measure of organizational religiosity. Likewise, it is appropriate to combine private religious practices such as prayer, Bible reading, watching religious TV, or listening to religious radio into a single measure of nonorganizational religious activity. However, it is not a good idea to combine frequency of religious attendance and frequency of private prayer into a single measure of "religiosity." The reason is that these dimensions may be related differently to health outcomes and may even cancel out each other's effects (i.e., religious attendance may be positively related to the health outcome, whereas prayer may be negatively related to it, with a net result of no effect). The subjective dimension of R/S may also require more refined categorization. I recommend breaking it down into R/S experience, R/S coping, importance of R/S, and intrinsic religiosity, since these subdimensions may also relate in different ways to health outcomes.

Admittedly, researchers have a variety of views on combining religious variables. Some would argue that if the researcher does not have specific hypotheses about specific measures of R/S, then it would be permissible to combine them into an index. This combination, they argue, would increase reliability, eliminate confusion like distortion and suppression, and address the issue of multicollinearity. However, for the reasons given above, I would not recommend combining R/S variables except those assessing a specific dimension of R/S. Some researchers use factor analysis or Cronbach's alpha to select religious variables to combine into scales, although I would recommend against doing that also. The "face validity" of the items should have the highest priority, rather than having this driven entirely by statistics. In other words, does it make logical, rational sense that the variables are all measuring the same aspect of R/S?

Correcting for Multiple Comparisons

Statistically Significant Findings

When multiple statistical tests are done, the p-value needs to be reduced to reflect the increased likelihood that a significant result will be found by chance alone even if there is no true relationship (Type I error). One way to address this problem is to adjust the significance level by using a simple Bonferroni correction. This would involve dividing the p-value 0.05 (the conventional level of statistical significance) by the number of statistical tests done. Therefore, if two statistical tests are performed to determine the relationship between R/S and two health outcomes (e.g., blood pressure and depressive symptoms), then the conventional significance level of 0.05 would be divided by 2, and the new significance level would be 0.025; if five statistical tests were done, then the new significance level would be 0.01, and so forth.

However, the consensus (backed by empirical justification) is that the Bonferroni correction is too conservative and therefore overadjusts the p-value, leading to Type II errors (failure to detect effects that are really present).[10] Many good reasons exist to avoid using conservative adjustments for multiple comparisons. First, no particular strategy to adjust for multiple tests is widely accepted. Second, there is no established threshold for "too many tests." Third, p-value adjustments can be arbitrary. For example, if the researcher wrote two papers (splitting the analysis in two), the number of tests would be noticeably reduced and there would be less concern about multiple comparisons. If, however, the researcher decided to present a comprehensive analysis in a single paper, conventional significance levels are somehow no longer appropriate. Finally, as noted above, although p-value adjustments reduce the probability of Type I errors, they significantly reduce power and inflate the probability of Type II errors. When there is any chance to help people who are suffering, many researchers prefer to risk a Type I error. Alternatives to the Bonferroni correction that have greater power and are flexible in their application to a range of statistical tests (e.g., t-tests, correlations, chi-squares) include the Sidak-Bonferroni approach and Hochberg's sequential method (see Olejnik and colleagues for a review).[11]

Researchers may also address the issue of multiple comparisons by arguing that the study involves "exploratory research" and is not a definitive test of the hypothesis, justifying a less rigid adjustment for multiple comparisons. Based on such arguments, many editors may accept papers that simply state that the significance level was lowered from 0.05 to 0.01 when five to ten comparisons are made, or to 0.005 for ten to fifteen comparisons. Bear in mind, however, that the impact of articles with multiple comparisons is less, and such articles are harder to get accepted. Thus, it is best to do repeated tests only when doing exploratory work. If the researchers want to mine their data for this purpose, then it would be best to use software designed to do an efficient job of that—a better job than one can do with repeated testing.[12]

> Always think carefully before doing a statistical comparison, recognizing that each additional statistical test may require downward adjustment of the significance level.

Bottom line: Always think carefully before doing a statistical comparison, recognizing that each additional statistical test may require downward adjustment of the significance level.

Trend Findings

Some journals (especially the better ones) do not allow reporting "trend level" or "marginally significant" findings, while other journals might. A trend-level finding is where the significance level (p value) of the parameter coefficient for a single statistical test is between 0.05 and 0.10 (after rounding). If multiple statistical tests are done, and the significance level is reduced to 0.01, then researchers could argue a trend level between 0.01 and 0.05 or, alternatively, between 0.01 and 0.10. Again, journal editors and reviewers vary on whether they accept this practice, and journals often publish specific instructions on what they allow.

SUMMARY AND CONCLUSIONS

I began this chapter by describing some fundamental rules for conducting statistical analyses that may help free researchers from an unnecessary dependence on statisticians and enable them to intelligently communicate with statisticians. I provided guidelines on how to take a systematic approach toward analyzing data by following an analysis plan and described steps to prepare a data set for analysis that increases accuracy and reduces error. I then made recommendations on how to analyze R/S variables in statistical models and provided suggestions on when and how to correct significance levels for multiple comparisons. Equipped with this background, the reader should be ready for the next chapter, which provides guidelines on how to choose the most appropriate statistical test based on study design and type of variable.

Statistics II: Statistical Tests and Approaches

OUTLINE

IN THIS CHAPTER I continue to introduce the reader to statistical language, describe the different variable types, review
the most appropriate statistical tests to use depending on
study design and variable type, briefly mention more advanced
statistical methods, and, finally, make recommendations on
when a statistician is needed. This key chapter includes some
complex material and may need to be reviewed several times.
However, researchers who plan to conduct their own statistical
analyses or wish to optimize their communication with statisticians should thoroughly absorb the material in this chapter.

LEVEL OF MEASUREMENT

As covered more thoroughly in Chapter 16, there are five basic
variable *classes*: predictors, moderators, confounders, mediators, and outcomes. The first four of these are also called *independent variables* or *covariates* (some researchers
simply call them *predictors*), and the last one (*outcome*) is called the *dependent variable*. Within each
of these variable classes, there are four *levels of
measurement*: categorical, continuous, ordinal, and
ratio. These variable types are distinguished from
each other based on the form that their response
categories take. Thorough familiarity by researchers with these
variable types is essential for choosing the correct statistical
tests to analyze their data. I focus here on categorical, continuous, and ordinal variables, the most common types that
researchers are likely to encounter.

> **Within each of these variable classes, there are four *levels of measurement*: categorical, continuous, ordinal, and ratio.**

Categorical Variable

A categorical variable (also called *nominal*) is one with discrete
response categories. Examples include gender (male, female)
and ethnicity (African-American, White—non Hispanic/Latino,
Hispanic/Latino, or Asian). Where there are two nominal categories for a variable (e.g., male and female), numeric coding is used, such as 0 and 1, and is arbitrary. Codes should be
chosen to facilitate communication of the results. When there
are more than two nominal categories, some analyses (regres-

sion) require coding the multicategory variable into k-1 binary "dummy" variables (where k is the number of categories). Other analyses (analysis of variance [ANOVA]) can use multicategory nominal variables as independent variables without recoding into dummy variables. An example of a variable that might require dummy coding for regression analyses is race. Response categories for race might be Caucasian, African American, Hispanic, and Asian. Creating dummy variables would allow the researcher to compare the effects of racial background on a health outcome. Caucasians might be considered the "reference group," to whom other racial groups would be compared (e.g., African American vs. Caucasians, Hispanics vs. Caucasians, and Asians vs. Caucasians).

The coding for these variables would proceed as follows: African Americans would receive a 1 on their dummy variable (call it AA), and everyone else would receive a 0; Hispanics would receive a 1 on their dummy variable (call it H), and everyone else would receive a 0; and Asians would receive a 1 on their dummy variable (call it A), and everyone else would receive a 0. Caucasians would not have a dummy variable because they are the reference group. Therefore, three dummy variables (AA, H, and A) would be included in the regression model. The regression output would produce a parameter coefficient (β) that describes each race's effects on the health outcome relative to the reference group (Caucasians), all within a single regression model.

Continuous Variable

A continuous variable (also called "interval level") is a characteristic such as age or blood pressure in which each unit difference (interval) on the response measure is equal to every other unit difference (e.g., a value of 2 for age is exactly twice the value of 1 for age, the value for age 4 is exactly twice the value of age 2, etc.). Unfortunately, the variables that interest psychologists and R/S researchers are not continuous. Researchers cannot measure something like spirituality with a ruler or scale, or use an instrument that gives nice, even response intervals. Researchers can give a test using questions they think are some measure of spirituality and see how many questions a participant gets "correct." This approach will result in a raw score that is an ordinal variable. Researchers can presume that someone who has a raw score of 16 has more spirituality than someone who has a raw score of 15, but how much more? Is the interval between a raw score of 15 and 16 the same as the interval between 25 and 26? Probably not.

If desired, researchers can convert the raw score to a scale score with equal intervals using the following statistical procedure. Take the mean score of the group that took the spirituality test and divide it by the population standard deviation of the group. This produces a Z-score, a type of scale score, which has equal intervals. Usually Z-scores are multiplied by some number and changed in other ways to make them easier to interpret. For example, the WISC-IV intelligence test that measures IQ sets the mean to 100, and each Z-score represents 15 IQ points.

Despite the fact that most variables of interest to R/S researchers are not continuous, parametric statistical tests (see explanation below) are often used to analyze them if the response distribution is not too far from the normal curve and the sample is fairly large. Sometimes, however, responses are not normally distributed around a mean, but instead are skewed in one direction or another. That is, when the responses are plotted against the familiar bell or normal curve, they do not fit the curve but instead skew to the left or the right. Since parametric statistical tests presume that the distribution around the mean is normal, these skewed distributions violate the central assumption of parametric tests. However, parametric tests have proved robust enough to give true results as long as the skewing is not too great. In cases of high skew, the data may need to be statistically "transformed" to create a more normal distribution, meaning a distribution that is a closer match to the normal curve (i.e., one in which 95 percent of subjects' responses lie within two standard errors of the sample mean). The most common way of doing this is to use a logarithm (log) or a square root transformation, although researchers differ on the approach.

Generally speaking, regression and analysis of variance are

> Despite the fact that most variables of interest to R/S researchers are not continuous, parametric statistical tests (see explanation below) are often used to analyze them if the response distribution is not too far from the normal curve and the sample is fairly large.

moderate to robust in handling violations of normality for the outcome (and there is no assumption made about the predictor variable distribution). With small sample sizes (e.g., fewer than thirty cases), more concern is warranted when responses to the data are not normally distributed. In general, because of the cost of transformation in terms of less obvious interpretation of the finding, transformation is usually not desirable. But some researchers/statisticians are more comfortable with transformations than others.

Ordinal Variable

An ordinal variable (also called "ranked") has responses that are ordered or ranked from high to low, similar to a continuous variable, but the difference between categories on the response measure is not equal like a continuous variable. In other words, the researcher can tell that some responses indicate more or less than others, just not how much more or less. An ordinal variable is also not like a categorical variable such as ethnicity because responses are in an order from low to medium to high, and each response is quantitatively higher or lower than another (not true for categorical variables). Examples of ordinal variables are grades on a test from F to A, self-rated health that ranges from poor to excellent, or self-rated pain that is rated from nonexistent to severe. This type of variable is very relevant to R/S and health research; many if not most religious variables are ordinal variables since response categories are ranked from low to high (and so are not categorical or continuous). I describe below how to handle such variables.

Statistical tests that examine continuous variables are called *parametric tests*, and those that measure categorical or ordinal variables are called *nonparametric tests*.[1] Parametric tests are often considered more powerful in detecting effects. Ordinal variables such as religious attendance, importance of religion, or intrinsic religiosity measured with Likert-type scales are often analyzed as continuous variables using parametric statistics under the assumption that the variables are

> Ordinal variables such as religious attendance, importance of religion, or intrinsic religiosity measured with Likert-type scales are often analyzed as continuous variables using parametric statistics under the assumption that the variables are normally distributed.

normally distributed. While technically not correct, since it may violate important assumptions in calculating confidence limits and p-values that require even intervals and normal distribution of data, this approach is often taken in the behavioral and social sciences. The reason for this approach is that the difference in results obtained using nonparametric statistics and parametric statistics are usually substantively identical.[2] For example, Spearman's rho and Pearson correlation are largely equivalent. Spearman's rho is really just a shorthand computational formula when ranks are used. Myers and Well offer a good discussion of when normality is a concern for analysis of variance (and by implication regression).[3] They show a small simulation where p-values are only adversely affected when distributions are very nonnormal and sample size is quite small (fewer than thirty cases). Furthermore, there are theoretical grounds (based on the central limit theorem) to justify using parametric statistics for ordinal data with five or more response categories.[4] Finally, when using regression models, R/S variables are usually predictors in the model, so their level of measurement doesn't really matter (it's the level of measurement of the health outcome that matters).

> The reason for this approach is that the difference in results obtained using nonparametric statistics and parametric statistics are usually substantively identical.

Choosing a Statistical Test

The kinds of statistical tests a researcher might choose to measure the relationship between a predictor and an outcome, or the effects of an intervention on an outcome, depend on (1) study design, (2) type of sample, (3) type of test, (4) type of variable (level of measurement), and (5) number of times the outcome is measured (see Table 15.1).

First, there are the two basic study designs: observational and experimental. Second, these study designs are divided into whether the study groups are either independent (subjects or groups unrelated to each other) or matched (subjects or groups related). Third, there are two types of tests, bivariate (those that examine a relationship between two variables) and multivariate (those that examine a relationship between two variables while controlling for other variables). Fourth, there are three

TABLE 15.1.

Common Statistical Tests

TYPE OF STUDY			TYPE OF TEST	
			Bivariate	Multivariate
Observational Studies				
Independent Samples				
Level of Measurement				
	Categorical (Nominal) Outcome			
		Cat predictor	Chi-square, Fisher's exact	Logistic regression
		Cont predictor	T-test, ANOVA	Logistic regression
		Ord predictor	Wilcoxon (< 5 level), ANOVA (> 4)	Logistic regression
	Continuous Outcome			
		Cat predictor	T-test, ANOVA	Multiple regression
		Cont predictor	Pearson correlation	Multiple regression
		Ord predictor	Gamma (< 5 level), Pearson (> 4)	Multiple regression
	Ordinal Outcome (< 5 levels)			
		Cat predictor	Tau-b, Wilcoxon, Kruskal-Wallis ANOVA	Ordinal logistic reg
		Cont predictor	Gamma	Ordinal logistic reg
		Ord predictor	Spearman, Kendall	Ordinal logistic reg
	Ordinal Outcome (> 4 levels)		(see Cont outcome)	(see Cont outcome)
Dependent Samples				
Level of Measurement				
	Categorical (Nominal) Outcome			
		Cat predictor	McNemar, Cochrane Q	Conditional log reg
		Cont predictor	Paired T-test, repeat meas ANOVA	Conditional log reg
		Ord predictor	Wilcoxon, Friedman ANOVA	Conditional log reg
	Continuous Outcome			
		Cat predictor	See text	See text, SEM
		Cont predictor	See text	See text, SEM
		Ord predictor	See text	See text, SEM
	Ordinal Outcome (< 5 levels)			
		Cat predictor	Loglinear	Loglinear
		Cont predictor	Repeated measures ANOVA	Loglinear
		Ord predictor	Friedman ANOVA	Loglinear
	Ordinal Outcome (> 4 levels)	(see Cont outcome)	(see Cont outcome)	(see Cont outcome)

continued on next page

Type of Study		Type of Test	
		Bivariate	Multivariate
Experimental Studies			
Within-Subjects (Single-Intervention, No Control Group)			
Level of Measurement			
	Categorical Outcome		
		Cat predictor	McNemar	Repeated measures logistic regression
		Cont predictor	—	Repeated measures logistic regression
		Ord predictor	—	Repeated measures logistic regression
	Continuous Outcome		
		Cat predictor	Paired T-test	Repeated measures ANOVA
		Cont predictor	—	Repeated measures ANOVA
		Ord predictor	—	Repeated measures ANOVA
	Ordinal Outcome (< 5 levels)		
		Cat predictor	Wilcoxon signed-rank test	Ordinal logistic reg
		Cont predictor	—	Ordinal logistic reg
		Ord predictor	—	Ordinal logistic reg
Between-Subjects (RCT—2 Groups)			
Level of Measurement			
	Categorical Outcome		
		Cat predictor	Chi-square, Fisher's exact	Logistic regression
		Cont predictor	—	Logistic regression
		Ord predictor	—	Logistic regression
	Continuous Outcome		
		Cat predictor	T-test, repeated measures ANOVA	Multiple regression
		Cont predictor	—	Multiple regression
		Ord predictor	—	Multiple regression
	Ordinal Outcome (< 5 levels)		
		Cat predictor	Wilcoxon rank sum, Kruskal-Wallis	Ordinal logistic reg
		Cont predictor	—	Ordinal logistic reg
		Ord predictor	—	Ordinal logistic reg

RCT = randomized clinical trial

Cat = categorical variable, Cont = continuous variable, Ord = ordinal variable, Reg = regression, Log = logistic, SEM = structural equation modeling, — = not applicable levels of measurement (categorical, continuous, and ordinal); for bivariate tests, level of measurement is important for both predictor and outcome, whereas for multivariate tests, level of measurement is only relevant for the outcome. Finally, the number of times the outcome is measured influences the choice of statistical test. Subjects may be assessed at baseline only (cross-sectional study), at baseline and at a single discrete follow-up, or at baseline and at several discrete follow-ups over time.

OBSERVATIONAL STUDIES, INDEPENDENT SAMPLES

These studies involve subjects or groups of subjects who are completely unrelated to each other—that is, they are independent. The following statistical tests cover most of the analyses that R/S-health researchers are likely to perform when analyzing data from such studies.

Bivariate, Categorical Outcomes

When predictor and outcome variables are measured as categories, and the researcher wants to determine the relationship between these two variables, then a *chi-square* (χ^2) *statistic* would be chosen.[5] The χ^2 test is the most commonly used statistical test. It examines whether two or more percentages are different from each other. An example of a research question that a χ^2 test could answer might be, "Is there a relationship between religious affiliation (yes, no) and marital status (married vs. not married)?" In other words, is the percentage of people with a religious affiliation different between those who are married and those who are not? Use of the χ^2 test depends on the number of subjects in the study. If there is only a small number of subjects (< 20), if the expected number of cases in any one cell is < 1, or if more than 25 percent of cells have < 5, then a *Fisher's exact test* would be used, although there is some debate about these conventional guidelines. The general consensus is that the Fisher's exact test is too conservative and that the <5 rule is too strict.[6]

When a predictor variable is continuous (like blood pressure) and the outcome variable is categorical (marital status), then an *independent* (*student's*) *T-test* would be used if the outcome variable consisted of two groups (i.e., married vs. not married), and a *one-way analysis of variance* (ANOVA) would be used if the outcome had more than two groups (i.e., married, divorced, widowed, never married). These are parametric tests. If the predictor variable is not normally distributed or is ordinal (like frequency of prayer or importance of religiosity), then the researcher would choose the *Wilcoxon rank sum test* or *Mann-Whitney U test* for an outcome with two groups, and the *Kruskal-Wallis ANOVA* for an outcome with more than two groups. These are nonparametric tests.

Multivariate, Categorical Outcomes

When an outcome variable is categorical, regardless of level of measurement of the predictor, and the researcher wants to control for other variables, then *logistic regression* would be chosen if the outcome variable had only two response categories (i.e., married vs. not married). If the outcome variable had three or more response categories (i.e., married vs. divorced vs. never married), then *multinomial logistic regression* would be chosen. In a prospective study where the researcher wants to examine the effect of a predictor (regardless of level of measurement) on time to a health event such as death and wants to control for other covariates, then a *Cox proportional hazards regression* would be used. The outcome in such a model is the occurrence of the event and the time to the event.

> When an outcome variable is categorical, regardless of level of measurement of the predictor, and the researcher wants to control for other variables, then *logistic regression* would be chosen if the outcome variable had only two response categories.

The regression models discussed above produce several kinds of results in their output for predictors and other covariates. Of particular importance are odds ratios (OR), risk ratios (RR), and hazard ratios (HR), along with their 95 percent confidence intervals. These statistics (equivalent to parameter coefficients discussed later in this chapter) are interpreted as follows. An OR is defined as the ratio of the odds of an event (e.g., a disease) occurring in one group to the odds of the event occurring in another group. A researcher might be comparing the odds of disease occurrence in a group of nonreligious persons with the odds of disease occurrence in a religious group.

An RR is the probability of an event (disease) occurring in a person exposed to a risk factor[7] (e.g., religion) relative to the probability of the event occurring in a person not exposed to the risk factor (e.g., no religion). OR and RR may be computed for either cross-sectional or longitudinal data. OR and RR are often quite similar when event rates are low; however, they become progressively different as the event rate increases.

Clinicians often quantify the effect of a risk factor on an outcome using the OR or RR since their interpretation is more intuitively meaningful than a correlation, chi-square, or other statistic of association. In health research, an OR is *the odds* of the outcome (disease) being 1 when the risk factor is 1 *compared* to the odds of the outcome being 1 when the risk factor is 0. The RR is *the probability* of the outcome being 1 when the risk factor is 1 ($P_{exposed}$) *compared* to the probability of the outcome being 1 when the risk factor is 0 ($P_{unexposed}$), that is,

$$RR = P_{exposed} / P_{unexposed}.$$

The relationship of the OR to the RR is:

$$RR = OR / [(1 - P_{unexposed}) + (P_{unexposed} \times OR)].$$

If $P_{unexposed}$ is very low (close to 0), then the RR approximates the OR. When interpreting an OR, the convention is to subtract 1 from the OR and multiply by 100 ($[OR - 1] \times 100$) to determine the percent increase or decrease in the odds of an outcome. The interpretation of an OR becomes tricky when researchers want to express it as a percentage increase or decrease in probability (P) of the outcome, which would require an algorithm in order to convert the OR into a probability— that is,

$$OR = (P_{exposed} / 1 - P_{exposed}) / (P_{unexposed} / 1 - P_{unexposed}).$$

Therefore, with an OR = 0.65, it is not correct to say there is a 35 percent decrease *in the probability* of the outcome (which many researchers have said, including myself). Instead, the correct interpretation for an OR = 0.65 is that it indicates a 35 percent reduction in the odds of the outcome being present

> Clinicians often quantify the effect of a risk factor on an outcome using the OR or RR since their interpretation is more intuitively meaningful than a correlation, chi-square, or other statistic of association.

> The correct interpretation for an OR = 0.65 is that it indicates a 35 percent reduction in the odds of the outcome being present when the risk factor is present compared to when the risk factor is absent.

when the risk factor is present compared to when the risk factor is absent. This is not the same as a RR of 0.65, which would indicate a 35 percent reduction *in the risk* of the outcome being present when the risk factor is present compared to when the risk factor is absent. Finally, while terms such "likelihood," "probability," and "risk" are often used interchangeably, there are subtle differences in their meanings (although too complex to explain here).

Similar to but not the same as the RR, hazard ratios (HR) are produced from Cox proportional hazards models and refer to the effect of a predictor variable on the hazard or rate at which an event takes place, taking into account whether an event occurs and how much time it takes for the event to occur. A Cox model is run when the outcome is "right-censored," which means the status on the outcome event (e.g., death) has not yet been determined for all participants during the observation period.

Bivariate, Continuous Outcomes

If a predictor variable is categorical and the outcome is continuous, the researcher would use the *independent T-test* if the predictor were binary (dichotomized) and use ANOVA if the predictor had more than two categories. If the predictor were ordinal with fewer than five categories and the outcome were continuous, then the *gamma* statistic would be used. When a predictor and outcome variable are both measured as continuous variables (or as ordinal variables with five or more categories) and the researcher wants to determine if there is relationship between them, then a *Pearson product moment correlation* (Pearson correlation or "r") would be chosen. The values for "r" range from +1.0 (which indicates perfect correlation) to 0 (which indicates no correlation) to −1.0 (which indicates a perfect inverse correlation). An example of a research question that such a test could answer might be "What is the relationship between percent of income given to religious causes (range = 0 to 100 percent) and systolic blood pressure (range = 90 to 240 mmHg)?" The larger the value of "r" and the larger the sample size, the more likely "r" is statistically significant. One can use the "r" and the sample size to look up significance levels (p values) in a table, or one can determine significance using a computer program.

In general, correlations (r) of 0.10 are considered small, 0.30 moderate, and 0.50 strong.[8] However, when dealing with psychosocial and behavioral variables such as R/S, which are difficult to measure precisely, are sometimes skewed in their distribution, and cannot be measured as continuous variables such as blood pressure or age, correlations in the range of 0.10–0.20 might be considered small, 0.20–0.30 moderate, and anything above 0.30 strong. Not everyone agrees with this opinion and may view it as encouraging bias; nevertheless, from what I've seen in studies looking at correlations between a psychosocial variable such as social support and mental health variables—variables that are known clinically to be strongly related—they seldom exceed 0.25–0.30. Any rules like this, though, are simply arbitrary and depend a great deal on the context. In other words, very small correlations in cancer prevention might be extremely important and affect many lives. Likewise, when studying a behavior such as R/S that is important to nearly 200 million people in the United States alone, even small correlations with health may translate into substantial public health importance.

Multivariate, Continuous Outcomes

When an outcome is measured as a continuous variable and the researcher wants to determine the relationship between a predictor (with any level of measurement) and the outcome, while controlling for other variables, then *multiple linear regression* would be chosen (also called ordinary least squares [OLS] regression). The regression output produces parameter coefficients[9] for the predictors and other covariates in the model, their standard errors, and the statistical significance of these coefficients.

> When an outcome is measured as a continuous variable and the researcher wants to determine the relationship between a predictor (with any level of measurement) and the outcome, while controlling for other variables, then *multiple linear regression* would be chosen.

Bivariate, Ordinal Outcomes

If the predictor is categorical and the outcome is ordinal, then the *tau-b* statistic would be used if the predictor were binary;

an alternative test to use with a binary predictor is the *Wilcoxon rank sum test* (aka *Mann-Whitney U*). If the predictor has more than two categories, then a *Kruskal-Wallis ANOVA* or a *tau-c* would be used. If the predictor is continuous and the outcome is ordinal, then a *gamma statistic* would be the choice. When a predictor and outcome variable are both measured as ordinal or ranked variables, then a *Spearman rank order correlation* (Spearman correlation or "ρ") or a *Kendall rank order correlation* ("τ") would be chosen; these are the nonparametric equivalents of the Pearson correlation ("r"). An example of a research question that a Spearman correlation (ρ) could answer might be, "What is the strength of the relationship between frequency of prayer (none, rare, occasional, often, very often) and subjective health (poor, moderate, good, very good)?" Unless the sample size is quite small and number of response categories for the variables is less than five, however, many researchers would simply use a parametric test (Pearson "r") for the correlation.

Multivariate, Ordinal Outcomes

> When an outcome is measured as an ordinal variable and the researcher wants to determine the relationship between a predictor (with any level of measurement) and the outcome, while controlling for other variables, then *ordinal logistic regression* would be the test of choice.

When an outcome is measured as an ordinal variable and the researcher wants to determine the relationship between a predictor (with any level of measurement) and the outcome, while controlling for other variables, then *ordinal logistic regression* would be the test of choice (also called *ordered logistic regression*). *Ordinal probit regression* is another popular approach for ordinal outcomes (if normally distributed). Many researchers, however, would simply use a parametric statistical method such as multiple linear regression (see discussion above). However, if the outcome had only a few ordinal categories (< 5) or sample size was small (< 50–100), many statisticians would probably avoid linear regression.

Summary

The detailed categorization above is meant to help researchers choose the statistical test that best matches their data. In reality, however, most statistical tests used by R/S-health researchers when analyzing data from observational studies where subjects are independent of each other can simply be divided into common bivariate tests (chi-square, T-test, ANOVA, and correlation) and common multivariate regression tests (linear regression or logistic regression). These categories cover the vast majority of statistical tests and measurement contingencies that researchers are likely to encounter. With regression techniques (both bivariate and multivariate), the level of measurement of the dependent variable (outcome) determines the type of test to be used, and the level of measurement of the predictor and other covariates does not matter.

> With regression techniques (both bivariate and multivariate), the level of measurement of the dependent variable (outcome) determines the type of test to be used, and the level of measurement of the predictor and other covariates does not matter.

OBSERVATIONAL STUDIES, DEPENDENT SAMPLES

Most situations requiring the analysis of data from dependent or matched samples involve case-control studies (where cases are not independent of controls since they are matched), studies involving couples or related subjects (twins), and longitudinal studies where several measures are taken on the same sample over time. Because of their importance in R/S and health research, I deal with longitudinal studies in a separate section below. Here, I focus here on analysis of data from case-control studies, where controls are matched to cases; these analyses may also be applied by analogy to couples, dyads, twins, or other samples of individuals associated with each other and therefore considered dependent. The outcome in case-control studies is usually a dichotomized categorical variable, case vs. control status, but may also involve more than one case and one control, and in that case may be either categorical or ordinal.

Bivariate, Categorical Outcomes

The *McNemar test* is used in case-control studies where researchers want to know if a dichotomized categorical predictor or risk factor[10] (e.g., atheism, yes vs. no) is more common among cases with a disease compared to matched controls without the disease. The McNemar test rather than the chi-square statistic is used because of the matching. For a dichotomized categorical risk factor that is being compared across three or more matched groups (cases1, cases2, controls) the *Cochrane Q test* is used. If the risk factor is continuous and the researcher wishes to compare cases and controls on that measure, then a *paired T-test* would be used. A *repeated measures ANOVA* would be chosen for a continuous risk factor if three or more matched groups were involved (cases1, cases2, controls). If the risk factor were ordinal or nonnormally distributed, then a *Wilcoxon signed rank test* (the nonparametric equivalent of the paired T-test) would be used for two matched groups, and a *Friedman two-way ANOVA* (the nonparametric equivalent of the repeated measures ANOVA) would be used for three or more matched groups.

An alternative method of comparing cases and controls would be to construct a bivariate *conditional logistic regression* model with only the risk factor in the model; this could be used to examine a risk factor with any level of measurement (categorical, ordinal, or continuous). If there were three or more matched groups (cases1, cases2, controls), then a bivariate *conditional multinomial logistic regression* might be used. If a survival analysis were desired (e.g., to examine if cases vs. controls live longer), then a bivariate *conditional proportional hazards regression* would be chosen.

Multivariate, Categorical Outcomes

If there are two matched groups as in a case-control study, then a multivariate *conditional logistic regression* is used to examine a risk factor at any level of measurement, while controlling for confounders at any level of measurement. If there are three or more matched groups (cases1, cases2, controls), then a multivariate *conditional multinomial logistic regression* is used. These

are simply extensions of the bivariate modeling procedures mentioned above. An alternative procedure
when examining a continuous risk factor between
three or more groups (cases1, case2, controls) would
be to do a *repeated measures ANOVA* with covariates
added. If a survival analysis were desired to compare two or more matched groups, a *conditional proportional hazards regression* would be chosen with
covariates added.

> If there are two matched
> groups as in a case-control
> study, then a multivariate
> *conditional logistic regression*
> is used to examine a risk
> factor at any level of mea-
> surement, while controlling
> for confounders at any level
> of measurement.

Bivariate and Multivariate, Continuous Outcomes

When comparing cases and controls, case-control status is the
outcome and cannot be continuous.

If the question is whether the relationship between a risk
factor and a continuous outcome is different in cases compared to matched controls, and the risk factor is a dichotomous
variable such as gender, then the researcher would do a *mixed
ANOVA* with one within-subjects factor (case vs. control) and
one between-subjects factor (gender), using a general linear
model procedure in SAS or SPSS. If the risk factor is a continuous variable, then things become more complicated. One could
use difference scores between cases and controls and predict
that with the continuous risk factor. Alternatively, one could do
separate regressions for cases and controls and compare the
two related / dependent regression coefficients;[11] this regression
technique could also be used to handle a dichotomized risk factor (e.g., gender). In both methods, covariates could be added to
the models to control for them. Alternatively, researchers might
simply use *structural equation modeling* (SEM) to handle such
situations.

Bivariate and Multivariate, Ordinal Outcomes

There may be a situation where there are more than two groups
of cases and controls and those groups are ordered. An example of ordered matched groups might be cases with diabetes,
cases with borderline diabetes, and controls without diabetes.

To compare categorical risk factors across these three ordered groups, *loglinear analyses* would be used. Continuous risk factors could be compared across two groups of cases and controls using a *paired T-test*. For three or more ordered groups of cases and controls, *repeated measures ANOVA* would be used. To compare ordinal risk factors across two groups of cases and controls, a Wilcoxon rank sum test would be used, and if there were three or more ordered groups of cases and controls, a *Friedman two-way ANOVA* would be chosen. Several possible ways are available to analyze such data, although many researchers would use a *loglinear* approach because it is quite general and flexible, and could be used to control for categorical covariates of any level of measurement.[12]

Miscellaneous

The analyses listed above for case-control studies (and, by analogy, other samples involving matched pairs) cover most situations, but some unusual situations not covered here could arise. In that event, the researcher should consult a statistician regarding the most appropriate test to use. A text by Card and colleagues provides an excellent review of statistical methods used with matched or dependent samples (including analyses involving twins, couples, or other pairs of subjects that are not independent of each other).[13]

Overall Summary

If the information above on statistical tests for analyzing independent and dependent samples seems overwhelming, researchers should remember one thing. All regression techniques can handle predictors of any level of measurement—categorical, ordinal, or continuous. What the researcher must do is match the regression technique with the appropriate level of measurement of the *outcome*. Bivariate relationships can be determined by simply including only the predictor variable (religion/spirituality) in the model without other covariates, and multivariate models can then

> **All regression techniques can handle predictors of any level of measurement—categorical, ordinal, or continuous.**

be run by including covariates to address confounding, mediation, and interactions.

Longitudinal Studies

As noted in Chapter 5, longitudinal studies are capable of establishing two of the three criteria necessary for causal inference (association and temporality). While they cannot establish the final criterion (nonspuriousness of association), statistical controls can help to address the concern that a third variable is responsible for the association. Therefore, longitudinal designs are far superior to cross-sectional studies in their contribution to internal validity (with respect to establishing a causal relationship between predictor and outcome). They are a high priority in R/S-health research.

> Longitudinal designs are far superior to cross-sectional studies in their contribution to internal validity (with respect to establishing a causal relationship between predictor and outcome).

Longitudinal studies involve the assessment of the same individuals repeatedly over time. Therefore, such analyses require statistical tests appropriate for "dependent samples," since the same individuals are being assessed repeatedly and thus are not independent of each other. For all researchers analyzing longitudinal data, I recommend a chapter by Jason Newsom, "Basic Longitudinal Analysis Approaches for Continuous and Categorical Variables,"[14] which outlines the most commonly used and best approaches for analyzing longitudinal data in a wide range of circumstances. Here I discuss approaches to analyzing longitudinal data depending on the level of measurement of the outcome variable, first examining outcomes that are continuous and then outcomes that are categorical or ordinal. This section ends with a brief exploration of ways to analyze longitudinal data involving matched pairs.

Continuous Outcomes

If the researcher was interested in making repeated assessments of a continuous outcome (such as blood pressure or depressive symptoms) in a single group of individuals to determine whether the outcome changes during the period of observation in a two-wave pre–post study design, then a *paired T-test* would be the test chosen. The paired T-test takes into account the fact that assessments are being made twice on the same individuals. Equally appropriate, and perhaps preferred because of its greater flexibility, would be to use a *repeated measures ANOVA*. The advantages of the repeated measures ANOVA are that it allows the examination of covariates (predictors, confounders, mediators, moderators) and can analyze data collected at more than two time points—neither of which are possible with the paired T-test.

If a repeated measures ANOVA is run without covariates in the model, the results would be interpreted as "the effect of time" or "differences due to time" on the outcome. In a two-wave study, the repeated measures ANOVA treats the two measures of outcome as different levels of one within-subjects factor, time. Such an analysis is often done to determine the natural rate of change in a health outcome over time and is important in observational studies when researchers want to know whether the follow-up period has been long enough to allow the outcome to change. The latter will directly impact the power of the study to detect whether a predictor (such as R/S) has an effect on a health outcome during that time. If the base rate of change in the health outcome during the observation period is too small, then researchers cannot expect a predictor to significantly affect the outcome during that time period and would have to redesign the study so that follow-up is long enough for sufficient change in the outcome to occur. Inadequate change in the health outcome during a too-short observation period is often the reason that R/S does not significantly predict health outcomes.

If sufficient time has elapsed and the health outcome does change significantly during the observation period, then the researcher may wish to examine the effects of predictors and other covariates on the outcome by adding them to a repeated measures ANOVA model. Besides being able to examine predictors and control for covariates, the repeated measures ANOVA can also handle data involving assessments of an outcome at more than two points in time. However, with three or more assessments, the analysis becomes more complex, and certain assumptions about the distribution of the data and time periods between data collection need to be met: the sphericity assumption, the compound symmetry assumption, and the nonadditivity assumption. Various statistical tests are used to determine whether these assumptions are met given the distribution of the data (see pp. 149–50 in Newsom's chapter cited earlier).

When the researcher is analyzing predictors of outcome in a two-wave longitudinal study, an even more common approach than repeated measures ANOVA is either lagged regression or regression using difference or change scores. Although standard regression techniques are used with these approaches, the procedure takes into account the dependent nature of the samples. With lagged regression (also called *conditional change, statistical equating, baseline adjusted*, or the *ANCOVA approach*), the effect of wave-1 predictors on a wave-2 outcome is examined while controlling for the wave-1 outcome. With the change score approach (also called *difference score regression*), standard regression is used to examine the effect of wave-1 predictors on a change score (wave-2 outcome minus wave-1 outcome). *Fixed regression* is an extension of difference score regression and may be used if researchers want to know whether change in a predictor has an influence on change in an outcome (e.g., whether an increase in church attendance from wave-1 to wave-2 correlates with a decrease in depressive symptoms from wave-1 to wave-2).[15] This approach could also be used to determine whether a baseline predictor such as R/S influences a health outcome while controlling for changes in other covariates (*time-varying covariates*). For example, when Strawbridge and colleagues examined the effects of baseline religious attendance in 1965 on survival twenty-eight years later (in this example, the outcome variable was categorical, i.e., alive vs. dead), they wanted to see if the effect on survival could be explained by changes in depressive symptoms, social support, exercise frequency, and other mediators; these variables are called time-varying covariates.

Lagged regression and difference score regression

> The lagged regression approach is often recommended because it is designed to rule out the explanation that the impact of the predictor on the wave-2 outcome is due to the initial association between the predictor and the wave-1 outcome.

do not always produce equivalent results. The reason is that difference scores tend to be related to the baseline or wave-1 score, whereas this is not a problem with lagged regression (see pp. 159–61 in Newsom's chapter). Thus, the lagged regression approach is often recommended because it is designed to rule out the explanation that the impact of the predictor on the wave-2 outcome is due to the initial association between the predictor and the wave-1 outcome. By controlling for baseline scores on the outcome, lagged regression also helps to address the problem of reverse causation (i.e., that the outcome variable is influencing the predictor rather than vice versa). Furthermore, lagged regression provides a parameter coefficient (the B for the wave-1 outcome score) that provides a measure of the stability of the outcome over time. What remains after accounting for this stability is the extent to which the outcome is unstable or changing during the period of observation (and is the variance that the predictor and other covariates will be capable of explaining). As stability in the outcome variable increases and the unexplained variance decreases, the likelihood that any predictor will significantly predict wave-2 outcome decreases—no matter how large an effect that a predictor has on the outcome. Establishing association and temporal precedence (two of the three criteria for causality), then, is dependent on the appropriate time lag between baseline and follow-up.

Unfortunately, there are drawbacks to the lagged regression approach as well. The most serious one is that it estimates the effects of predictors on the outcome by forcing all individuals to begin with the same baseline score on the outcome. In many instances this is not the case, especially if there is a relationship between the predictor and the health outcome at baseline (which often occurs in R/S-health research since the effects of previous R/S activity have already influenced the health outcome prior to the baseline assessment). Furthermore, regression techniques used in lagged regression cannot address nonlinear changes over time, requiring either transformation of the data or use of other approaches.

For longitudinal studies involving three or more waves of data, many researchers today analyze their data using multilevel models that estimate both fixed effects and random effects (see below). Particularly useful are *growth curve models* (a special type of multilevel model) that allow researchers to examine individual trajectories of change for each subject as well as examine predictors of between-subject variation in those trajectories (see below). *Generalized estimating equations* (GEE) is also increasingly used for multiwave designs in health research (and also allows for the examinination of time-varying covariates). GEE is a limited version of multilevel modeling where slopes are not random (and use somewhat different algorithms for estimating regression coefficients). In any case, increasing attention has been paid to longitudinal studies in recent years and, as a result, many advances have taken place in methods used to analyze these data.

> For longitudinal studies involving three or more waves of data, many researchers today analyze their data using multilevel models that estimate both fixed effects and random effects.

Categorical and Ordinal Outcomes

Newsom notes that much less attention has been paid to the analysis of longitudinal data involving "discrete" health outcomes. When the outcome is a dichotomized outcome variable (disease present vs. absent), the simplest test of change in status over time is the *McNemar* test or the *Cochran-Mantel-Haenszel* test.[16] For example, a researcher examines a sample of patients with depressive symptoms for change in status regarding the presence of major depression during a five-year observation period (baseline = present vs. absent; follow-up = present vs. absent). The research question is whether there has been a significant change in major depression status from baseline to follow-up—that is, the change in status more than would be expected by chance alone? Bear in mind that when sample sizes are less than 30, the McNemar test does not produce exact p-values and so an "exact" test is needed (e.g., binomial test or Liddell test).

An alternative approach to use with two waves of data is a *conditional logistic regression* model, which can also examine predictors of change and control for other covariates. An extension of this method, the Rasch model, is useful for examining three or more waves of data.[17] Conditional logistic regression uses a difference score as the outcome by subtracting pretest from post test status, resulting in difference scores of –1, 0, and +1, with the model run without an intercept. For longitudinal studies involving outcome variables with more than two categories of response (e.g., yes, no, undecided), Newsom suggests using *loglinear models*; these models can handle either nominal or ordinal outcome variables.

Just as discussed for continuous outcomes, the lagged regression approach can also be employed for categorical outcomes involving two waves of data using *logistic regression*. This method predicts the change in probability of an outcome occurring at wave-2 after controlling for the probability of the outcome at wave-1. Likewise, the difference score approach can also be used, with possible outcome values being –1, 0, and +1, depending on changes in the status of the outcome over time; this can then be analyzed using an *ordinal logistic regression* (if responses are rank-ordered) or a *multinomial logistic regression* (if responses are nominal). Changes in predictor or covariates (time-varying covariates) can also be examined using a fixed regression approach by constructing a *conditional logistic model* as discussed in the previous paragraph.

> The lagged regression approach can also be employed for categorical outcomes involving two waves of data using *logistic regression*.

Similarly, lagged regression can be used to assess changes over two waves in outcome variables that are ordinal or ranked (e.g., no depression, minor depression, major depression, major depression–severe). This works the same way as the multiple regression for continuous outcomes or logistic regression for nominal outcomes, but using *ordinal logistic regression*. The same applies to examining difference scores, although Newsom has noted some potential problems with this approach for ordinal data.

> Lgged regression can be used to assess changes over two waves in outcome variables that are ordinal or ranked.

Matched Pairs Approaches

Much less frequently, researchers might wish to conduct longitudinal studies involved matched pairs (e.g., case-control studies, twin studies, couples or marital dyads). Researchers may wish to compare longitudinal relationships among predictors and outcomes between cases and controls or between members of other matched pairs. *Structural equation modeling* (SEM) is probably the best statistical method for such study designs. Alternatively, Cook and Kenny discuss the use of social relations models that are suitable for repeated measures and paired data (e.g., actor-partner effects).[18] Growth curve models can also be used to analyze data involving matched pairs.

EXPERIMENTAL STUDIES

Up to this point I have been discussing observational studies, where the purpose is to observe, not intervene or in any way affect the natural history of events. Because of the nature of R/S variables, observational studies are often the only way to investigate relationships with health. Only experimental data, however, can conclusively identify the nature of a relationship—that is, determine which variable is actually affecting the other. Even in the best-designed observational study, researchers can never be sure that they have selected the correct predictors, confounders, and mediators (or that they could ever know all of them), and then measure these variables perfectly without error. Researchers are still speculating about which variables account for the relationship between R/S and health.[19] Other challenges involve defining R/S and measuring it accurately and precisely (see chapters 12 and 13). These concerns, characteristic of all observational studies, underscore the importance of testing interventions. Although experimental studies involving R/S and health are difficult to design and challenging to successfully carry out, with ingenuity and effort they have been done and are a high priority for future research.[20]

Experimental studies consist of two types. In the first type (within subjects design), an intervention is applied to all members of a single group and baseline, and follow-up measures of the outcome (assessed at a single discrete point or multiple points after the baseline) are examined to determine if

> Even in the best-designed observational study, researchers can never be sure that they have selected the correct predictors, confounders, and mediators and then measure these variables perfectly without error.

> Although experimental studies involving R/S and health are difficult to design and successfully carry out, with ingenuity and effort they have been done and are a high priority for future research.

any change results.[21] In the second type of experimental study (between-subjects design), the outcome (assessed at a single discrete point or multiple points after the baseline) is compared between one group that receives the intervention and a control group that does not. The outcome variable type determines the kinds of statistical tests used for both within- and between-subjects designs. I first review statistical tests for within subjects designs and then describe tests for between-subjects designs, each by outcome variable type.

Within Subjects Design

In the within subjects design, an intervention is applied to all members of a single group. This involves comparison of matched pairs that are not independent—but, in this instance, a pair consists of a subject at baseline and the same subject at follow-up, where the subject serves as his own control. This is also called a *single group experimental study* or *single group design*. This study design has a low level of internal validity, since many other extraneous factors besides the intervention could cause a change in the outcome from baseline to follow-up, including various historical events or simply the passage of time. Statistical analyses for this type of design are identical to those chosen to analyze data from observational longitudinal studies where subjects are repeatedly assessed and researchers wish to determine whether a significant change in the outcome occurs over time.

> In the within subjects design, an intervention is applied to all members of a single group. This involves comparison of matched pairs that are not independent—but, in this instance, a pair consists of a subject at baseline and the same subject at follow-up, where the subject serves as his own control.

Categorical Outcomes

If the researcher wants to know whether an intervention administered to everyone in a single group has an effect on a dichotomized categorical outcome measured at baseline and at a single time point after the intervention, then a *McNemar* test would be the statistical test chosen. For example, a researcher may ask, "Is prayer an effective strategy for reducing fear in children prior to an operation?" For this example, the health outcome is fear and it is assessed categorically as a binary outcome (fear present or absent) both at baseline before the prayer (intervention) and at follow-up after the prayer. If the researcher wanted to control for confounders, then a *repeated measures logistic regression* could be used. In general, though, covariates are rarely controlled in experiments of this kind. For this design to be a true experiment there would have to be no other factors affecting the change in the outcome or that covary with the treatment—conditions that are rarely true for this type of design.

Continuous Outcomes

If the researcher wants to know whether an intervention administered to everyone in a group has an effect on a continuous outcome, and the outcome is measured at baseline before the intervention and at a single point after the intervention (pre- and post-assessments), then a *paired T-test* would be the statistical test of choice. For example, consider the research question, "Does prayer prior to surgery lower blood pressure among older adults during surgery?" Blood pressure (outcome) is measured as a continuous variable at baseline before the prayer intervention and at follow-up during the surgery. A paired T-test is used then to determine whether the average blood pressure is significantly different before the prayer compared to after the prayer during surgery. Alternatively, a *repeated measures ANOVA* might be used, which treats the assessments of outcome as different levels of one within-subjects factor, time. This test would also be used if the researcher wanted to control for confounders or mediators (again, rarely done in experiments of this kind). The latter would be accomplished by adding between-subjects factors to the repeated measures ANOVA. Alternatively, lagged regression or difference score regression might be used (see "Longitudinal Studies" above).

Ordinal Outcomes

If the researcher wants to know whether an intervention administered to everyone in a group has an effect on an ordinal outcome, and the outcome is measured at baseline before the intervention and at a single point after the intervention, then a *Wilcoxon signed-rank test* would be chosen. For example, consider the research question, "Does prayer increase self-rated health among disabled persons in rehabilitation?" Self-rated health (outcome) is measured as an ordinal variable (poor, moderate, good, very good) at baseline before prayer and at follow-up after prayer. The above statistical test would be used to determine if the prayer intervention caused a significant increase in self-rated health. To control for confounders or mediators, some type of loglinear or probit model would be used, such as *ordinal logistic regression*, using a lagged regression or difference score regression approach.

Between Subjects Design

In the *between subjects design*, the effect of an intervention in one group is compared to changes in a control group that does not receive the intervention (where both groups are completely independent of each other and determined by randomization). This is also called a *randomized clinical trial* (RCT).

Categorical Outcomes

If a researcher conducts an RCT to compare the effects of an intervention against a control group (two independent groups) on a binary categorical outcome (i.e., 1 = improved, 0 = same) assessed at a single fixed point in time and there are no differences between the two groups at baseline, then the simplest statistical test to assess the intervention's effects would be a *chi-square statistic*. Again, the chi-square test is not suitable when the expected values in any of the cells of a contingency table are below 5; instead, use a *Fisher's exact test* (although see earlier discussion regarding concerns with limiting cell numbers to < 5). If there were three or more groups (intervention1, intervention2, control), then a chi-square statistic would also be used. If the researcher were concerned about baseline differences between an intervention and a control group, then a *logistic regression* would be chosen to control for those baseline covariates.[22] If there were three or more groups, then a *multinomial logistic regression* would be used to control for baseline differences. If the researcher wanted to consider the time it takes for an outcome event to occur, as well as control for baseline differences between groups, then a *Cox proportional hazards regression* would be used. In a Cox regression, if the goal were to compare two survival curves that described the time to an event in an intervention and in a control group, then a *log rank test* is used.

Continuous Outcomes

If a researcher conducts an RCT to compare the effects of an intervention against a control group (two independent groups) on a continuous outcome assessed at a single fixed point after the intervention and there were no group differences at base-line, then the statistical test chosen would be an *independent T-test* (unpaired T-test or two-sample student's T test). If there were three or more groups (intervention1, intervention2, con-trol), then a *one-way analysis of variance* (ANOVA) would be used. If the outcome were assessed at more than one follow-up (e.g., three months, six months, nine months), then a *mixed-fac-torial ANOVA* would be the test of choice (an extension of the repeated-measures ANOVA to include a between-subjects com-parison). Even better, *growth curve models* could be used as a further refinement of the mixed-factorial ANOVA. Growth curve models include random coefficient models and latent growth models that are considered special cases of multilevel mixed models.

If the researcher is concerned about baseline differences between intervention and control subjects on covariates known to be associated with the outcome (confounding), then the sta-tistical test chosen would depend on the number of intervention and control groups and how often the outcome is measured. For a two-wave study, researchers would either (a) use a *lagged multiple regression model* (for a baseline [wave-1] measure-ment and a single outcome measurement [wave-2], researchers would predict the wave-2 outcome controlling for wave-1 base-line score and other covariates), or (b) use a multiple regression model to predict change scores (take the difference between baseline wave-1 and follow-up wave-2 outcome scores). *Analysis of covariance* (ANCOVA) could also be used to equalize base-line outcome scores and covariates between treatment groups. If there were more than two outcome measurements (or more than two treatment groups), then covariates could be added to a *mixed factorial* ANOVA; alternatively (and preferably), these data could be analyzed using a *growth curve model*.

Ordinal Outcomes

If a researcher conducts an RCT to compare the effects of an intervention against a control group (two independent groups) on an ordinal outcome assessed at a single fixed point after the intervention and there are no group differences at baseline, then the statistical test chosen to assess the intervention's effects would be a *Wilcoxon rank sum test* (or *Mann-Whitney U test*). If there were three or more groups (intervention1, intervention2, control), then a *Kruskal-Wallis ANOVA* would be used. If the researcher were concerned about baseline differences (confounders) between intervention and control subjects that might affect the outcome in a 2-wave, prepost design, then *ordinal logistic regression* would be chosen to adjust for those baseline differences (e.g., use a *lagged* ordinal logistical regression model to predict the wave-2 ordinal outcome, controlling for wave-1 ordinal outcome score and confounders, as described for continuous outcome above). Ordinal logistic regression could also be used if there were multiple interventions or if the outcome was measured at multiple time points after the intervention. In general, because randomization is intended to balance all known and unknown confounders, some statisticians don't like to do too many adjustments (whether the outcome is continuous or ordinal), especially if the trial is large.

Advanced Statistical Tests

There are even more advanced statistical approaches that can take into account measurement error and missing data points, and can examine individual trajectories of change in a health outcome over time. I now briefly describe these.

Structural Equation Modeling[23]

A statistical method for taking into account measurement error is *structural equation modeling* (SEM). Because measurement errors attenuate correlations, accounting for them in predictive models can provide more accurate estimates of relationships among variables. SEM is similar to multiple regression but it has the ability to model interactions, nonlinearities, correlated independent variables, measurement error, correlated error terms, multiple latent independent variables, and one or more latent dependent variables. A latent variable (unobserved) is one that is inferred from other measured variables (observed) and could be a predictor such as religion/spirituality. SEM models combine path analysis with factor analysis. As such, SEM models have two components. The first component, a measurement model, resembles a factor analysis and produces a set of latent factors from observed variables. The second component, a structural model, resembles a path analysis and estimates regression coefficients for the factors produced in the measurement model. These models are ideal when (1) most or all of the measures are multi-item indices and (2) the researcher wants to test the plausibility of a hypothesized causal model consisting of multiple mediators and complex causal processes. SEM is considered a more powerful alternative to multiple regression, time series analysis, and analysis of covariance.

> A statistical method for taking into account measurement error is structural equation modeling (SEM). Because measurement errors attenuate correlations, accounting for them in predictive models can provide more accurate estimates of relationships among variables.

Mixed Models[24]

Mixed models are used to analyze longitudinal data with repeated measurements of predictors and outcomes (usually three or more waves). The primary function of this approach is to take into account clustered or hierarchically structured data that typically violates independence assumptions of ANOVA or regression analysis. By using only within-individual variation to estimate regression effects, mixed models effectively control for all stable characteristics (i.e., characteristics that don't change). Mixed models offer an advantage over more traditional repeated measures analyses in that they allow available data to be used even if data from some time points are missing.

> Mixed models are used to analyze longitudinal data with repeated measurements of predictors and outcomes (usually three or more waves). The primary function of this approach is to take into account clustered or hierarchically structured data.

In general, a mixed model can handle random effects and fixed effects. As inferred above, these models for repeated measures or nested data take into account correlation within and between units. An example of nested data might include patients at different hospitals. In the education world, an example would be student test scores that might be correlated within classes, schools, or school districts. With a mixed model the researcher can estimate the differences between individual students and between the groups to which they belong.

Growth Curve Modeling[25]

A major advantage of *growth curve models* is that they focus on individual change. Growth curve models are special cases of the hierarchical structuring that mixed models deal with— that is, repeated measurements nested within individuals. While standard lagged dependent variable regression models are well suited to predict change in outcomes over two points in time, those models are limited to indirect assessments of change across more than two waves. In contrast, growth curve analyses directly describe and explain individual change over three or more waves of data. These techniques can be particularly useful when change is not linear. Not only is an average increase or decrease over time assessed, but the individual variation of change is also captured. Thus, these models are useful for exploring why some individuals increase rather than decrease or remain constant over time. For example, a researcher might want to examine changes in muscle strength over a lifetime and factors which predict that change. Growth curve analysis can be used to examine this in a two-stage model of change. In the first stage, an individual's repeated measures (e.g., muscle strength scores) are modeled as a function of an individual growth trajectory. In the second stage, individual growth trajectories (e.g., regression coefficients) are permitted to vary as a function of individual background characteristics (e.g., predictors such as age or frequency of exercise). Growth curve modeling does not refer to a particular statistical method, but to numerous methods[26] that

> Growth curve analyses directly describe and explain individual change over three or more waves of data. These techniques can be particularly useful when change is not linear.

are used to generate a curve that matches change in an outcome (growth or decline) as closely as possible. There is a lot of overlap between growth curve models and mixed models; both are mixed models and both can handle nonlinear data. In some disciplines they are called *mixed* or *multilevel models*, and in other disciplines they are called growth models.

Insufficient space is available here to describe in detail the advanced statistical methods above, so I've provided references that the reader can consult for more information.

Website for Statistical Calculations

The Internet is a wonderful resource for researchers seeking to better understand statistical tests, and may provide a number of statistical calculations free of charge. Daniel Soper's Statistical Calculations website[27] includes functions related to (1) calculating simple statistical tests such as chi-square and ANOVA; (2) in clinical trials, calculating a-priori sample size for a student T-test given effect size, power, and significance level; (3) in observational studies, calculating sample size for a multiple regression analysis given effect size, power, significance level, and number of independent variables (the general rule is fifteen subjects per independent variable); (4) in clinical trials, calculating post-hoc statistical power[28] for a student T-test given effect size, sample size, and significance level; (5) in observational studies, calculating statistical power for a multiple regression or hierarchical multiple regression model given sample size, significance level, number of independent variables, and amount of variance explained by model (r^2); (6) in observational studies, calculating indirect effects, given regression coefficient (B) between predictor and mediator and regression coefficient (B) between mediator and outcome (and calculating its significance level, i.e., Sobel test); and (7) a number of other simple statistical calculations that avoid the need for complex statistical software.

StatSoft, a data analysis and software company, offers a free, electronic statistical textbook at http://www.statsoft.com/text

> The Internet is a wonderful resource for researchers seeking to better understand statistical tests, and may provide a number of statistical calculations free of charge.

book/. This is the only Internet resource about statistics recommended by Encyclopedia Britannica. A printed version of the same book sells for eighty dollars on Amazon.

When a Statistician Is Needed

A statistician is a professional, often someone with a background in mathematics or science, who analyzes data and looks for patterns to explain relations between attitudes or behaviors and health outcomes (if working in the social and behavioral sciences). When a statistician is involved in a study from the beginning, including survey development, the statistician can ensure the validity and usefulness of the data collected and then choose the appropriate statistical tests to analyze that data. A statistician possesses at least a master's degree in the field of statistics or epidemiology, if not a PhD or DrPH (doctor of public health).

> When a statistician is involved in a study from the beginning, including survey development, the statistician can ensure the validity and usefulness of the data collected and then choose the appropriate statistical tests to analyze that data.

Many readers may think, *Well, I needed a statistician several pages ago*. However, with a little motivation, access to one of the statistical texts recommended in Table 14.1, and perhaps an online course or two in basic statistics, about 90 percent of the statistical analyses that R/S-health researchers need to do can be done without the assistance of a statistician.[29]

Beginning researchers, however, should stick to the simpler statistical tests that they understand. The attitude of B. F. Skinner, the famous psychologist, was that if you needed a sophisticated statistical test to detect some effect, you didn't have much of an effect anyway. It is always important, though, to know when a statistician is needed.

Writing a Grant

A statistician is needed when writing a grant. Period. Exclamation mark. Statistics (as the reader may appreciate after the previous section) is like a foreign language, and unless the researcher can speak that language fluently, then it is wise not to try to write the statistical analysis section of a grant. Why?

The reason is that at least one person reviewing the grant will be a statistician. If that person reads the statistical analysis section of the grant and doesn't immediately recognize the fluent language of a statistician, then the grant will probably not get a good review (and there is no room for error these days; see Chapter 20 on funding). The statistician is often considered by other reviewers to be the most powerful and influential person in the group, and unless the statistician gives the grant a blessing, others probably won't either.

So, how does a researcher obtain a statistician to write the statistical analysis section of a grant that has not yet been funded? Statisticians often agree to write the statistical analysis section of the grant if they are included for a percentage of their salary during each year of the grant (usually about 10 percent), and so will not expect any money upfront for doing this.

> **A statistician is needed when writing a grant. Period. Exclamation mark.**

Writing a Paper for a Top Journal

A statistician is needed when writing a paper for *JAMA*, the *American Journal of Psychiatry*, *Journal of Consulting & Clinical Psychology*, *Journal of Gerontology*, and other highly competitive peer-reviewed journals, since most nonstatisticians are not capable of writing the analysis section for submissions at this level. This is especially true for psychology, sociology, and epidemiology journals, and is also true when the statistical analysis is relatively complex. There is a lesson here. Medical, psychiatric, and nursing journal editors often do not send the paper to a statistician for review if the analysis is relatively simple. Therefore, nonstatisticians should not try to impress the editor or reviewers by using statistical techniques that are complicated or novel. If they do and the journal editor doesn't readily understand the statistical method, then that editor will likely send the paper to a statistician for review. The statistician then will recognize that a novice has done the analysis and give it a thumb's down or recommend changes in the statistical approach that may be difficult for a nonstatistician to make. If a nonstatistician is writing the analysis section of a research report, it pays to make the statistical analysis simple and obvious. If the analyses are complex, then get a statistician to review the section and offer that person authorship on the paper in return.

Summary and Conclusions

In this chapter I discussed levels of measurement involving independent and dependent variables, a key factor in choosing a statistical test. Based on this and the type of study design, I recommended specific statistical tests for analyzing data in observational studies involving independent samples, observational studies involving dependent or matched samples, longitudinal studies with repeated measurements, and experimental studies without and with control groups. More advanced statistical tests were also briefly mentioned and references provided on where to find more in-depth information. I concluded this chapter with a discussion of when a statistician is needed, which may be sooner rather than later for some researchers depending on their training and level of experience. This chapter covered some complex but critical issues in statistics with which all R/S researchers should be familiar.

CHAPTER 16

Confounders, Explanatory Variables, and Moderators

A S THEY CONDUCT their studies and analyze their results, researchers need to distinguish the different classes of variables with which they work. If they fail to do so they may misinterpret their findings and draw erroneous conclusions about the relationship between religion/spirituality (R/S) and health. Although I've mentioned in earlier chapters the various classes of variables and the differences between them, I go into greater depth in this chapter. In particular, I describe the problems that can result when variable classes are not distinguished from each other, focusing on confounders and explanatory variables. I then recommend how to handle these variables when conducting statistical analyses of data collected from observational studies.

The five classes of variables that I examine here are predictors, outcomes, confounders, explanatory variables, and moderators. Every study focuses on the relationship between a predictor and an outcome. Controlling for confounders helps to determine if the relationship is true and nonspurious. Once it is established that the relationship is true, it is useful to elaborate this basic association by exploring mediation (or suppression) and moderation. Mediators and suppressors help us to understand why predictors are associated with outcomes. Moderators help us to understand when or under which conditions the relationship between predictor and outcome is more or less pronounced.

PREDICTORS AND OUTCOMES

Predictors

A predictor is also known as an *independent variable*, an *exposure variable*, or a *risk factor*. An investigator usually wants to know whether a predictor is related to an outcome variable, and in particular, whether it has a causal relationship to that outcome. In other words, if the predictor changes, does the outcome variable change as a direct result of the change in the predictor? While such causal effects are most directly demonstrated by experimental studies, most studies on R/S and health are observational. Observational studies can contribute information toward the determination of causality but cannot establish it.

For our purposes, the primary predictor variable being examined is R/S, and the question is whether R/S is a true causal risk or protective factor for health or simply a "marker" for good health (for example, is religious attendance simply a marker for physical functioning or mobility?). A marker is associated with the outcome, but is not causal, and altering a marker does not affect the outcome. Critic Richard Sloan gives the example of the relationship between risk for heart disease and having a crease in the earlobe.[1] For some unknown reason, those at higher risk for heart disease have this crease. Clearly, the crease in the earlobe does not cause heart disease and cutting off the earlobes of those with the crease does not cure their heart disease. The earlobe crease, then, is simply a marker of heart disease, not part of the causal mechanism that leads to the disease.

> As they conduct their studies and analyze their results, researchers need to distinguish the different classes of variables with which they work. If they fail to do so they may misinterpret their findings and draw erroneous conclusions.

> The question is whether R/S is a true causal risk or protective factor for health or simply a "marker" for good health.

Outcomes

Researchers are interested in the relationship between a predictor and an outcome. An outcome variable may also be called a *dependent* or *criterion variable*. In R/S-health research, the outcome of interest is health. Health could mean physical health, psychological health, social health, or even community health. Delinquency, crime rates, violence, teenage pregnancy, and substance abuse could all be considered aspects of individual or community health. Health is the primary outcome that interests us as health professionals, and we are interested in R/S only because of its possible relationship to health (which distinguishes health professionals from religious professionals).

> Health is the primary outcome that interests us as health professionals, and we are interested in R/S only because of its possible relationship to health (which distinguishes health professionals from religious professionals).

CONFOUNDERS

Confounders are variables that are related to both a predictor variable and an outcome variable that partially or completely account for the relationship between the two, but are not along the causal chain that leads from predictor to outcome (as an explanatory variable would be). In other words, confounders are spurious factors—factors that predict both the predictor and the outcome. If confounders are not measured, the predictor stands in for these variables, and the result is a misleading association between predictor and outcome. One way to determine that a predictor may be a causal factor (which if altered would change the outcome) and not simply a marker for the outcome is to statistically control for confounders. If the relationship between predictor and outcome goes away when confounders are controlled, then this suggests that the predictor is a marker and not part of the causal pathway that leads to the outcome.

> If the relationship between predictor and outcome goes away when confounders are controlled, then this suggests that the predictor is a marker and not part of the causal pathway that leads to the outcome.

For example, if an investigator finds a statistically significant relationship between religious attendance (predictor) and longevity (outcome), this may be partially or entirely due to confounding by gender.

It is known that women attend church more often than men, *and* that women live longer than men (gender is related to both religious attendance and longevity). Thus, controlling for gender in the statistical analysis may cause the relationship between attendance and longevity to weaken or disappear completely. Likewise, baseline physical health status might also confound the relationship between religious attendance and longevity. The ability to attend religious services may be dependent on a person's physical ability to get to religious services, and so attendance may simply serve as a marker for physical mobility. Good physical mobility, in turn, is known to predict greater longevity.[2] Controlling for baseline physical mobility in the statistical analysis, then, will help to determine whether religious attendance is simply a marker for good physical mobility or an independent causal factor leading to greater longevity.

Thus, before concluding that R/S is a causal risk or protector factor for a health outcome and therefore a potential target for intervention to improve health, we need to determine whether adjustment for confounders might reduce or eliminate the association with health. Strictly speaking, this requires that all confounders (both known and unknown) are controlled for *and* are measured with 100 percent precision. Both of these goals, of course, are difficult to achieve in observational research of any kind. This is equally true for other psychosocial and behavioral predictors of health, not just R/S predictors, and is a known weakness of observational studies. As mentioned in Chapter 8, all possible confounders of the R/S-health relationship are not known, and even the ones that are known may not be measured with perfect precision. In randomized clinical trials, the process of randomization at least theoretically handles this problem by equally distributing confounders between the intervention and control groups. Randomized clinical trials, however, are not without problems of their own, which I described in Chapter 9.

Therefore, when examining relationships between R/S variables and health outcomes, it is important to be as comprehensive as possible in measuring confounders as precisely as

> When examining relationships between R/S variables and health outcomes, it is important to be as comprehensive as possible in measuring confounders as precisely as possible and controlling for them in statistical analyses.

possible and controlling for them in statistical analyses. Variables that could confound the R/S-health relationship include age, race, gender, education, socioeconomic status, possibly baseline health status (see discussion below), and probably some unknown factors as well. We know that those who are more R/S tend to be older, female, African American or Hispanic, less educated, and of lower socioeconomic status. We also know that poor health is related to being older, male, African American, less educated, and of lower socioeconomic status. Thus, failure to control for any one of these confounders can result in either an underestimation or an overestimation of the relationship between R/S and health.

Explanatory Variables

Explanatory variables help to explain why predictors affect outcomes, and refer to both mediator variables and suppressor variables.[3]

Mediator Variables

Mediation is established in four steps as described by Baron and Kenny:[4] first, the researcher must show that the predictor is related to the outcome; second, the researcher must show that the predictor is related to the mediator; third, the researcher must show that the mediator is related to the outcome, while controlling for the predictor; and fourth, if the explanatory variable completely mediates the relationship between predictor and outcome, then the relationship between the predictor and outcome after controlling for the mediator should be reduced to zero. This determines a mediator. Mediation may be complete (as above) or partial, where the relationship between predictor and outcome weakens but does not disappear entirely.[5]

The following is an example of mediation. Suppose a researcher wants to find out whether hurricanes cause damage to houses along the coastline. In this case, the predictor variable would be the hurricane, and the outcome variable would be damage to houses. When correlating these two variables, a positive relationship would likely be found. Besides simply determining the correlation, however, the researcher might want to measure other factors that could explain how this positive correlation came about (i.e., identify factors that lie along the causal chain from the hurricane to the damage). Therefore, she might decide to measure the wind speed, the rainfall, and the stability of buildings along the coast. Each of these variables would be called *mediators* since they could help to explain how or why hurricanes cause damage to houses along the coastline. If these three factors are mediators of the relationship, then adding them to a statistical model with the predictor (hurricane) and the outcome (damage) would cause the positive relationship between the hurricane and damage to diminish in strength or even disappear. If that was the case, then the researcher could conclude that these three variables help to explain how hurricanes cause damage. Said in another way, the wind speed, rainfall, and building stability mediate the relationship between the occurrence of a hurricane and the damage it causes. Researchers would not, however, conclude that hurricanes aren't causing any damage just because they no longer predict damage when wind speed, rainfall, and building stability are controlled for. Hurricanes are a fundamental element of the causal process.

In a similar manner, R/S (predictor) might lead to good physical health (outcome) by following the theoretical causal models described in the next chapter (Chapter 17). In this case, the mediating variables might be human virtues, health behaviors, positive emotions, negative emotions, mental disorders and substance abuse, social connections, and physiological functions. When studying the effects of religious attendance on longevity, then, we would expect that controlling for these mediators in a statistical model might cause an initially positive relationship between attendance and longevity to weaken or even disappear. This would occur because these variables might partially or completely explain the relationship between attendance and longevity.

When studying the effects of religious attendance on longevity, then, we would expect that controlling for these mediators in a statistical model might cause an initially positive relationship between attendance and longevity to weaken or even disappear.

Suppressor Variables

A suppressor variable is a variable that helps to explain a relationship between a predictor and a health outcome, but operates differently than a mediator. The suppressor variable covers up a relationship between predictor and outcome, and controlling for that suppressor variable in a statistical model changes that relationship. An exaggerated form of suppression is called *distortion*, where controlling for the distorter variable actually reverses the direction of the original relationship (from positive to negative or from negative to positive). In R/S-health research, this becomes a real problem when R/S variables are confused with mediators that are proximally related to health outcomes. For example, consider a study that is examining the relationship between R/S and depression and is measuring R/S using the Spiritual Well-Being Scale (SWBS). The SWBS consists of two subscales, a religious well-being (RWB) subscale that measures relationship with God and an existential well-being (EWB) subscale that measures psychological well-being (literally the inverse of depression). When RWB and EWB are included in the same statistical model examining relationships with depression, EWB acts as a distorter variable, suppressing the inverse relationship between RWB and depression. This is because EWB (as an indicator of well-being) is so strongly related to depression. The beneficial effect that RWB is having on depression is acting primarily through its effect on enhancing EWB, and if one statistically removes that effect, then RWB becomes either unrelated to depression or may even become positively related to it (see Chapter 18).

When a predictor has an effect through a mediator or a suppressor variable on an outcome, this is called an "*indirect* effect," which is in contrast to the effect that the predictor has on the outcome that is independent of mediators or suppressors, which is called a *direct* effect (see Chapter 18 for a complete discussion of direct and indirect effects).

> When a predictor has an effect through a mediator or a suppressor variable on an outcome, this is called an "*indirect* effect," which is in contrast to the effect that the predictor has on the outcome that is independent of mediators or suppressors, which is called a *direct* effect.

Moderators

A *moderator* is a variable whose value changes the strength of the relationship between a predictor and an outcome. When a significant relationship is more or less pronounced at certain levels of a third variable, the third variable is called a *moderator*. For example, when religious coping only affects depression in the presence of high psychological stress, psychological stress is considered a moderator. When a moderator influences the effect of a predictor on an outcome, then the moderator is said to interact with the predictor (in the example above, stress interacts with religious coping in its effects on depression). While moderation in its original meaning implied a weakening of a causal effect, a moderator can amplify, weaken, or even reverse the effect of the predictor. Similar to predictors and outcomes, a moderator may be a categorical variable (such as ethnicity or gender), a continuous variable (such as age or income), or an ordinal variable (such as social support or stress level).

> A *moderator* is a variable whose value changes the strength of the relationship between a predictor and an outcome.

Mediators and moderators often get confused, partly because the names sound so much alike. In contrast to mediation (as described earlier), *moderation* is established when an interaction term (predictor × moderator) is included in a regression model with the predictor, moderator, and outcome, that is, $Y = b_0 + b_1x_1 + b_2x_2 + b_3(x_1 \cdot x_2) + \varepsilon$, where x_1 is the predictor, x_2 is the moderator, b_0 is the intercept, b_1 and b_2 are the parameter coefficients that indicate the size of the predictor's and moderator's independent effects on the outcome Y, and ε is the error term. The parameter coefficient b_3 provides the strength of the effect of the interaction term. If b_3 is statistically significant, then this establishes x_2 as a moderator. In order to interpret what the interaction means, the researcher might conduct a stratified analysis, analyzing the relationship between predictor and outcome at different levels of the moderator.[6]

For example, if the interaction term is significant between religious coping and psychological stress in a regression model where the outcome Y is depression, then the researcher might stratify the analysis by stress level and examine the relationship between religious coping and depression separately in those with low stress and in those with high stress. However, in order to justify stratifying the analysis like this, the parameter coefficient (b_3) for the interaction term must be statistically significant (or close to it). To make things even more complicated, as noted earlier, the moderator may also be a confounder and/or a mediator.

Several variables are known to interact with R/S in its relationship to health. As noted in Chapter 14, these variables include age, gender, ethnicity, education status, income, stress level, and others as well. Thus, R/S appears to have a stronger association with health in older adults, women, African Americans and Hispanics, those with lower socioeconomic status, and those with high stress levels.

CONFUSING CONFOUNDERS AND EXPLANATORY VARIABLES

I now discuss a subject of crucial importance for interpreting results from observational studies, a subject that has particular relevance for R/S-health research. In reviewing studies on R/S and health for the two editions of the *Handbook*, I found that researchers often confuse confounding variables and explanatory variables. This is especially true for vocal critics of the R/S-health field such as Richard Sloan and his colleagues, who claim that research in this field is weak and inconsistent.[7]

> **Researchers often confuse confounding variables and explanatory variables.**

The purpose of adjusting for confounders is to isolate a true relationship between a predictor and an outcome, not to explain why that relationship exists. The confusion between confounders and explanatory variables is not only common among critics but also among R/S-health researchers who sometimes lump confounders and explanatory variables into the confounder category. When this is done and all those so-called confounders are controlled in a statistical model, an initially positive relationship between R/S and health often weakens or goes completely away. Researchers may interpret this finding as indicating that no true relationship exists between R/S and health, and thereby dismiss the possibility that R/S might be related to health. However, recall the above example of how explanatory variables such as wind speed, rainfall, and building stability explain how hurricanes cause damage to houses. If the researchers considered these explanatory variables as confounders when examining the effect of a hurricane on coastal damage, they would likely conclude that hurricanes cause no damage to houses (just like the critics above claim that R/S has no relationship to health).

Sloan and colleagues demonstrate this faulty approach in the only original study (to my knowledge) that this research group has ever published on the relationship between R/S and health.[8] That study examined religious attendance as a predictor of mortality in the Established Populations for Epidemiologic Studies in the Elderly (EPESE) cohort (n = 14,456) that was followed over six years. Covariates that were measured included demographics (age, gender, marital status, education, job status), physical health (three separate measures of physical functioning, and individual measures of self-rated health, number of chronic conditions, and nursing home residence), health behaviors (cigarette smoking), social support (visits by close relatives, visits by close friends, whether living with someone or not, club/organization membership), and mental health (depressive symptoms, cognitive functioning). All covariates—both confounders and explanatory variables—were lumped together into a single Cox proportional hazards model and then conclusions made based on those findings. Despite this faulty approach (failure to distinguish confounders from explanatory variables), weekly religious attendance still predicted a significant 22 percent (RR = 0.78, 95% CI 0.70–0.88) reduction in mortality for the overall sample.

To get around this finding, investigators then stratified the analysis by the four EPESE sites (East Boston, Iowa, New Haven, and Duke), reporting separate results by each site. Based on those analyses they concluded that the relationship between religious attendance and mortality was weak and inconsistent since frequent religious attendance significantly predicted mortality in only two of the four sites. Careful analysis of their results, however, reveals that when only confounders are controlled (i.e., demographics and the six measures of baseline physical health), frequent attendance predicted significantly lower mortality in *all four sites*, decreasing mortality by 19 to 33 percent. Only after controlling for the explanatory variables (health behaviors, social support, mental health) did the relationship in two sites lose statistical significance. Bear in mind that these investigators are the R/S-health field's most strident critics, and yet this is the best they could do to minimize the attendance-mortality findings. Their own research indicates that the effect of religious attendance on mortality is statistically significant overall and at all four sites—stronger than marital status, education, self-rated health, social factors, depression, or cognitive functioning—an effect on mortality that is equivalent to being an older adult who is healthy and active enough to be employed in a paying job (even after conservatively controlling for six measures of baseline physical health). Such a finding, in my estimation, is anything but weak and inconsistent.

If an initially positive relationship between R/S and a health outcome disappears after controlling for confounders, then it is correct to conclude that no true relationship exists between R/S and the health outcome. If researchers report that an effect weakens or disappears after controlling for explanatory variables, however, I would not agree that there is no relationship. The true relationship between R/S and the health outcome is the magnitude of the association after controlling for confounders. Once this relationship is determined, the job of researchers then becomes to determine how this relationship between R/S and health came about—that is, to explain the relationship. This is accomplished by including explanatory variables in the statistical model along with R/S variables and confounders. If the researcher controls for all variables that explain how R/S could affect health, then he should expect the R/S-health relationship to weaken or approach zero, since the relationship is now fully explained. In summary, explanatory variables explain a relationship but don't explain it away, as confounders do. I now provide more examples from other published studies below.

Researchers sought to examine the relationship between self-rated religiosity and longevity in 993 participants in the Terman Life-Cycle Study.[9] The results of this analysis indicated

> The true relationship between R/S and the health outcome is the magnitude of the association after controlling for confounders. Once this relationship is determined, the job of researchers then becomes to determine how this relationship between R/S and health came about—that is, to explain the relationship.

that women who viewed themselves as more religious around the age of forty had a significantly lower risk of premature mortality during a forty-one-year follow-up period. Also measured were social involvement, alcohol use, and cigarette smoking, which were related to premature mortality. When social involvement was added to the model, the relationship between religiosity and mortality weakened only slightly and remained significant. When alcohol use and cigarette smoking were added, however, the relationship between self-rated religiosity and mortality was reduced to nonsignificance. The researchers concluded (correctly) that self-rated religiosity predicted lower premature mortality in women, which could be explained by their refraining from drinking alcohol and smoking cigarettes.

In another example, Gillum and colleagues examined the relationship between religious attendance and mortality in a national random sample of 8,450 adult Americans.[10] Results indicated that those who never attended religious services had the highest mortality during a nine-year follow-up period. After the researchers controlled for baseline confounders (age, gender, ethnicity, education, geographic location, self-rated health, health problems, and mobility), not attending religious services continued to predict significantly greater mortality (vs. attending weekly or more). This, then, was their main finding. Next, investigators sought to explain the relationship by adding explanatory variables to the statistical model (social support, smoking, alcohol use, exercise, seeking regular medical care, body mass index, C-reactive protein, and systolic blood pressure). After adding these explanatory variables to the model, the effect of not attending religious services on mortality weakened to nonsignificance. The researchers concluded (correctly) that not attending religious services predicted greater mortality, and that lower social support (not being married), worse health behaviors, and abnormalities in physiological function explained the relationship.[11]

CRITICS' RESPONSE

Critics have responded to our concerns by arguing that it is difficult to distinguish explanatory variables from confounders due to the difficulty in establishing that a variable is on the causal pathway between the predictor and outcome (i.e., that a variable is part of the mechanism by which a predictor affects the outcome). They are correct in maintaining that in observational studies it is difficult to differentiate confounders from explanatory variables, and that this decision "must often rely on common sense, intuition, background knowledge, or one's theoretical or ideological persuasion."[12] Furthermore, when dealing only with cross-sectional data, such a determination may not be possible.[13] However, plenty of longitudinal evidence is available to show that R/S is related to human values, health behaviors, positive and negative emotions, mental disorders, substance abuse, and social connections (see Chapter 1), and there is also good rationale for suspecting that these relationships are causal (based on the doctrinal teachings and health practices that religious traditions promote). Furthermore, there is ample evidence that these intermediary constructs are associated with basic physiological functions that affect susceptibility to disease and risk of mortality, and good reasons for suspecting that these relationships are likewise causal (based on known mind-body effects from experimental studies). Therefore, biological plausibility along with "common sense, intuition, and background knowledge" would all argue that these constructs are explanatory variables, not confounders.

> In observational studies it is difficult to differentiate confounders from explanatory variables, and this decision "must often rely on common sense, intuition, background knowledge, or one's theoretical or ideological persuasion."

Critics and their statistical colleagues do acknowledge that treating explanatory variables as confounders can be problematic. This problem, well known in the epidemiological literature,[14] is *overadjustment* leading to a false conclusion that a putative risk factor is not causally important to the outcome or an underestimation of the effect that the risk factor is having on the outcome.[15] For example, including an explanatory variable such as social support as a confounder (rather than an explanatory variable) in a model examining the relationship between R/S and health will likely reduce the power of R/S as a predictor, which could result in the false conclusion that R/S is not causally important. Therefore, investigators might never test the possibility that interventions directed at R/S could improve health outcomes.

One of the best examples of a situation where it is not clear if a variable is either a confounder or an explanatory variable is baseline health status, especially when studying the relationship between religious attendance and longevity. Most critics would say that baseline measures of mobility (or physical function) should be controlled for as confounders when studying this relationship. They argue, as I stated in an earlier example, that attendance at religious services is actually measuring the physical ability to get to religious services, so religious attendance is only a marker, not a cause of physical health. While this makes sense, it ignores the possibility that religious attendance prior to the baseline evaluation was a contributor to that baseline physical health (mobility). Indeed, if religious attendance increases longevity by having positive effects on physical health (as we hypothesize), then it is likely to have had a positive influence on subjects' health status over the years prior to the baseline health assessment. This is not taken into account, however, when investigators control for baseline health status as a confounder.

Critics also acknowledge that if a risk factor provides a constant exposure over years on health status—that is, the risk factor is stable and does not change—then there is a greater likelihood that the risk factor will have affected the baseline health status[16] (and so might push investigators toward treating baseline health as an explanatory variable rather than a confounder). Is there any evidence that religious involvement (as a risk factor for longevity) is stable and changes little over the years? Although religious involvement does change substantially from adolescence to young adulthood (i.e., decreases),[17] once it stabilizes in young adulthood research indicates that religious involvement remains relatively stable across the lifespan. For example, Wink and Dillon examined changes in religiousness over a forty-year period from ages thirty to seventy, finding that the correlation between religiosity assessed in the mid-thirties and again in the mid-forties was 0.75, from mid-forties to mid-fifties/early sixties was 0.82, and from late-sixties to mid-seventies was also 0.82. Overall, religiosity assessed in the mid-thirties and again in the mid-seventies was correlated at 0.67.[18] These high correlations provide strong evidence for stability. Furthermore, religiousness may be especially stable among those with high religious involvement, as shown by McCullough and colleagues, for subjects followed from ages twenty-seven to eighty,[19] and high religiousness (weekly attendance or more) is most likely to affect health status. Thus, those with high religiousness at baseline, particularly when that baseline is determined in middle age or later life, are likely to have been religious for many years prior to that, during which religiousness may have contributed to that baseline health status.

Finally, critics may acknowledge that R/S is related to better physical health, but dismiss the finding on grounds that those who are more R/S are simply more socially active, live healthier lifestyles, and are more health conscious (claiming, then, that it has nothing to do with religiosity). This argument, however, ignores the possibility that the reason that R/S individuals are less socially isolated, avoid cigarette smoking, don't use drugs, drink less alcohol, and pay more attention to their health is *because they are more R/S*. Loving thy neighbor and avoiding self-destructive activities that may harm the "temple of the Holy Spirit" are behaviors that all major religious traditions strongly endorse. Again, I would argue that these variables explain *how* R/S affects physical health and should not be used to explain away the effects, as critics are prone to do.

RECOMMENDATIONS FOR HANDLING CONFOUNDERS AND EXPLANATORY VARIABLES

When examining the relationships between R/S (predictor) and health (outcome) in quantitative observational studies, researchers should identify the variables that are likely to confound that relationship and the variables that are likely to explain it. They should then measure those confounders and explanatory variables as accurately and precisely as possible. In the first step of the analysis, after examining the relationship between R/S and the health outcome, researchers should control for confounders (as noted in the last chapter). The result of that analysis is the main finding on the relationship between R/S and health that should then be reported. If statistically significant ($p < 0.05$ for a single comparison), then the association meets the criterion used by the scientific community to say that a relationship probably exists that is not due to chance alone and not due to confounding. If the association is not statistically significant after controlling for confounders, then researchers should conclude that there is no true relationship between R/S and the health outcome.[20]

If the relationship remains statistically significant after controlling for confounders, the researcher's job is then to explain how that relationship came about. Explanatory variables should then be entered into the model. If one or more of these is statistically significant and the strength of the relationship between R/S and the health outcome weakens, then this is evidence that the explanatory variables are explaining the R/S-health relationship. If the R/S-health relationship diminishes to nonsignificance after controlling for explanatory variables, then the researcher can conclude that the R/S-health relationship has now been fully explained (but not explained away).

If the health outcome being studied is physical health (mortality, medical event, progression of illness, etc.), and the study is a prospective one, then I would recommend controlling for baseline physical health as a confounder. However, physical health should be examined in a separate step of the analysis, not combined with other confounders (i.e., examine other confounders in one step and then in a second step add baseline physical health). Treating baseline physical health as a confounder will likely result in a "conservative" estimate of the effect of R/S on the physical health outcome—that is, doing this will probably underestimate the strength of the relationship between R/S and that outcome (especially if baseline health is assessed after age thirty-five). If,

> If the R/S-health relationship diminishes to nonsignificance after controlling for explanatory variables, then the researcher can conclude that the R/S-health relationship has now been fully explained (but not explained away).

> Treating baseline physical health as a confounder will likely result in a "conservative" estimate of the effect of R/S on the physical health outcome.

after controlling for other confounders and baseline physical health, the relationship between R/S and the health outcome remains statistically significant, then researchers can tentatively conclude that an independent relationship exists between the R/S predictor and the health outcome (bearing in mind the assumptions made earlier).

If, after controlling for baseline health, the relationship between R/S and the health outcome diminishes to nonsignificance, then researchers may conclude that no relationship between R/S and health is present; however, they should point out that this lagged regression approach is a pretty rigorous standard and that if the R/S variable had affected the health outcome prior to the baseline evaluation (quite likely), then controlling for baseline physical health may have resulted in an underestimation of the relationship between R/S and the health outcome. This is especially true in prospective studies where the follow-up period is relatively short (less than five years) and the baseline evaluation occurs when subjects are middle-aged adults or older (given the stability of religious involvement and the likely effects on health prior to the baseline evaluation).

Finally, when the dependent variable is highly correlated over time (such as health), one may need extra statistical power to detect significance of predictors when the baseline outcome is controlled. Because researchers are looking for predictors of something that does not change much, one needs greater sensitivity to predict the small degree of change. Furthermore, having the appropriate time lag is important. Just like researchers would not expect smoking to lead to lung cancer only six months after starting to smoke or expect a stressful day at work to result in a major depression a month later, one should not expect that attending religious services for a few months would substantially extend longevity.

> When the dependent variable is highly correlated over time (such as health), one may need extra statistical power to detect significance of predictors when the baseline outcome is controlled.

SUMMARY AND CONCLUSIONS

In this chapter I described the different classes of variables that investigators use in quantitative observational studies to examine relationships between R/S and health. These include predictors (risk or protective factors), outcomes (dependent variables), confounders, explanatory variables (mediators or suppressors), and moderators. In the rest of the chapter, I focused on the problem of distinguishing confounders from explanatory variables, and made recommendations on how to proceed when analyzing confounders and explanatory variables and on how to handle baseline physical health in prospective studies.

While it is important to comprehensively identify and precisely measure confounders, it is also important to carefully separate confounders from explanatory variables (rather than lump them all into a single category). Treating all covariates like confounders (as critics in this field seem eager to do) will likely result in an underestimation of the relationship between R/S and health. The true independent relationship between R/S and health results when confounders alone are controlled. If that relationship is statistically significant, then investigators should seek to identify the reasons for the relationship and so would then control for explanatory variables. Admittedly, distinguishing between confounders and explanatory variables, especially when working with cross-sectional data, may be difficult at times. It may also be difficult in prospective studies that examine the effects of R/S on health to determine whether health status at baseline should be treated as a confounder or an explanatory variable.

Experts disagree over whether a variable is considered a confounder or an explanatory variable, and the decision rests on many factors, including having a rationale based on a theoretical model, biological plausibility, common sense, intuition, background knowledge, and other factors. I believe there is sufficient evidence (reviewed in Chapter 1 and based on two editions of the *Handbook of Religion and Health*) to argue that positive psychological traits, health behaviors, positive emotions, social support, negative emotions, mental disorders, and substance abuse are explanatory variables that may be causally related to both R/S and to physiological functions that affect the risk of physical disease and mortality.

R/S must affect health through some type of mechanism. I am not claiming that this happens via miracles or other kinds of Divine intervention, which cannot be studied using the methods of science. If R/S influences physical health in a way we can study, then it must do so through psychological, social, and behavioral pathways, which can be examined using the tools available to us in the social and behavioral sciences.

CHAPTER 17

Models and Mechanisms

UNDERSTANDING HOW RELIGION/SPIRITUALITY (R/S) can impact health is essential for identifying research questions, designing research studies to answer those questions, and especially, setting up statistical analyses to examine relationships between R/S and health. Such understanding is also important for the design and testing of R/S interventions directed at improving health. In this chapter I emphasize the importance of identifying the first cause or initial source that initiates the health effects that R/S may have. I also stress the need to specify clearly the nonoverlapping constructs that lie along the pathway that leads from that initial cause to physical health and longevity. I then discuss a theoretical causal model of how R/S might impact physical health and longevity both directly and indirectly through human virtues (positive psychological traits), daily decisions, health behaviors, social connections, positive and negative emotions, and the basic physiological pathways affected by these intervening variables. I first describe a model developed from a Western religious perspective and then adapt that model to Eastern and secular humanistic perspectives. After describing these models, I discuss the roles that genetic, environmental, and epigenetic factors serve in setting up the playing field on which R/S, psychological, social, behavioral, and physiological factors act. My hope is that these models help explain how R/S affects health and clarify the discussion of explanatory variables presented in the last chapter.

Primary Source of the Effect

A deeper understanding of causal pathways is essential for identifying predictors, confounders, moderators, and explanatory variables in observational studies, where the ultimate goal is to learn enough about health and the risk factors that affect it so that interventions can be developed to improve health. Identifying the initial cause or primary source of the effect is crucial in understanding the causal pathways by which R/S affects health. Let me illustrate by an example.

> Identifying the initial cause or primary source of the effect is crucial in understanding the causal pathways by which R/S affects health.

Understanding the initial cause of pneumococcal pneumonia is important in determining treatments that can be directed at that cause. The cause (pneumococcus bacteria) sets into motion a series of changes in the body that, if not arrested, eventually result in death. Without an adequate understanding of the pathway from the cause to the outcome, interventions may be directed at the wrong point in this pathway. In this case, fever, fatigue, cough, and shortness of breath are symptoms associated with pneumonia. They are the body's response to the cause (bacteria), *but they are not the cause.* Treatments directed only at the symptoms of pneumonia do not affect the underlying pathological process. The primary cause of the pneumonia needs to be identified and then treatments directed at that cause to favorably influence the outcome. The root cause of this particular pneumonia has been identified through careful research to be a bacterial infection. When we treat that infection with the right antibiotics, then the other symptoms associated with the pneumonia (fever, cough, fatigue) automatically get better.

We face the same dilemma when studying the relationship between R/S and health. The way we define our constructs and attribute importance to them is essential for correctly understanding the basis for this relationship. This is particularly challenging, as noted in chapter 11, given the broadness of terms used today, such as "spirituality." If our goal as researchers and health professionals is to improve health, then we need to know what it is about spirituality that affects health. This understanding will allow us to give specific instructions, grounded in each person's particular faith tradition, on the types of cognitions, experiences, and behaviors in that tradition likely to improve health. The right instructions depend on a thorough understanding of the causal pathways that lead from R/S to health. If an intervention is contemplated, then it is important to identify what initiates the sequence of events that affect the health outcome.

What, then, stands at the head of the causal pathway that leads from R/S to physical health and greater longevity? What is the origin or "first cause"? We know that the first cause of pneumococcal pneumonia is a certain kind of bacteria, so we direct our interventions at that. Many characteristics are associated with R/S (like the many manifestations of pneumonia) which may not be the first cause that initiates the sequence of events leading to better or worse health. As I argued in Chapter 11, constructs such as meaning and purpose, hope, connectedness with others, peacefulness, or existential well-being (often used to measure spirituality) are not R/S itself but rather the consequences of R/S (i.e., by analogy they represent the fever, cough, etc., associated with pneumonia). Said differently, rather than lying at the head of the causal pathway, these constructs lie somewhere downstream from the first cause that eventually starts the process moving toward health. We already know that having meaning and purpose, hope, and so on, are on the pathway that leads to better mental health, which in turn can affect physical health through mind-body pathways via immune, endocrine, and cardiovascular systems. What is not clear, however, is what initiates this process.

Saying that meaning and purpose, hope, social connectedness, or another factor is the primary cause provides very little information on what to intervene on to improve health. We can't just tell suffering patients to get peaceful, or be hopeful, or have meaning in their lives, any more than we can do away with the bacterial infection in pneumonia by treating the fever and cough. Unless we can tell patients

> Saying that meaning and purpose, hope, social connectedness, or another factor is the primary cause provides very little information on what to intervene on to improve health.

how to maintain hope, meaning, and purpose, the suggestion only adds frustration to suffering. *Where* do chronically ill disabled people get meaning and purpose? *Where* do they get hope or peace or well-being? What makes them want to connect with others? Simply knowing that a person lacks meaning or purpose or peace in life does not help in deciding on what to do in order to increase that meaning, hope, and purpose. Similarly, knowing that a person has a fever doesn't help choosing a treatment for the underlying cause. The fever is the result of something else that must be identified and treated in order to stop the disease. The person should be encouraged to take acetaminophen or aspirin, which will help to relieve the fever and make the person feel better, but the fever will keep coming back and the disease causing the fever will continue to get worse and worse.

> There are basically two causes that stand at the beginning of the pathway that leads to these positive psychological and social states, which in turn lead to good mental and physical health.

So, what is the initial cause of the positive psychological and social states (peacefulness, harmony, connectedness, and meaning) that ultimately influence physical health outcomes? I would argue that there are basically two causes that stand at the beginning of the pathway that leads to these positive psychological and social states, which in turn lead to good mental and physical health: religious causes and secular causes. The basic question in R/S-health research is whether religious causes are any more effective at stimulating this process than secular causes. Secular causes might include having an outgoing, extroverted personality, or high intelligence; having a good job or exciting hobby; experiencing physical pleasure (eating, sex, thrill-seeking activities); having a good education or adequate finances; or having a humanistic philosophy to guide life. These are certainly sources of meaning and purpose, hope, peace and harmony, and happy relationships with others. But, all things considered, are they as effective as or more effective than R/S causes?

From a health-care professional's perspective (the one taken in this chapter), if secular causes are equally as effective as religious causes and if religious causes are not harmful, then there is no need to consider religious factors as relevant to health care. There is also no need for a field of R/S and health, and we health-care professionals should direct our energies elsewhere.

Causal Models

I summarize here theoretical causal models that were originally presented in the *Handbook of Religion and Health*.[1] These models describe how R/S in Western, Eastern, and secular humanistic faith traditions influence physical health. Figure 17.1[2] describes this process from a Western monotheistic religious worldview. Those faith traditions view God as personal and separate from creation. This model is then adapted for an Eastern religious worldview (Figure 17.2), making a rather large leap and assuming that the causal mechanisms underlying the health effects of the Eastern faith traditions involve the same psychosocial, behavioral, and physiological pathways that operate for Western religions. The final model (Figure 17.3) presents the pathways by which a secular humanistic perspective, one that views the world without reference to the transcendent, might influence health outcomes. While based on a considerable amount of indirect research (see *Handbook*) and at least one recent study,[3] these models remain largely theoretical, and their pathways need further verification (or refutation) through additional systematic research. I am most confident about the first model as it applies to Western faith traditions. Admittedly, I have some uneasiness about adapting that model to Eastern religious and secular traditions, but we have to start somewhere.

Western Monotheistic Model

I begin by identifying what I think is the initial cause or driving force that leads to R/S experiences and practices that ultimately influence, directly and indirectly, the constructs that lie along the pathway that lead to physical health and longevity. I am assuming that there is *something* that comes before the positive character traits/human virtues, positive emotions (purpose and meaning, peacefulness, harmony), and positive social interactions that prevent or neutralize negative mental health states that adversely affect physiological functions influencing susceptibility to disease and mortality. Because this initial cause may vary depending on religion, we find clues about its nature by examining the core teachings of each of the Western religious traditions and seeing what these traditions focus on. Consider the following verses taken from the sacred writings of Islam, Judaism, and Christianity.

The Holy Qur'an

And yet there are people who choose to believe in beings that allegedly rival God, loving them as [only] God should be Loved: whereas those who have attained to faith Love God more than all else. (Al-Baqara 2:165)

And worship God [alone], and do not ascribe divinity, in any way, to aught beside Him. (An-Nisa 4:36)

The Torah

I am HaShem thy G-d, who brought thee out of the land of Egypt, out of the house of bondage. Thou shalt have no other gods before Me. Thou shalt not make unto thee a graven image, nor any manner of likeness, of any thing that is in heaven above, or that is in the earth beneath, or that is in the water under the earth; thou shalt not bow down unto them, nor serve them; for I HaShem thy G-d am a jealous G-d, visiting the iniquity of the fathers upon the children unto the third and fourth generation of them that hate Me; and showing mercy unto the thousandth generation of them that love Me and keep My commandments. (Shemot 20:2–6)

Hear, O Israel: The HaShem our G-d, The HaShem is One. And thou shalt love HaShem thy G-d with all thy heart, and with all thy soul, and with all thy might. And these words, which I command thee this day, shall be upon thy heart; and thou shalt teach them diligently unto thy children, and shalt talk of them when thou sittest in thy house, and when thou walkest by the way, and when thou liest down, and when thou risest up. And thou shalt bind them for a sign upon thy hand, and they shall be for frontlets between thine eyes. And thou shalt write them upon the door-posts of thy house, and upon thy gates. (Devarim 6:4–9)

The Jewish Bible

Only for G-d wait thou in stillness, my soul; for from Him cometh my hope. (Tehilim 62:6)

I will lift up mine eyes unto the mountains: from whence shall my help come? My help cometh from HaShem, who made heaven and earth. (Tehilim 121:1–2)

For My people have committed two evils: they have forsaken Me, the fountain of living waters, and hewed them out cisterns, broken cisterns, that can hold no water. (Yermiyah 2:13)

The New Testament

Thou shalt love the Lord they God with all thy heart, and with all thy soul, and with all thy mind. This is the first and great commandment. (restated in three of the four Gospels: Matthew 22:37; Mark 12:30; Luke 10:27)

In the Islamic-Judeo-Christian tradition, then, belief in/attachment to and love of God stand at the head of the pathway, together representing the initial driving force that leads to purpose and meaning in life, hope, peace, existential well-being, and forgiveness, and which enables people to unconditionally love and connect with others. This is what for Muslims, Jews, and Christians must be remembered, practiced, supported, and nourished.

The primary question, again, is whether religious causes—beginning with belief in, attachment to, and love of God—are more powerful sources of positive psychological and social states and ultimately better mental and physical health, compared to secular causes. Such a question can be subject to scientific research by defining the constructs, measuring them, and then observing what happens or by intervening to see if health changes (assuming for now that intervening here is possible and ethical). This is not to say that designing such studies is simple. Using clear, nonoverlapping

> In the Islamic-Judeo-Christian tradition, then, belief in/attachment to and love of God stand at the head of the pathway, together representing the initial driving force.

constructs and correct statistical modeling of those constructs along causal pathways, however, are critical if such research is to produce meaningful results.

I now examine and explain the theoretical causal model presented in Figure 17.1. In that figure, I capitalize the word "God" as is done when referring to the deity in the major Western religious traditions. In these traditions, God is viewed as lying outside of and separate from the created universe, which is in contrast to the Eastern religious traditions, where God is viewed as everything in the universe and beyond. In Western religious traditions, God is perceived as having the characteristics of a person, someone who can be related to just like any other person, and who experiences emotions such as love, anger, and disappointment, just like people do, since people were made in God's image in the creation account.

Attachment to God is expressed by the theological virtues of faith in God, hope in God, and love of God (theological virtues as distinct from human virtues). These reflect a relationship to and dependence on God. Such notions about the nature of God are formed within a faith community which has beliefs that help to socialize members of the community into that faith tradition. Belief in and attachment to God, formed within the faith community, then give rise to public and private religious practices and religious experiences. Attachment to God, expressions of that attachment in the theological virtues, and the resulting religious practices and experiences all form the construct that I refer to as *religion/spirituality* (R/S).

Although the effects in this causal model are likely bidirectional to some extent, I present here pathways that describe the predominant effect as going from left to right. Thus, R/S influences physical health both directly and indirectly through a set of mediating psychological, social, and behavioral factors. The psychological and social factors are (a) positive psychological traits (i.e., human virtues), (b) positive emotions, (c) social connections, and (d) negative emotions/mental disorders. Human virtues involve constructs such as forgiveness, honesty, courage, self-discipline, altruism, humility, gratefulness, patience, and dependability. Some investigators have actually included these traits in the definition of R/S itself, which I think is incorrect and confusing, since these traits are really downstream from R/S—that is, are a result of R/S involvement (not R/S itself). R/S beliefs, practices, and rules of conduct help to nourish and support the development of human virtues.

Human virtues, in turn, enhance social connections, promote positive emotions, and help to counteract negative emotions, prevent emotional disorders, and guard against substance abuse. Social connections involve relationships with friends, family, and others with whom people work, play, or interact. Human virtues lead to satisfying, supportive relationships, and form the basis for stable, long-term social connections. Practice of the human virtues also promotes positive emotions such as feelings of well-being, happiness, hope, optimism, and a sense of meaning and purpose in life. As they enhance social connections and positive emotions, human virtues help to prevent or neutralize negative emotions. Negative emotions include mental disorders such as depression, anxiety, tendency toward suicide, and consumption of drugs and alcohol that may be used to relieve negative emotions. Positive emotions, social connections, and negative emotions, then, are seen as causing physiological changes that ultimately affect risk of physical disease and mortality.

Besides acting through human virtues, R/S also influences physical health through another mediating pathway having to do with daily decisions, health habits, and health-related behaviors. R/S affects the choices that people make when confronted with situations that demand a decision. These decisions are made on a day-by-day, hour-by-hour, and minute-by-minute basis, affecting the social connections people have with others, positive and negative emotions, and vulnerability to health problems. R/S helps to guide those decisions in a direction that are prosocial, less risky, and generally more health promoting. Some of those decisions have to do with health habits and behaviors that directly influence mental and physical health such as exercise, diet, weight, sexual behaviors, cigarette smoking, delinquent or criminal activities, and accident risk. Health-related behaviors also include participation in

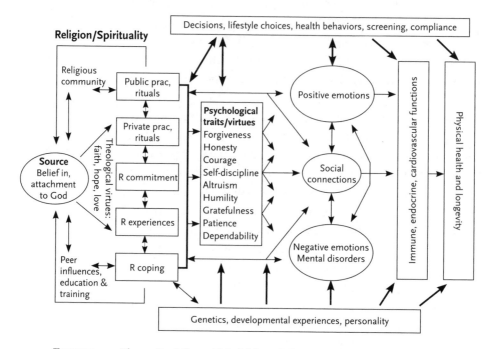

FIGURE 17.1. Theoretical Causal Model from Western Religious Perspective

disease-screening activities (mammography, blood pressure or blood glucose checks, prostate or colon cancer screening) and compliance with treatments prescribed by health professionals. R/S beliefs directly influence such decisions and indirectly influence them through the human virtues and positive emotions they promote. Finally, the physiological changes known to occur as a result of psychological, social, and behavioral influences include immune, endocrine, and cardiovascular functions, which in turn have a direct impact on risk of disease (see *Handbook* for research documenting these associations).

The implication of the above model is that R/S always has positive effects on psychosocial and behavioral mediators that lie along the pathway that leads to physical health. Negative effects, however, are also possible depending on the setting and the content of R/S beliefs. For example, negative or conflicted attachments to God would be expected to affect health in the opposite direction of those associated with positive attachments. A relationship with God may be filled with anger, distrust, and fear, based on a view of God as distant, judgmental, and persecutory rather than as loving, merciful, and understanding. Admittedly, R/S struggles are often involved as a relationship with God grows and matures, and so may be characteristic of early and sometimes even later stages of such a relationship (consider the stories of Job, Noah, and David in the Bible). Religious struggles characterized by feeling punished or deserted by God or questioning God's power, especially if those struggles are not resolved, place a person at risk for worse mental health[4] and early mortality.[5] Thus, R/S beliefs may not always lead to positive health outcomes, especially if persons remain stuck in a turbulent and disharmonious relationship with God (or with a faith community).

> The implication of the above model is that R/S always has positive effects on psychosocial and behavioral mediators that lie along the pathway that leads to physical health. Negative effects, however, are also possible depending on the setting and the content of R/S beliefs.

Eastern Model

I now describe a model that explains how R/S based within an Eastern religious worldview might likewise influence physical health through an identical set of mechanisms (see Figure 17.2). This model simply replaces God with Brahman (the Divine Ground of all matter, energy, time, space, and being) and other lesser gods in the Hindu tradition, and Buddha or Ultimate Reality (the cause of all existence, ground of being, and foundation of reality) in the Buddhist tradition. For Hinduism, the attachment to Brahman (equivalent to faith, hope, and love of God) is manifested by Dharma, meaning "that which upholds or supports," and referring to a way of life that involves performing one's righteous duty. For Buddhism, the attachment to Buddha or Ultimate Reality is manifested by the Four Noble Truths: (1) there is suffering, (2) craving or desire is a cause of suffering, (3) there is the cessation of suffering in nirvana, and (4) living according to the Eightfold Path can lead to a cessation of suffering. These core R/S beliefs, then, lead to R/S behaviors and experiences just as described in the Western monotheistic model, and consequently influence lifestyle choices and health behaviors, promote human virtues, and affect psychological and social health, which ultimately influence physiological states and physical health outcomes.

Given my lack of knowledge about and experience in the Eastern religions, again, I am much less certain about this causal model as an explanation of how R/S affects physical health in these traditions. I would imagine that while the model I have presented is a start, it will require major revision by those who are more knowledgeable about the Eastern religions and the cultures in which they have arisen. Both Western and Eastern models presented here follow the definitions of R/S in Chapter 11.

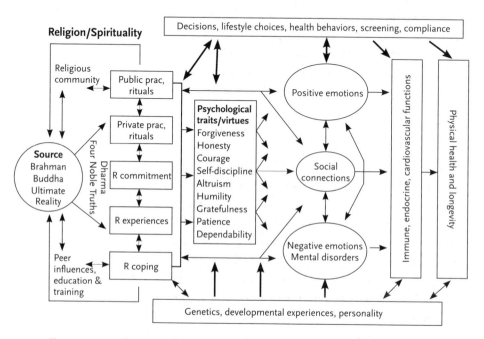

FIGURE 17.2. Theoretical Causal Model from Eastern Religious Perspective

Secular Model

There is yet a third model described in Figure 17.3 against which the health benefits of Western and Eastern religions might be compared. The beliefs and philosophy of life involved in secular humanism may affect health through the same or similar pathways described for the religious models. The secular model is identical to the Western and Eastern models, except that the initial cause (source) is characterized by a commitment to the human self and to the human community, and is manifested by reason, a view of the world through the eyes of science, and without reference to the transcendent. This stance, rather than resulting in R/S practices and experiences, instead produces a focus on the present life, the public good, a search for truth, and an emphasis on ethics and justice. These manifestations of secular humanism, then, affect decision-making, health behaviors, human virtues, social connections, and positive and negative mental health, causing changes in physiological functions and vulnerability to disease and death, all in a similar manner as described for R/S.

Future research will help determine which model (Western, Eastern, or secular) is more or less likely to have health benefits, depending on the particular setting and particular culture in which they operate. All three models, however, must be understood as acting within the context of a complex set of genetic and environmental influences.

> The secular model is identical to the Western and Eastern models, except that the initial cause (source) is characterized by a commitment to the human self and to the human community, and is manifested by reason, a view of the world through the eyes of science, and without reference to the transcendent.

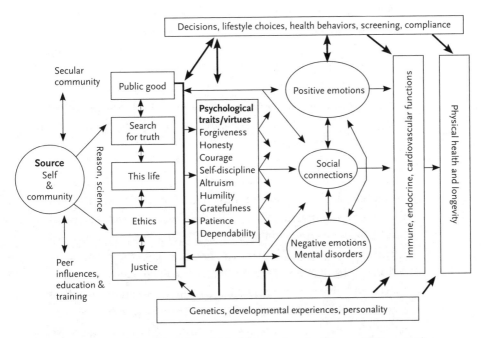

FIGURE 17.3. Theoretical Causal Model from Secular Humanist Perspective

Genetic, Environmental, and Epigenetic Influences

Each of the three models rests upon a base of genetic, environmental, and gene-environmental influences. In other words, R/S and secular mechanisms act within a context that is determined by an inherited biology and the circumstances in which individuals find themselves. This applies to all levels of the models presented here, from R/S (or secular humanism) to daily decisions, virtues, and health behaviors; to positive emotions, sociability, and mental disorders; to immune, endocrine, and cardiovascular pathways; to vulnerability to physical diseases and mortality. Every one of these constructs is affected by genetic, environmental, and epigenetic influences.

> R/S and secular mechanisms act within a context that is determined by an inherited biology and the circumstances in which individuals find themselves.

Genetic

Positive psychological traits or virtues are almost certainly influenced by genetic factors related to temperament and personality,[6] and there is good evidence that positive emotions (happiness, for example),[7] vulnerability to stress,[8] the tendency to be sociable,[9] and mental disorders such as depression or anxiety[10] are impacted by genetic factors as well. It is now widely accepted that immune, endocrine, and cardiovascular functions, as well as most disease states and longevity itself, have strong genetic influences.[11]

Tendencies toward R/S involvement itself may be influenced by genetic factors.[12] While it is easy to understand the influences that environmental factors during childhood and the teen years might have on the development of R/S beliefs, practices, and commitments, there is also evidence that genetic factors may influence the likelihood that individuals will engage in R/S practices and have reinforcing R/S experiences. Certain inherited genetic polymorphisms are known to increase emotional sensitivity to negative life events,[13] and in this way either increase sensitivity to R/S experiences or increase the need for them. For example, the short allele (S) of the serotonin transporter-linked promoter region (5-HTTLPR) has been associated with higher scores on the Telegen Absorption Scale,[14] which in turn has been associated with higher levels of intrinsic religiosity.[15] Likewise, a polymorphism of the 5-HT1A (serotonin) receptor gene has been linked to higher scores on the spiritual acceptance subscale of the Temperament and Character Inventory (TCI),[16] which has also been associated with lower 5-HT1A receptor binding in the brain that suggests greater emotional sensitivity in those who are more R/S.[17] The DRD4 gene (dopamine) also appears to be associated with higher scores on the TCI's spiritual acceptance subscale, which is supported by the theory that R/S experiences are mediated by the release of dopamine.[18] Finally, many twin studies find that identical twins (with the same genetic makeup) raised apart are more likely to engage in religious practices than are fraternal twins (with different genetic makeup) raised apart.[19]

> Genetic factors may influence the likelihood that individuals will engage in R/S practices and have reinforcing R/S experiences.

Environmental

Environmental factors during early childhood, the teen years, and throughout life are also likely to affect the constructs in these models. For example, intrauterine factors (maternal stress, depression, or substance abuse),[20] poor maternal-infant "fit" during the first year of life,[21] absence of care and love from parents during childhood, experiences with siblings and peers during the school years, and traumatic experiences in adulthood that are outside of the individual's control (emotional and physical assaults or trauma from accidents) almost certainly influence the development of R/S beliefs, positive psychological character traits, positive life decisions, health behaviors, the development of social bonds, the ability to experience positive emotions, and the risk of developing mental disorders—which in turn affect vital health-preserving physiological systems and ultimately increase or decrease disease risk.

> Environmental factors during early childhood, the teen years, and throughout life are also likely to affect the constructs in these models.

Epigenetic

Not only do genetic and environmental factors have separate and individual influences, but interactions between these factors may also have effects. Scientists are only now beginning to fully appreciate the effects of gene-environment influences, which have the potential to influence constructs at every level of these causal models. For example, animal studies demonstrate that mother rats that nurture their newborn babies by licking them actually alter the genetic makeup of those babies (adding methyl groups to histones in the chromatin makeup of their DNA), changes that can then be passed down through generations from the babies to their own children and grandchildren.[22] Those changes affect the regulation of genes that control responsiveness of hypothalamic-pituitary axis to stress. Environmental factors like nurturing, then, may influence whether genes controlling physiological responses to stress are turned off or on.

> Not only do genetic and environmental factors have separate and individual influences, but interactions between these factors may also have effects.

Epigenetic influences have also been identified in humans. For example, Hicks and colleagues argue that environmental adversity amplifies the genetic risk for mental disorders such as antisocial behavior and substance abuse,[23] and Sing and colleagues claim that environmental stress may lead to an early expression of genes coding for diabetes, hypertension, and other cardiovascular disorders.[24] Epigenetic influences add to the complexity of the causal models described earlier, since such effects may be operating in both directions—that is, while gene-environmental interactions may influence constructs in our models, including tendencies toward R/S involvement, R/S factors—perhaps by promoting nurturing behaviors, lowering stress levels, and increasing successful coping—may also moderate the effects of environmental adversity and thereby affect genes that regulate the expression of various diseases.

What is the bottom line here? The causal effects that R/S (or secular humanism) may have on health are occurring within a context where many other factors—genetic, environmental, and epigenetic—are affecting mental, social, behavioral, and physical health components in these pathways. If the above models accomplish nothing else, they underscore how complex the relationship between R/S and health really is.

So What? Importance of Specifying a Causal Model

Identifying a model that accurately illustrates the causal pathways that connect R/S with physical health outcomes has many benefits. First, a model that describes how R/S affects health will help researchers ask better research questions, choose better study designs that are capable of answering those questions, and analyze the results in a way that fully captures both the direct and indirect effects of R/S on health (see chapters 16 and 18). Second, having a solid understanding of how R/S affects health will help inform the development of R/S interventions on the individual and community level, interventions directed at impacting health behaviors, positive and negative psychological states, and social health that could prevent or more effectively control disease. Third, understanding how R/S affects physical health should increase our understanding of how the mind influences the body—that is, how a psychosocial factor such as R/S can influence physiological systems and disease states, thus contributing to general scientific knowledge in the social and behavioral sciences. Finally, having a naturalistic, rational explanation for how R/S influences health may encourage mainstream medical researchers to study R/S influences just like they now study psychological, social, and behavioral factors related to disease onset and course.

> The causal effects that R/S (or secular humanism) may have on health are occurring within a context where many other factors—genetic, environmental, and epigenetic—are affecting mental, social, behavioral, and physical health components in these pathways.

Summary and Conclusions

I have emphasized the need to have clear and non-overlapping constructs in order to develop a causal model for understanding how R/S affects health. Such a model is important for specifying research questions, designing research studies to address

> Identifying a model that accurately illustrates the causal pathways that connect R/S with physical health outcomes has many benefits.

them, and setting up statistical analyses that fully capture the effects that R/S may be having. I have presented a theoretical causal model developed from a Western religious perspective that explains how R/S may influence physical health through direct and indirect influences on positive psychological traits, lifestyle choices, health behaviors, psychological and social states, and basic physiological functions. That model, with some uncertainty, has been adapted for Eastern religious and secular humanistic perspectives. I have also emphasized the influences that genetic, environmental, and epigenetic factors have on constructs at every level of these models, underscoring the tremendous complexity of the R/S-health relationship.

Statistical Modeling

WHEN EXAMINING RELATIONSHIPS between religion/spirituality (R/S) and health using observational research, it is crucial to build statistical models that accurately and completely identify the relationships that are present. Failure to heed this advice can result in misinterpretation of what the results mean. Having clear, nonoverlapping definitions of constructs (Chapter 11), avoiding measurement contamination (Chapter 11), following a plausible theoretical model (Chapter 17), and *especially*, considering both direct and indirect effects (Chapters 16 and 18) will assist in this regard. In this chapter, I describe studies that illustrate what happens when investigators fail to address these issues. I then contrast this with studies where researchers have modeled R/S variables so that results can be interpreted correctly. Finally, I make recommendations using graphic illustrations of the optimal way of modeling R/S variables, explanatory variables, and health outcomes.

Examples of Modeling Errors

While the examples that follow below do not involve incorrect modeling per se, the conclusions drawn from these models are not correct because they did not consider the possibility of indirect effects. Furthermore, the use of R/S measures contaminated with the health outcome and the failure to distinguish the authentic R/S components of those measures from contaminated components led to further confusion in the interpretation of results. In order to preserve the privacy of my colleagues, I do not provide citations that reveal the identity of researchers in the examples below.

Example #1: SWB Scale

A highly respected team of investigators from several Ivy League universities analyzed cross-sectional data on a systematically identified sample of 918 adults in New England. The aim of the study (published in a high-profile medical journal) was to examine the relationship between religiosity, spirituality, and the likelihood of having major depression. Frequency of attendance at religious services (RA) was the measure of religiosity and was dichotomized into "any attendance" vs. "no attendance" for analysis. The twenty-item Spiritual Well-Being (SWB) Scale was the measure of "spirituality." Investigators noted that the SWB scale consisted of two subscales, the ten-item religious well-being (RWB) and the ten-item existential well-being (EWB) scales. In bivariate analyses, the researchers found that any attendance at religious services was associated with a 35 percent reduction in the odds of major depression (OR = 0.65, 95 percent CI = 0.49–0.86); RWB was unrelated to depression; and EWB was strongly inversely related to depression (compared to those with low EWB, those with moderate EWB had a 52 percent lower odds of depression [OR = 0.48, 95% CI = 0.34–0.77], and those with high EWB had a 72 percent lower odds [OR = 0.28, 95% CI = 0.19–0.40]).

Next, investigators entered all three R/S variables (RA, RWB, EWB) into a single logistic regression model predicting major depression, controlling for age, income, race, marital status, and gender. Results indicated that the odds of major depression were 29 percent lower in those who attended religious services (OR = 0.71, 95% CI = 0.51–0.99, barely statistically significant); 49 percent lower in those with moderate EWB (OR = 0.51, 95% CI = 0.35–0.74); and 72 percent lower in those with high EWB (OR = 0.28, 95% CI = 0.18–0.42). However, with all variables in the model, the odds of major depression were now 50 percent *higher* in those with moderate or high compared to low RWB (OR = 1.50, 95% CI = 1.03–2.18). Based on these findings, the investigators concluded that "although religious service attendance and existential well-being were protective, religious well-being was associated with increased odds of MDE [major depressive episode]. To our knowledge, this is the first study to examine all three of these religiosity and spirituality factors together with the risk of MDE and also the first study to report a positive association between higher levels of religious well-being and the presence of a psychiatric illness." They also go on to state, "Other researchers have interpreted the stronger association of existential well-being with MDE, compared to religious well-being, to mean that one's own purpose in life is more important than the relationship with a higher being [ref]." Investigators then discussed what the finding of greater depression in those with higher RWB might mean, raising the possibility that those who are more depressed are more likely to rely on religious coping, and that religious coping might be positive or negative. Furthermore, they pointed out that higher levels of religiosity might be a marker for insecure attachment, a risk factor for mental health problems. Thus, much of the discussion was aimed at trying to figure out why those with higher RWB were at greater risk for major depression.

However, what did the investigators really find? Did they find that depression is more likely in those with higher compared to lower religious well-being? Did they find that depression is more common among those with a stronger relationship to a higher being (i.e., God)? Let's take a closer look at their constructs and the way they modeled them. First, EWB was an aspect of "spirituality" that investigators examined and controlled for in logistic regression models. Recall from Chapter 11 that EWB is simply a measure of emotional well-being and has very little to do with anything distinctively spiritual. The finding that those with higher emotional well-being are less likely to have major depression is not earthshaking news. Why should it be surprising that depressed people lack emotional well-being and that those with high emotional well-being are not depressed? This simply describes a tautological association.

Second, the positive relationship between RWB and depression only surfaced *after* investigators included both RWB and EWB in the same statistical model. In fact, without EWB in the model, those with higher RWB actually had 20 percent *lower* odds of depression compared to those with low RWB (OR = 0.80, 95% CI = 0.54–1.16). What happened here? How did the association between RWB and depression go from negative to positive? When investigators controlled for EWB (which you'll recall is actually an indicator of high well-being or low depression), the relationship between RWB and depression reversed from negative (less likely) to positive (more likely). This is called "distortion" or a "distorter variable" (where a third variable, in this case EWB, reverses the direction of the original relationship). This is an exaggerated form of "suppression" (see Chapter 16).

Thus, the claim of a positive association between RWB and depression in the example above was simply the result of overlapping construct definitions, less than complete statistical modeling (a path model would have provided information on indirect effects), and inaccurate interpretation. Instead, investigators should have considered that the positive relationship between RWB and depression did not fit a consistent mediation pattern and instead could have resulted from the distorter effects of EWB on the inverse correlation between RWB and depression. This distorter effect was suggested by the fact that the direct effect of RWB on depression was positive (OR = 1.50) and indirect effect of RWB on depression through EWB was negative (due to a fairly robust positive corre-

> The claim of a positive association between RWB and depression in the example above was simply the result of overlapping construct definitions, less than complete statistical modeling (a path model would have provided information on indirect effects), and inaccurate interpretation.

lation between RWB and EWB, e.g., $r = +0.35$, $p < 0.001$, and a strong negative correlation between EWB and depression).

Example #2: SWB Scale

Researchers at another major medical center in the U.S. examined the cross-sectional relationships between spiritual well-being, emotional well-being, and quality of life (QOL) in a sample of ninety-five cancer patients. Investigators used hierarchical multiple regression models to examine relationships between spirituality (measured using the twenty-item SWB scale comprised of RWB and EWB subscales) and anxiety/depression, quality of life, and overall symptoms of psychopathology. EWB was added first to the models, which (not surprisingly) explained 30 to 40 percent of the variance in anxiety/depression and overall symptom severity and 11 percent of the variance in QOL. They then added RWB to the model with EWB, which explained an additional 4 percent of the variance in anxiety/depression and overall symptom severity, and 0 percent of the variance of QOL. Researchers concluded that the existential aspect of spirituality (EWB) was most important to the emotional health and QOL of cancer patients, and that future research should focus on the broader aspects of spirituality rather than on the religious aspects.

Again, it is not surprising that EWB—an indicator of emotional well-being—explains so much of the variance in emotional well-being (again a circular association), and that RWB ends up explaining very little of the variance in mental health and quality of life. Here again, EWB likely served as a suppressor variable. As in Example #1, no effort was made to examine the indirect effects of RWB through EWB on emotional well-being (e.g., RWB was likely a primary source of EWB). Unfortunately, the authors did not report the relationship between RWB and EWB, although most studies (as in Example #1 above) have found that relationship to be strong. Therefore, the researchers' conclusions were misleading and provided little direction for clinicians or patients. Telling depressed and anxious patients that they need to have more meaning and purpose, hope, and optimism in life does very little good unless clinicians can suggest a source for these positive psychological and emotional states beyond the actual states themselves.

Example #3: FACIT-Sp

In this third example, rather than use the SWB scale, investigators used the FACIT-Sp-12, which was described in Chapter 11 and consists of an eight-item meaning and peace subscale and a four-item faith subscale. This was a cross-sectional study of 237 cancer survivors, in which researchers sought to examine the relationships between spirituality and health-related quality of life (HRQOL). The mental and physical health subscale scores of the SF-12 were used to measure HRQOL. First, researchers wished to see whether the meaning and peace subscale of the FACIT-Sp (which they called EWB) mediated the relationship between the faith subscale of the FACIT-Sp (the religious component) and the mental health component of HRQOL (B = +0.19, p < 0.01), using hierarchical regression to examine this. Not only did the results suggest that EWB mediated the relationship between the faith subscale and mental health, but when EWB was added to the model with the faith subscale, the parameter coefficient for the faith subscale's relationship to HRQOL changed from +0.19 to −0.14 (p < 0.05) (another example of distortion, just like in Example #1). The researchers concluded that greater religious faith as indicated by higher scores on the faith subscale of the FACIT-Sp was related to worse mental HRQOL. In fact, they even indicated that this religious component of the FACIT-Sp actually counteracted the positive impact that the EWB component of spirituality was having on HRQOL, implying that spirituality was good and religion was bad in these cancer patients.

Again, the conclusion is an erroneous one, based on confusion over the definition of spirituality, contamination of the EWB measure of spirituality with indicators of emotional well-being, and a purely tautological relationship between EWB and HRQOL. Good emotional health (as indicated by high scores on the EWB subscale) is indeed related to good mental health (as indicated by high scores on the mental health subscale of the HRQOL measure). It is not surprising that *after* EWB "sucked" all of the emotional well-being out of mental health (when investigators controlled for it in the model), researchers found that religious faith was no longer related to good mental health (and even became inversely related to it). These investigators did not consider the possibility that a primary source of EWB was the religious faith component of the FACIT-Sp, and consequently ignored the indirect effects that the faith subscale was having on HRQOL through EWB. Indeed, the faith subscale and EWB subscale were highly correlated ($r = +0.51$, $p < 0.001$) in this study. Instead, investigators emphasized the importance of the EWB component of spirituality on HRQOL and how this should be the focus of study, not the religious or faith aspects. Again, this places the focus on the outcome itself, emotional well-being, rather than on a primary source of emotional well-being, religious faith.

Example #4: FACIT-Sp

In many other studies, the FACIT-Sp has been used to measure spirituality in cancer patients, and the conclusion was that the nonreligious aspects of spirituality are the most important in determining quality of life. Here's another example. In a study of 222 patients with prostate cancer, researchers examined relationships between spirituality and disease-specific HRQOL, general HRQOL, anxiety, symptom distress, and emotional well-being. The overall FACIT-Sp score was positively related to every aspect of higher QOL, lower anxiety, less symptom distress, and greater emotional well-being. However, when the two subscales were examined together in a regression model, controlling for psychosocial and biomedical covariates, only the meaning/peace subscale (EWB) was related to mental health outcomes (it was significantly associated with every one of the nine mental health outcome measures). With meaning/peace in the model, however, there was no relationship between the faith subscale (religious) and any outcome, causing investigators to conclude that "the peace and meaning subscale is responsible for the improvement in HRQOL, as opposed to the faith component.

The health benefits of spirituality, at least in low-income men coping with prostate cancer, may be related to a sense of harmony and purpose beyond spiritual beliefs expounded on in organized religion."

The conclusion is incorrect because investigators did not examine the indirect effects of the faith subscale acting through the meaning/peace scores on QOL outcomes. From where do researchers think the patients are getting peace and meaning? Saying that those with high levels of meaning and a deep sense of peace have high quality of life is completely circular. Where does one enter into the circle to change things?

Example #5: FACIT-Sp

Finally, in a study published in the *Lancet* (a medical journal with one of the highest impact factors in the world), investigators examined relationships between spirituality measured using the FACIT-Sp and hopelessness, desire for a hastened death, and suicidal ideation in 160 terminally ill cancer patients. In bivariate analyses, both the meaning/peace and the faith subscales of the FACIT-Sp were strongly inversely correlated with all three outcomes. However, when both subscales were included in a single regression model, the faith (religious) subscale lost significance in predicting desire for a hastened death and suicidal ideation, and only the peace/meaning subscale remained significant. Much ado was made in the article about the finding that patients who had greater peace and meaning in their lives were less suicidal. Is not such a result obvious? Based on this finding the authors concluded, "The ability to find or sustain meaning in one's life during terminal illness might help to deter end-of-life despair to a greater extent than spiritual well-being rooted in one's religious faith." Of course, no attempt was made to examine the indirect effects that the faith measure had *through* peace/meaning on suicidal thoughts (which was likely substantial, given the strength of the bivariate correlation).

The investigators in the studies above were quick to dismiss any effects that religious faith may have, and editors/reviewers were quick to accept that explanation.

The scientific community in general has long held quite negative views toward religion, but in contrast, quite positive views toward "spirituality"—especially spirituality that has been neutered of any aspect of religion. As a result, it is not surprising that the investigators in the studies above were quick to dismiss any effects that religious faith was having, and editors/reviewers were quick to accept their explanations.

EXAMPLES OF APPROPRIATE MODELING

In contrast to the above, there are also examples of research that has examined relationships between R/S and health outcomes in a comprehensive way and interpreted the results appropriately. I now describe a number of studies that have modeled the direct and indirect effects of R/S on health outcomes, giving credit where credit is due. Here, I gladly provide citations for these reports.

Example #1: Religion, Hopelessness, and Depression

In a study of 271 persons diagnosed with clinical depression, investigators at Loyola College examined the relationships between religious beliefs/practices, depression, and hope.[2] They hypothesized that religious involvement would be associated with less severe depression and that this relationship would be mediated by a greater sense of hope. Religious measures were religious belief (using a religious well-being scale), attendance at religious services, and private religious practices. Hope was measured using a hopelessness scale (the opposite of hope), and depression was assessed using the Beck Depression Inventory. Controlling for a generous list of confounders (age, gender, race, employment status, living situation, marital status, and education), researchers found that religious beliefs were inversely related to depression ($\beta = -0.22$, $p < 0.01$). Religious beliefs were also inversely related to hopelessness ($\beta = -0.45$, $p < 0.001$) (i.e., positively related to hope). Investigators then constructed a path model that examined whether hopelessness might explain the relationship between religious belief and depression. After controlling for hopelessness in the model, the inverse relationship between religious belief and depression was reduced and actually switched directions so that religious belief was now positively related to depression (β = +0.17, p < 0.01). However, researchers examined the indirect effect of religious belief on depression through hopelessness, and found it to be significant (β = −0.32, p < 0.001), yielding a total effect that reflected an inverse relationship between religious belief and depression. They correctly concluded that the pathway by which religious belief reduced depression severity was by increasing a sense of hope.[3] Investigators did not dismiss religious belief as an unimportant factor just because the effect was explained by hope, nor did they claim that only hope was necessary rather than religious belief (as some researchers in previous examples did).

> Investigators did not dismiss religious belief as an unimportant factor just because the effect was explained by hope, nor did they claim that only hope was necessary rather than religious belief.

Example #2: Religion, Compassion, and Depression

Researchers at Brigham Young University examined the relationship between religiosity, compassionate attitudes and behaviors, depressive symptoms, perceived stress, and life satisfaction in a sample of 126 adults.[4] In the part of the study that addressed depressive symptoms, religiosity was inversely related to depression (r = −0.34, p < 0.0001), religiosity was positively related to compassionate attitude (r = +0.41, p < 0.0001) and compassionate behavior (r = +0.44, p < 0.0001), and compassionate attitude and behavior were inversely related to depression (r = −0.51, p < 0.0001, and r = −0.34, p < 0.001, respectively). Controlling for compassionate attitude and behavior, investigators found that the relationship between religiosity and depressive symptoms was reduced to nonsignificance (r = −0.14). Therefore, while there was no direct relationship between religiosity and depression, the indirect relationship of religiosity through compassion on depressive symptoms was substantial. The investigators correctly concluded that compassion explained the relationship between religiosity and depression. Again, there

> There was no attempt to dismiss religion as being unimportant; instead, researchers emphasized that it was through compassion that religiosity was affecting depression.

was no attempt to dismiss religion as being unimportant; instead, researchers emphasized that it was through compassion that religiosity was affecting depression.

Example #3: Religion, Self-Actualization, and Job Satisfaction

In a study of 215 hospice interdisciplinary team members, researchers at the University of South Florida examined relationships between R/S beliefs, R/S integration, self-actualization, and job satisfaction.[5] Initially, there was a relationship between R/S beliefs and greater job satisfaction ($r = +0.28$, $p = 0.001$), a relationship between R/S beliefs and both R/S integration ($r = +0.34$, $p = 0.001$) and self-actualization ($r = +0.50$, $p = 0.001$), and a relationship between job satisfaction and both R/S integration ($r = +0.429$, $= 0.001$) and self-actualization ($r = +0.274$, $p = 0.001$). When a multiple regression analysis was used to examine the relationship between R/S beliefs and job satisfaction with both R/S integration and self-actualization included in the model, the significant association between R/S beliefs and job satisfaction became nonsignificant ($\beta = -0.06$) (suggesting that R/S integration and self-actualization mediated the relationship between R/S beliefs and job satisfaction). Structural equation models were then created to examine relationships between all variables simultaneously so that both direct and indirect effects between R/S beliefs and job satisfaction could be accounted for. As expected, the model with the best "fit" was one in which R/S beliefs had indirect effects through R/S integration ($\beta = +0.13$) and self-actualization ($\beta = +0.09$) on job satisfaction, but had no direct effect. Researchers correctly concluded that job satisfaction is more due to the transformation of one's R/S beliefs into the process of integrating R/S at work and self-actualization, and less due to any direct effects of R/S beliefs on job satisfaction. Investigators acknowledged that R/S beliefs were important in explaining job satisfaction, but saw R/S as acting indirectly through these other intervening variables.

> Investigators acknowledged that R/S beliefs were important in explaining job satisfaction, but saw R/S as acting indirectly through these other intervening variables.

Example #4: Religion, Conventional Peers, and Substance Abuse

Investigators at the University of Georgia examined relationships between religiosity and substance abuse in 318 African American high school dropouts.[6] There were significant inverse relationships between religiosity and both marijuana ($r = -0.18$, p < 0.01) and alcohol use ($r = -0.15$, p < 0.05); positive relationships between religiosity, positive life orientation ($r = +0.13$ to $+0.14$, p < 0.05), and conventional peers ($r = +0.13$ to $+0.20$, p < 0.01); and a strong inverse relationship between conventional peers and substance use ($r = -0.19$ to -0.26, p < 0.01). Structural equation modeling showed that there was no direct relationship between religiosity and substance use, but there were indirect effects for religiosity through a positive life orientation ($\beta = -0.05$) and conventional peers ($\beta = -0.17$). Researchers correctly concluded that religiosity influenced substance use indirectly by facilitating a positive life orientation and increasing affiliation with conventional peers.

Example #5: Testing the Overall Model

Finally, researchers at the University of Cincinnati recently examined the effects of R/S on physical functioning through intervening variables in 345 patients with HIV infection.[7] Direct and indirect effects of R/S were examined using structural equation modeling, with the aim of testing an earlier version[8] of the model I presented in Chapter 17. The best-fitting model was the one where R/S predicted religious coping, which predicted higher social support, which predicted lower depression, which predicted higher energy levels, which predicted increased physical functioning. Investigators concluded that their data were consistent with an expanded version of the Koenig model, which accurately described the relationships between R/S and self-reported physical health (operating primarily by indirect effects through intervening variables).

In each of these five examples, investigators modeled the effects of R/S variables on health by examining both direct effects on health and indirect effects through explanatory variables. None of these studies dismissed R/S as being irrelevant or less important than intervening variables, but instead recognized that R/S was acting indirectly through those intervening variables, something that investigators in the first five examples failed to acknowledge. Path analysis using regression or structural equation modeling was useful in identifying (and determining the significance of) direct and indirect effects in these studies.

> None of these studies dismissed R/S as being irrelevant or less important than intervening variables, but instead recognized that R/S was acting indirectly through those intervening variables.

Direct and Indirect Effects[9]

Figure 18.1 illustrates the direct and indirect effects of an R/S predictor on a health outcome (depression) through a single explanatory variable (existential well-being[10]) (upper model). The second model (lower) generalizes the situation so it applies to *any* explanatory variable, where the explanatory variable may be a human virtue (i.e., forgiveness, gratefulness, altruism), social support, or a health behavior (following the hypothetical causal models described in Chapter 17). If the health outcome was physical illness or mortality, then the explanatory variable might be depression or a physiological function. Genetic and developmental factors, along with demographic variables, would serve as control variables in such models.

Figure 18.2 illustrates a more complex model that includes more than one explanatory variable, and while the math is more complex, the principles are the same. The R/S variable is acting directly on the health outcome, indirectly on the health outcome through each of the explanatory variables, *and* indirectly on the health outcome through the effects that the explanatory variables are having on the health outcome through each other. All of these direct and indirect effects must be considered when interpreting the total effect that R/S is having on the outcome.

Computer programs that run path models or structural equation models (AMOS, EQS, Mplus, LISREL) produce parameter coefficients for direct, indirect, and total effects in their outputs, controlling for confounders. Using such computer programs is the easiest way to determine the direct, indirect, and total effects and their significance levels. However, the researcher

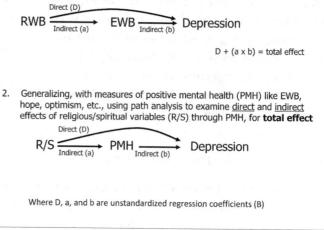

1. Religious well-being (RWB) & existential well-being (EWB) on depression using path analysis to identify <u>direct</u> and <u>indirect</u> effects of RWB through EWB, for **total effect**

   Direct (D)

   RWB ⇄ EWB → Depression
   Indirect (a)   Indirect (b)

   D + (a x b) = total effect

2. Generalizing, with measures of positive mental health (PMH) like EWB, hope, optimism, etc., using path analysis to examine <u>direct</u> and <u>indirect</u> effects of religious/spiritual variables (R/S) through PMH, for **total effect**

   Direct (D)

   R/S ⇄ PMH → Depression
   Indirect (a)   Indirect (b)

   Where D, a, and b are unstandardized regression coefficients (B)

FIGURE 18.1.
Path Analysis with
Single Explanatory
Variable

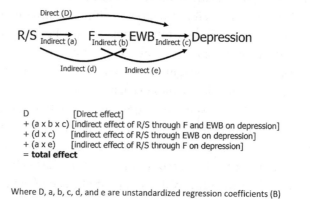

Religion/spirituality (R/S), forgiveness (F), and existential well-being (EWB) on depression using path analysis to identify <u>direct</u> and <u>indirect</u> effects of R/S on depression, for **total effect**

Direct (D)

R/S → F → EWB → Depression
Indirect (a) Indirect (b) Indirect (c)

Indirect (d)   Indirect (e)

D   [Direct effect]
+ (a x b x c) [indirect effect of R/S through F and EWB on depression]
+ (d x c)   [indirect effect of R/S through EWB on depression]
+ (a x e)   [indirect effect of R/S through F on depression]
= **total effect**

Where D, a, b, c, d, and e are unstandardized regression coefficients (B)

FIGURE 18.2.
Path Analysis with
Multiple Explanatory
Variables

may also accomplish this by running two regression models (for a single mediator) as follows: Run a regression model that contains only the predictor variable (X), confounders (C), and the outcome (Y). The "total effect" is the B_t of the predictor variable X in the model (and the p-value for B_t gives the significance level for the total effect). Next, add the explanatory variable (M) to the model. The B_d for the predictor variable X in the resulting model is the "direct" effect (and the p-value for the B_d gives the significance level for the direct effect).

Determining the B for the "indirect" effect (B_{id}) is a little more complicated. This can be accomplished by running two regression models, where X is the predictor, C is the confounders, M is the mediator, and Y is the outcome. In the first model, M is regressed on X (e.g., $M = B_0 + B_1X + C + e$); in the second model, Y is regressed on M and X (e.g., $Y = B_0 + B_2X + B_3M + C + e$). The indirect effect is the product of B_1 and B_3 from these models ($B_{id} = B_1 \times B_3$). Note that the indirect effect can also be calculated by simply subtracting the direct effect from the total effect ($B_{id} = B_t - B_d$).[11] Determining the significance level (p value) of the indirect effect is a bit more complicated. The standard error (SE) for the indirect effect can be calculated by hand using the standard errors from these regressions, but there has been considerable debate about the best way to do it.[12] Fortunately, Kristopher Preacher has an online calculator (http://www.people.ku.edu/~preacher /sobel/sobel.htm) that does it automatically if the researcher inputs the unstandardized Bs and their standard errors, producing the indirect effect, standard error, and significance level calculated in three different ways (Sobel, Aroian, Goodman). The summation of the Bs of the direct and the indirect effects should equal the B of the total effect if relationships are linear ($B_t = B_d + B_{id}$).

There is some question of whether unstandardized B or standardized beta (β) coefficients should be used in these calculations (see Glossary for definitions of unstandardized B and standardized beta coefficients). Most statisticians recommend using the unstandardized Bs.[13] However, this method applies only when the mediator and outcome variables are continuous (and possibly ordinal). When the mediator or the outcome variable is dichotomous (as in logistic regression), David A. Kenny recommends standardizing the coefficients before computing indirect effects.[14] An alternative to standardizing coefficients as Kenny recommends is to use the Clogg test, which tests for the change in the magnitude of the unstandardized coefficient before and after controlling for the mediator.[15] When adding the

> Computer programs that run path models or structural equation models (AMOS, EQS, Mplus, LISREL) produce parameter coefficients for direct, indirect, and total effects in their outputs, controlling for confounders.

> The total *effect* is the effect of the R/S predictor on the health outcome after confounders are controlled. A *direct* effect is the effect of the R/S predictor on the health outcome after confounders and explanatory variables are controlled. *Indirect* effects are the effects that R/S is having on the health outcome through intervening explanatory variables (mediators/suppressors).

mediator, the effect of the predictor usually becomes smaller in magnitude. The Clogg test tests whether this change in the predictor coefficient is significantly different from zero (and the test can also be used for continuous mediators and outcomes).

For R/S-health researchers, then, the total *effect* is the effect of the R/S predictor on the health outcome after confounders are controlled.[16] A *direct* effect is the effect of the R/S predictor on the health outcome after confounders *and* explanatory variables are controlled. *Indirect* effects are the effects that R/S is having on the health outcome through intervening explanatory variables (mediators/suppressors). When path analysis is done using regression models, the direct and indirect effects are represented by the unstandardized B coefficients for each path obtained from the regression output (assuming variables are continuous). If the Bs of the direct effect and indirect effect are either both positive or both negative, then the explanatory variable is considered a mediator; if the Bs of the direct and indirect effects are the opposite (one positive and one negative), then the explanatory variable (such as existential well-being) is considered a suppressor variable. If the addition of a covariate leads to a significant total effect that was not significant before, this would be another indication that a suppressor variable was affecting the relationship. For more information on direct and indirect effects, mediation and suppression, I refer the reader to a very accessible and informative paper.[17]

Summary and Conclusions

In this chapter I provided several examples of published research where investigators did not model their variables in a comprehensive way (e.g., did not examine all the hypothesized pathways between predictor and outcome), resulting in an underestimation of the effects that R/S factors were having on a health outcome and an incorrect interpretation of the findings. I also provided several examples of published studies where investigators considered both the direct effect of R/S on the outcome and the indirect effects through intervening explanatory variables, and recognized R/S as the source of the effect. I also provided illustrations of how to model the effects of an R/S predictor on a health outcome, first with a single explanatory variable (mediator or suppressor) and then with more than one explanatory variable. In conclusion, it is important to (1) understand the differences between R/S variables that are the source of the effect on health, the variables that confound the relationship between R/S and health, and the explanatory variables that explain how R/S affects health, and (2) model these variables so that both direct and indirect effects are considered when explaining and interpreting the effect that R/S is having on health.

It is important to (1) understand the differences between R/S variables that are the source of the effect on health, the variables that confound the relationship between R/S and health, and the explanatory variables that explain how R/S affects health, and (2) model these variables so that both direct and indirect effects are considered when explaining and interpreting the effect that R/S is having on health.

PART 5

Publishing and Funding Resources

Publishing Results

THIS CHAPTER DEALS with writing up a research study for publication, submitting it to an academic peer-reviewed journal, responding to reviewers' critiques, resubmitting to that journal, and responding if the paper is rejected. I also discuss other ways of publishing research such as in online journals, in book chapters, or in books. I begin this chapter by discussing why publishing is important. I am saddened by the fact that many R/S-health researchers expend huge amounts of time and effort in designing, managing, and writing up the results of their research, yet never get those results published so that others can learn about that work. One of reason for my success as an academician is that I try to publish anything I ever do or say.

WHY PUBLISHING IS IMPORTANT

Researchers should make every effort to publish their findings, for many reasons. These reasons include sharing results with the scientific community, enhancing one's curriculum vitae, acquiring tenure or securing a job, increasing chances of getting a grant, and acquiring professional and public recognition for work done.

Sharing Discoveries

One of the major reasons for publishing research findings is to share them with other researchers. New discoveries—including those in the R/S-health area—are contributing to a worldwide scientific knowledge base on which future discoveries will be grounded. In this way, researchers contribute to the ongoing process of scientific discovery and advancement that we hope will ultimately lead to better health and well-being for everyone. Investigators cite studies published many decades earlier that have made a significant or seminal contribution. Published research discoveries may, in fact, enable researchers to leave their mark on history.

Building Curriculum Vitae

Publishing is so important that most curriculum vitae (CV) are structured based on academic publications. Immediately following educational background and previously held and current academic positions comes the listing of peer-reviewed publications. Here is the order in which those publications are typically listed on a CV:

1. Original data-based publications
2. Reviews or meta-analyses of others' original data-based publications
3. Invited commentaries
4. Book chapters
5. Books
6. Articles in the popular literature

The first three listed above are peer-reviewed, whereas the last three are not. The prestige of a publication is much higher if it has been carefully reviewed by peers, and then a journal editor has decided that the findings are important enough to take up precious journal space.

Achieving Tenure

If a college or university values research and academic productivity, then tenure is often determined by a faculty member's number of original first-author, data-based, peer-reviewed publications. "Publish or perish" is a well-known phrase in academia, and there is a lot of truth in it. The researcher's publication record is evidence of her ability to carry out a research study from start to finish—and the finish line is the peer-reviewed publication that results from the data that has been collected. When a researcher is looking for a job or switching to a new position at an academic institution, one of the first things interviewers look at is number of publications.

> "Publish or perish" is a well-known phrase in academia, and there is a lot of truth in it.

Getting Grants

One reason job interviewers are particularly interested in a researcher's publication record is that it reflects how productive he has been based on the funding support he has received. In particular, the publication record reflects his potential to obtain funding support in the future. A past history of success is always the best predictor of future success, and grant reviewers know this. If the principal investigator has many publications in high-quality peer-reviewed journals, especially if those publications are focused in a particular area, then this says to reviewers that the researcher is someone worth investing in.

Professional and Public Recognition

Publication of original data-based research may provide the researcher with acclaim in professional societies and academic circles, as well as stimulate invitations to speak about or teach on the subject of the research. Academic journal publications often mark investigators as experts in their particular field. As a result, they may be called on by hospitals or even government agencies to lend their expertise. The public media (newspaper, television, radio) are also interested in new research findings that are applicable to the population at large and will engage the public's interest. Religion/spirituality (R/S) and health is a topic that carries with it enormous public interest, and the media know it.

LEARNING TO WRITE WELL

Before researchers can publish their findings, however, they need to learn to write. Writing is a skill that is learned through study and improved with practice. First, writing requires knowledge about the rules of written communication—that is, English grammar, word choice, sentence structure and length, and so forth. The researcher should consider either taking a review course on writing or at least purchasing a time-tested book on writing and studying it. Perhaps the most widely used book in the world on writing is *The Elements of Style*,[1] which has sold over 10 million copies since it was first written in 1918. The book focuses on learning how to write better, and has become required reading in high schools and colleges around the country. Rudolf Flesch wrote a series of books on writing that have been around more than fifty years, including *How to Write Better* (1951),[2] *The Art of Readable Writing* (1949),[3] and *The ABC of Style* (1964).[4]

The Flesch Reading Ease and the Flesch-Kincaid Grade Level

> Before researchers can publish their findings, they need to learn to write. Writing is a skill that is learned through study and improved with practice.

tests are widely used to assess how easy a person's writing is to read and the grade level necessary to comprehend it. The Flesch Reading Ease score or readability index is calculated using the formula: 207 *minus* (total words *divided by* total sentences) *minus* 85 *times* (total syllables *divided by* total words). The higher the score, the easier it is to read the material (90–100 is sixth-grade level reading, 60–70 is high school freshman reading, and 0–30 is college graduate reading). *Readers Digest* has a readability index score of 65, *Time* magazine has a score of 52, and the *Harvard Law Review* has a score in the low 30s. The highest possible score (most easily read) is 120, where every sentence consists of only two one-syllable words.[5]

The Flesch Reading Ease score and Flesch-Kincaid Grade Level test are available in Microsoft Word (Word 2000 onward, at least) and can be used to check how easy a document is to read. The procedure is as follows: go to Tools, Spelling & Grammar, then Options and ensure that "Show readability statistics" is checked; next, go through the entire document clicking "ignore all" until a box comes up that reads, "The spelling and grammar check is complete." Then click "OK," and the readability statistics immediately come up with the Flesch and Flesch-Kincaid scores. For example, this chapter has a Flesch Reading Ease score of 45.2 and a Flesch-Kincaid grade level of 11.5 years. Compare this with the Flesch Reading Ease score for Chapter 15 on examining statistical tests, which is 30.4. Specific sections of a document can also be highlighted, and then only that section checked for readability.

The bottom line is that writing sentences with fewer words and words with fewer syllables increases readability. The researcher's goal is to write in a way that is easily read, but which uses the scientific language and terminology expected by peers in their field. Remember that if researchers' writing skills aren't up to speed yet, especially if English is not their first language, and they have done some good research and don't want to wait until they possess the writing skills to publish it, they can bring on an English expert to help them develop the article. Many top researchers in the R/S and health field now do this. However, doing so can be expensive and is usually only a tempo-

> The researcher's goal is to write in a way that is easily read, but which uses the scientific language and terminology expected by peers in their field.

rary solution since researchers need eventually to develop these writing skills themselves.

How to Write a Research Report

Many investigators have a problem with writing. They may not know how to write, lack writing experience, or have a fear of writing. Writer's block is not uncommon even among academicians. A sign of writer's block is that the person can't get started. How can one get all the information from a study that may have taken months or years to complete into a short, concise, publishable paper? The task may simply seem overwhelming. There may also be fear of rejection or critique.

> Many investigators have a problem with writing. They may not know how to write, lack writing experience, or have a fear of writing.

A general rule is that the more people write, the better they write and the easier it gets. Because of this, R/S-health researchers need to write and write and write. How can inexperienced writers or those with writer's block get started? As I indicated earlier, first read about writing or take a course on how to write. Once that is done, here is a suggestion. First, outline a draft of the paper. Simply type the words "title," "abstract," "introduction," "methods," "results," and "discussion" on separate blank pages. This is the structure that the researcher needs to follow. Next, fill out each page—disregarding grammar, spelling, and organization. Just get all the information down, whether writing it down on paper or typing it into a computer document. Then begin to mold and shape each section of the paper by editing, rewriting, organizing and reorganizing, and adding material as necessary.

Why get everything down like this? *It is much easier to edit something than to create it from scratch.* Once the writer gets everything written down, the resulting feeling of accomplishment helps keep the writer going. Doing so, however, is likely to produce a paper that is way too long and detailed for publication in a journal, but at least it's all down there. Deleting or shortening unnecessary sections that are repetitive or less important is again a lot easier than trying to write a concise report on the first try.

STRUCTURING A RESEARCH REPORT

The structure of a research report is similar across the medical, social, and behavioral sciences, even though some journals may have specific requirements that vary. The following are the primary sections of a research report that I discuss here:

Title page
Abstract
Introduction
Methods
Results
Discussion
Tables
Figures
References

> The structure of a research report is similar across the medical, social, and behavioral sciences, even though some journals may have specific requirements that vary.

Title Page

At the top of the title page is the title of the article. The title should be in the same type size as the rest of the paper, is usually capitalized throughout, and should be no more than ten to twelve words at most. Some journals may also request a "running title" that is an abbreviated version of the complete title and about one-third its length. Next come the names and affiliations of the authors. These are centered on the page consecutively from first author to last author. Included here should be the full name with middle initial and degrees, the author's academic title (professor of . . .), the name of the institution, and the location (city and state). After the list of authors should appear the phrase "word count" on the left side of the page that gives the number of words in the text (not including references or tables or abstract). At the bottom of the page should be the address and contact information for the corresponding author (usually the first author), the funding source for the research (including grant number if NIH, e.g., R01-MH00012), and indication of any conflicts of interests that the authors may have.

Abstract

The abstract summarizes the Objective of the study, the Methods, the Results, and the Conclusions, and is usually structured in this way (structure may vary, however, by journal, so this should be verified in the journal's "Information for Authors"). The abstract is important because it presents the essence of what investigators want to communicate to their audience. This abstract will likely have a much greater circulation than the full article since the abstract will be available worldwide for free on the Internet, whereas readers may have to pay a fee to get the full article. Unfortunately, the length of the abstract is only about 100 to 250 words, so researchers need to be very concise and selective about what goes in here: one sentence for the objective, several sentences for the methods, several sentences for the findings, and one sentence for the conclusions. The study design, sample size, and response rate (or dropout rate) should be included in the methods. Of particular importance is including percentages and numbers in the Results, along with the statistic (odds ratio, correlation, p-value) that indicates the strength of the finding. Again, the reason is that this information will be available to the world via online databases (Medline, PubMed, etc.) so that other researchers may cite the study based on the abstract alone, especially if they cannot get the full article. The more citations that a researcher's paper gets, the better and more highly valued it is. Furthermore, citations are sometimes used as a basis for awarding tenure. The abstract is concluded with three to five keywords (chosen carefully) by which the study will be indexed, along with a word count for the abstract.

Introduction

The introduction should establish the significance of the topic being studied, indicate what is known, and cite relevant previously published research. The researchers need to make clear here how the present study is adding to what is already known. The length of this section varies depending on discipline; for major medical journals, only one double-spaced page of introduction may be necessary (without subheadings); sociology and psychology journals, however, are usually interested in the theory behind the study, so the length in those journals may be ten double-spaced pages or more (with subheadings). The introduction should end with the research questions/hypotheses that are being tested, presented under a subheading titled "Hypotheses" or "Research Questions." In general, the introduction should be no longer than one-quarter the length of the paper. Unfortunately, reviewers often do not pay much attention to the introduction, but rather focus on the methods and findings.

Methods

The methods section should begin with a description of the study design (cross-sectional, prospective, clinical trial), the population being studied, how the sample was acquired (sampling method), the procedure for collecting the data, and who collected it (including their training). If a clinical trial, then the intervention should be described in detail as well as what the control group received. Next, there should be a separate section (with subheading) that describes the measures used in the study for assessing the independent and dependent variables, including a citation for each measure and information on reliability and validity. How much detail about measures to include here depends on the type of journal. Psychology and sociology journals want lots of information about measures, whereas medical and psychiatric journals require less information. The methods section should end with a paragraph titled "Statistical Analysis," where the order and types of statistical tests and software are described, along with any adjustments in significance level as a result of multiple comparisons. The methods section should be about one-third of the paper.

Results

Begin with a description of the sample size, response rate, and sample characteristics (age, gender, race, diagnoses, education, socioeconomic status, etc., perhaps with a table). This is also the place to describe nonresponders or dropouts and compare their characteristics with those of responders (hopefully, there are few differences) For a clinical trial, a table comparing the subjects in the intervention and control groups at baseline, and a detailed description of dropouts in each group should be provided. Next, describe the results of the study by hypothesis. Specifically, begin a new paragraph, restate the first hypothesis, underline it, and then provide the results; repeat this for each hypothesis. Refer to data tables in discussing the results. Describe important findings in detail in the text, although don't repeat everything in the tables. For the major findings, provide the statistical details—mean values for measures, standard deviations, the statistical test and result, standard error, 95% confidence intervals, degrees of freedom, and significance level (even if already in a table).

Discussion

Lead off with how this study is unique, its major finding, and why that finding is important. Don't simply restate the results, but rather integrate the finding into what other studies have reported (with relevant citations). Next, explain and hypothesize what the study results mean. Provide several possible alternative explanations, and indicate the most likely explanation with justification for it. Next, present a separate paragraph with the subtitle, "Limitations." Describe here the weaknesses of the study and the limitations of the findings based on those weaknesses. At the end of this paragraph the researcher should describe the strengths of the study, explain why the strengths outweigh the weaknesses, and why the weaknesses of the study do not invalidate the results. The discussion section should end with a separate paragraph with the subtitle, "Conclusions." Briefly summarize the findings and their importance in this section, and end with a discussion of the clinical implications of the results. The discussion section should be no longer than about one-quarter of the paper.

Tables

After the discussion should come the data tables. Most papers have up to a maximum of five tables; three tables are ideal depending on the size of the study. Usually, the first table describes the sample (means, standard deviations, percentages, N's). The second table may present a correlation matrix of all variables, or simply provide the bivariate relationships between the outcome and the predictors, confounders, and mediators. The third table usually describes the multivariate models (controlled analyses). Tables should be labeled with short, descriptive titles. Define any abbreviations used in the table at the bottom of the table. Type size should be the same as that used in the text. A general rule is to make tables simple with lots of white space—not crammed or excessively busy-looking.

Figures

Following the tables, the researcher may include one or two figures. If the study is a complex one and subjects come from multiple sources, then a figure describing subject flow may be useful to readers. If a clinical trial, the figure should illustrate subjects in the intervention and control groups that started the study, dropped out, and completed it. A figure may also be used to describe the theoretical model being tested in the study, especially for psychology, sociology, or nursing journals. The most important figure, however, is the one that graphically illustrates the most striking finding. That finding does not have to be the results for the primary hypothesis, but could be from a secondary hypothesis or even a post-hoc analysis (i.e., exploratory findings not hypothesis driven). As with tables, figures should use the same type size throughout and be simple and easy to understand (i.e., short title, figure labels, not busy-looking, and all abbreviations defined).

References

Last come the references cited in the paper. Most journal articles reporting original data include twenty to forty references, although review articles may have one hundred or more. Always cite peer-reviewed articles that report original data. A book or website might be occasionally cited but not more than one or two per paper; popular articles should not be cited. Every journal has its own distinctive reference style and format, so it is important to examine the Information for Authors to determine what that format is. Many researchers use a reference manager (EndNote, RefWorks, Reference Manager, etc.) to store and organize their references, as well as easily convert references for one journal format into another.

Length of Report

The length of a paper (text only) varies from eight to eighteen double-spaced pages for medical and psychiatric journals. For clinical journals, the article length should probably not be over fifteen double-spaced pages or three thousand words. Remember that *the length of the paper is directly proportional to the likelihood of acceptance.* Some psychological, sociology, and nursing journals may accept longer articles, up to thirty or more pages in some cases, although these are usually comprehensive review articles, not reports of original research. Additional recommendations about article format are to double-space text, use one-inch margins throughout the document, use 12-point type (Times Roman), and do not outline (always write in paragraph form).

> Remember that *the length of the paper is directly proportional to the likelihood of acceptance.*

SUBMITTING REPORT TO JOURNAL

Once all the coauthors contribute to and review the article, it is ready for submission. Go to the journal website and read the Information for Authors carefully regarding length, copyright procedure, and method of submission. Next, prepare a short letter to the editor indicating that the researcher would like to submit the article (state the full title) for consideration for publication in the journal. Indicate that the article is not submitted elsewhere (only submit to one journal at a time, unlike grant submissions). If the journal asks that authors provide a list of recommended reviewers, then this letter is the place for that information. No other information should be included in the letter.

Before an article is sbmitted to a journal, the paper should be as polished as possible. The first submission makes the greatest impression on the editor and reviewers and will determine if a revise-and-resubmit request is offered (vs. rejection). Some researchers may actually hire an editor to go over their paper to ensure that grammar, sentence structure, and spelling are correct. Errors like this bother reviewers and lower the paper's chances of acceptance.

> Before submitting an article to a journal, the paper should be as polished as possible. The first submission makes the greatest impression on the editor and reviewers.

REVISING AND RESUBMITTING

The journal responds by either rejecting the paper or indicating that the authors need to make corrections in response to reviewers' comments and resubmit the paper for reconsideration; journals rarely accept papers without revisions. If the editor sends a revise-and-resubmit letter, the author should read it carefully to get the editor's general feelings about the manuscript. How much enthusiasm do the editor and reviewers display regarding the paper? Any show of enthusiasm at all is usually a good sign. If there is no enthusiasm and many, many pages of reviewer critique, then it may not be worth the time to revise the paper for resubmission to this journal. If, however, the editor and reviewers are somewhat positive about the paper and not a huge amount of corrections are demanded, then it is worth addressing the reviewers' concerns. A specific procedure for doing this follows:

A. Read each reviewer's comments carefully.

B. In the letter to the editor, state that the reviewers' concerns have now been addressed and the paper is stronger and clearer. Following that statement, the researcher should provide a detailed description of how and where she did what each reviewer suggested and where in the paper the changes were made. For example,

> The researcher should provide a detailed description of how and where she did what each reviewer suggested and where in the paper the changes were made.

Reviewer #1

1. *Authors did not control for socioeconomic status in their model.*

Response: We have now controlled for socioeconomic status, and the results can be found in Table 2. A discussion of these results can be found in the text on p. 10, second paragraph, 4th line.

2. *Authors should have described their measure of religiosity more clearly.*

Response: We have now described our intrinsic religiosity measure more clearly, and this description can be found in the text on p. 8, third paragraph, lines 8–12.

Reviewer #2
1. *Investigators overstated their conclusions.*

Response: We have now revised our conclusions so that they are now more conservative and less far-reaching. The changes can be found in the text on p. 12, 1st paragraph, lines 4–10.

C. Never be defensive in responses to reviewers' comments, no matter how insulting or inaccurate those comments are. Even if the authors are absolutely in the right and the reviewer is dead wrong, the authors should admit that the problem was their fault because they were not clear enough. The explanation should then be given, and location in the text provided where changes were made, all in a friendly and humble tone.

> Never be defensive in responses to reviewers' comments, no matter how insulting or inaccurate those comments are.

D. Authors should probably respond to at least 80 percent of the reviewers' concerns. If there are lots of reviewers' concerns, and the authors respond "strongly" (i.e., did what reviewers suggested and described this in detail) to 80 percent of the concerns, then they can probably ignore the remaining 20 percent—particularly those that are difficult to address. Reviewers' concerns can be quite idiosyncratic, especially when it comes to R/S-health research. Don't ignore concerns, however, if the editor requests that the authors address the concern or if more than one reviewer has the same concern.

E. The letter of response described under B above should be written so that it can stand alone. In other words, after reading the letter, the editor should have a good idea of how the authors changed the paper, where in the paper the changes were made, and whether to accept or reject the paper based on the information provided.

RESPONDING TO A REJECTION

If a journal rejects the paper, then authors should respond as follows:

A. Deal with the pain of the rejection. This is not easy for anyone (including this author!).

B. As difficult as it may be, read the comments made by reviewers.

C. Respond to reviewers' concerns by altering the paper. *This applies only to changes that are easy and quick to make.* As noted above, reviewers' comments are often very idiosyncratic when reviewing research on R/S and health. The fact is that people often have strong views about religion, either for it or against it, which also applies to reviewers. The next set of another journal reviewers' concerns when submitting to another journal could be entirely different from the concerns of previous reviewers, so why make the changes unless they contribute to the likely acceptance of the article?

D. Resubmit quickly to another journal. The pain of the rejection will subside considerably once the paper is again under review and the hope of publication is revived.

> The pain of the rejection will subside considerably once the paper is again under review and the hope of publication is revived.

RECOMMENDED JOURNALS

Below is a list of recommended journals for R/S-health researchers. I present them in order from the most to the least prestigious (based on their "impact factor"[IF]).[6] I also indicate those that are particularly receptive to research on R/S-health (*somewhat, **moderately, ***highly). Researchers should always shoot a little high when submitting to journals, since there is always a chance that the journal reviewers will like the paper. Shooting excessively high, however, is a waste of time.

General Medical

TIER 1

New England Journal of Medicine (IF = 47.050)
Lancet (IF = 30.758)
Journal of the American Medical Association (IF = 28.899)
Annals of Internal Medicine (IF = 16.552)

TIER 2

Archives of Internal Medicine (IF = 9.813) *
American Journal of Medicine (IF = 4.466) *
Journal of General Internal Medicine (IF = 2.654) *
Academic Medicine (IF = 2.338)
Journal of Family Practice (IF = 1.426)*

TIER 3

Southern Medical Journal (IF = 0.924)***
International Journal of Psychiatry in Medicine
    (IF = 0.909)***

Specialty Journals

TIER 1

American Journal of Psychiatry (IF = 12.522)*
Journal of Consulting & Clinical Psychology (IF = 4.461)*
American Journal of Epidemiology (IF = 5.589)*
American Journal of Public Health (IF = 4.371)*
American Heart Journal (IF = 4.357)

TIER 2

Journal of the American Geriatrics Society (IF = 3.656)**
American Journal of Geriatric Psychiatry (IF = 3.535)**
Annals of Behavioral Medicine (IF = 3.145)**
Journals of Gerontology, biological (IF = 3.083)*
Journals of Gerontology, psychology (IF = 2.094)*

TIER 3

Gerontologist (IF = 1.880)**
Journal of Nervous & Mental Disease (IF = 1.771)***

Research on Aging (IF = 1.474)*
American Journal of Nursing (IF = 0.685)

Sociology of Religion / Psychology of Religion / Pastoral Care Journals
TIER 1
Journal for the Scientific Study of Religion (IF = 0.929)***
Mental Health, Religion and Culture (IF = 0.545)***

TIER 2
Journal of Religion and Health (IF = 0.320)***
Journal of Psychology and Theology (IF = 0.311)***
International Journal of the Psychology of Religion (IF = not rated [NR])***
Journal of Psychology and Christianity (IF = NR)***
Journal on Jewish Aging (IF = NR)***
Journal of Muslim Mental Health (IF = NR)***
Religions (online Open Access) (IF = NR, too recent)***

TIER 3
Journal of Religion, Spirituality & Aging (IF = 0.195)***
Journal of Pastoral Care (IF = NR)***
Journal of Healthcare Chaplaincy (IF = NR)***

ONLINE PUBLISHING (FOR A FEE)

Several online journals publish research-based papers for a fee. The advantage of these journals is that the peer-review process is less rigorous, articles can get published more quickly by this route, and when published as Open Access, the entire article is usually available for free in PDF form to anyone who wants to download it. For example, BiomedCentral.com has literally hundreds of open access online journals in virtually every field of medicine and science. The fees, however, are pretty steep. For example, if an article is accepted for publication in BMC Psychiatry (IF = 1.832), the "article processing charge" is $1,760 (similar for most of the online journals published by this group). Another online publishing group is PloS ONE, which also publishes academic jour-

> **Several online journals publish research-based papers for a fee.**

nals in dozens of areas in medicine and science and claims a 69 percent acceptance rate. It is also Open Access and has a publishing fee of $1,350 per article. I'm not sure whether grant funds can be used to pay for publishing, but these fees could certainly be paid out of departmental funds or flexible-fund accounts. The journal names sound quite legitimate, and when a citation appears on the researcher's CV it may be difficult to distinguish from articles published in regular mainstream print journals.

OTHER WAYS OF PUBLISHING RESEARCH

If researchers are having difficulty publishing their original research through conventional peer-review routes, they can always publish their findings in a book chapter, a book, or even on a personal website.

Book Chapter

> If researchers are having difficulty publishing their original research through conventional peer-review routes, they can always publish their findings in a book chapter, a book, or even on a personal website.

When asked to contribute a chapter to a book, the researcher is free to report original data and discuss it as part of the overall topic. Doing so accomplishes several goals besides circumventing the usual peer-review process. First, it documents the research finding and attributes it to the researcher. Second, the researcher can then cite the book chapter in other articles published in the mainstream literature or even in a grant application (if the research findings are from pilot data).

Book

If the researcher is not fortunate enough to have colleagues who ask him to write a chapter in a book, then what? He could decide to publish the research in his own book. There is no peer-review process for books[7] and there is no limitation on the length of the manuscript (as with a research article). There is only one caveat. The researcher needs to find a publisher willing to publish the book. Finding a willing publisher can be a challenging task these days when people are not buying books as much as in previous years. Publishers are now much more selective in what they publish. Even if the researcher cannot find a publisher to publish his book, however, all is not lost. With a little cash, he can simply publish the book himself.

Self-Published Book

Many publishing companies now exist that allow individuals to self-publish a book for a fee. A researcher can conduct a study, write up the findings, and publish those findings in a book—without ever having to deal with peer reviewers, write book chapters for colleagues, or woo conventional book publishers into accepting the manuscript. The self-published book will be literally impossible to distinguish from other books published by conventional routes. Publishing companies involved in self-publishing will create a nice book cover, edit, and print the manuscript in paperback or hardcover in easy-to-read type, and will even market the book through online distributors such as Barnes & Noble or Amazon. Of course, there is a fee, which can range from three hundred dollars to over five thousand dollars depending on the services desired. Examples of self-publishing groups include Publish America, Outskirts Press, and many others. However, I suggest the author be cautious when choosing a self-publishing group, since they may vary in their reputation and some are difficult to work with; it pays to do some homework when selecting from the many companies out there. Self-published e-books[8] are also becoming quite popular. Amazon.com allows authors to publish, market, and sell their own e-books that can be read using Kindle, iPad, and other e-readers.

Personal Website

What if the researcher is just out of graduate school and has no money, no financial support, and may be burdened with loans to pay off? The situation is still not hopeless. She can simply create a website for free and place the unpublished research report on the site. For example, Yola.com allows anyone with access to the Internet to create a personal website for free (there are others too, such as Wix.com and Webs.com). Once the website is created, the researcher can upload a PDF of the research report onto the site, which will be available for anyone to read, download, and print. Furthermore, the researcher can cite the title of the research report and the website address when writing articles (or even research grants) related to the topic.

In general, all researchers should consider developing a website that highlights their published and unpublished research so that it will be accessible to others. They should also consider blogging on established websites such as *Psychology Today* in order to get the word out about good, interesting research they and others have done in spirituality and health. Publicity departments at universities and hospitals (i.e., media relations, or office of news and communications) are also good vehicles for publicizing research so that it gets into mainstream print and online media.

SUMMARY AND CONCLUSIONS

In this chapter I discussed why publishing is important for R/S-health researchers, provided resources on learning how to write, discussed how to structure a research report, described how to submit a research report to a journal, provided detailed instructions on how to respond to journal reviewers, recommended what to do when a paper is rejected, suggested academic journals to publish in, described how to publish via online Open Access journals, and suggested other ways of getting research findings into print and accessible to others (book chapter, traditional book, self-published book, or personal website). No matter how much effort researchers put into a study (designing it, funding it, executing it, and analyzing results), it will be for naught unless the research is published somewhere. Getting research published is a skill that can and must be learned.

Funding for Research

FINDING MONEY TO support research is essential for carrying out successful projects that provide new discoveries and advance scientific knowledge. Funding support frees up investigators' time to conduct research and allows them to hire the right people for a research team with the expertise necessary to execute a research project. The purpose of this chapter is to give religion/spirituality (R/S)–health researchers ideas on where to acquire resources to support their research. First, I address the challenge of obtaining outside funding for R/S-health research. I then discuss ten strategies for obtaining resources to conduct research, running the gamut from doing research without funding to obtaining funding from NIH, private foundations, individual donors, and other sources.

CHALLENGES

Obtaining outside support for R/S-health research can be a challenge. In this section I discuss what it takes to secure outside grant support to conduct research. In order to obtain successful funding, researchers need a novel research question and solid design, a record of prior successes conducting research, affiliation with an academic institution, a research team and optimum research environment, promising pilot data, connections with influential people in the funding agency, considerable time, lots of energy, and tolerance for rejection. Yes, it is a tall order.

> In order to obtain successful funding, researchers need a novel research question and solid design, a record of prior successes conducting research, affiliation with an academic institution, a research team and optimum research environment, promising pilot data, connections with influential people in the funding agency, considerable time, lots of energy, and tolerance for rejection.

First, in order to get a research grant from a government agency (National Institutes of Health [NIH], Centers for Disease Control [CDC], etc.) or a private foundation (Templeton, Fetzer, etc.), it requires not only an interesting, novel, relevant, and feasible research question, but also a convincing record of success in conducting research, publishing the findings, and often, prior grants. NIH does offer research grants for new investigators, but these grants are highly competitive and most require evidence of prior success in research (e.g., first-author publications of original research). Many junior investigators obtain this research experience by doing a postdoctoral fellowship, when they focus on learning research methods and applying them, often working on the team of a senior researcher who may also serve as a mentor.[1]

Second, getting a grant usually requires that the researcher be affiliated with an academic institution (usually a research university) as a full-time faculty member. This is not always true, especially for foundation grants. The NIH and other government agencies also have a number of mechanisms for obtaining support for industry-related research and even for small private businesses involved in research related to public health. Nevertheless, most principal investigators who submit such grants usually have an academic affiliation. The reason is that the academic institution takes responsibility for monitoring the grant and for the research that the grant supports.

Third, success at obtaining research grants usually requires the existence of a research team and an environment that is conducive for research. The research team needs to be in place at the time of submission even before the grant is received. By "research team," I mean a principal investigator and co-investigators at the same institution who contribute expertise to the project, a statistician, consultants with expertise from outside the institution, and a variety of research personnel (a project coordinator, research assistants, data technicians, interviewers, etc.). Likewise, the environment must be ideal for conducting the research—that is, computer facilities, office space, ready access to subjects, ready access to other researchers, and so forth. In many ways, the entire system is set up in a way that supports ongoing research by investigative teams that have already been funded (and after the discovery of interesting new findings on which investigators are now building). The research team and environment need to be established and just waiting to begin the research that will provide the next key piece of new information to advance the field.

Fourth, successful grant applications almost always require pilot data (see Chapter 21). Pilot data are evidence from prior research, usually a study that is much smaller than the proposed study, that shows promise. Pilot data (also called "preliminary findings") provide evidence that the researcher has experience with the methodology being proposed, access to the necessary populations, able to successfully manage a research project (even though small) through to completion, and able to publish the findings. Most important, those findings must be suggestive that further research along the lines proposed in the grant is needed and likely to produce new, important information.

Fifth, getting a grant requires connections—in other words, whom do you know? Researchers need to have ongoing relationships with key individuals in the funding agency. For NIH or government-funded grants it helps to know and have a good relationship with project officers. These individuals are familiar with the agency's priorities and how to pitch a proposal. They may even be helpful in finding small pots of money that could be used to support a particular research project. Likewise, knowing and having a good relationship with foundation officers or

> The process of thinking through, writing up, and submitting a grant application with a chance of getting funded takes at least twelve months on average and may take longer these days.

foundation board members is also helpful in securing successful grants from these foundations.

Sixth, successful grants require time and energy. The process of thinking through, writing up, and submitting a fundable grant application takes at least twelve months on average and may take longer these days.[2] That time must be taken away from other job duties for which the investigator may be responsible. Therefore, it will take long hours, often hours that are usually spent outside the office with family or friends, requiring considerable commitment on the researcher's part as well as physical and emotional stamina.

Finally, to get a grant funded, the researcher needs considerable tolerance for rejection. Even with a good research idea, experience conducting research, prior peer-reviewed publications, academic affiliation, a research team and ideal research environment, promising pilot data, personal connections, and a lot of time and energy, grant applications are often not funded the first time around. Those who received support from NIH are almost always rejected the first time and require resubmission. Before the two-strike rule at NIH became effective, successful grants almost always required several prior submissions.

NIH grant applicants now have only one chance to revise their proposal in response to reviewers' concerns and then resubmit for a final decision. The Templeton Foundation, on the other hand, allows only one submission, which is either accepted or rejected. NIH and even many private foundations such as Templeton fund only around 10 to 15 percent of grants submitted, and many of the grant applications that are not funded have fulfilled most or all of the requirements that I described above. The bottom line: getting outside grant support for research in R/S and health is not easy (not impossible, but pretty darn difficult).

> Getting outside grant support for research in R/S and health is not easy (not impossible, but pretty darn difficult).

SOURCES OF SUPPORT

The heart of this chapter involves identifying resources of support for R/S-health research. I divide this section into ten parts: (1) doing research without funding, (2) funding your own research, (3) NIH, (4) other federal government sources, (5) national health organizations, (6) industry/corporations, (7) local, community, or state grants, (8) institutional grants, (9) private foundations, and (10) individual donors.

Doing Research without Funding

Given the difficulty of obtaining outside research support, especially when just starting out in the area, most R/S-health researchers should expect to do a lot of initial research without any external funding. In fact, most published research on R/S and health has been done exactly this way. Investigators have used data from mentors' projects or existing public data sets, or surveyed their own patients (if clinicians) or the students in their classes (if teachers). Much of this research was observational in nature (responses to questionnaires) and cross-sectional, and so did not require much support. In order to do research without funding support, a person needs four things: time, data, statistical skills, and the ability to write.

> Most R/S-health researchers should expect to do a lot of initial research without any external funding. In fact, most published research on R/S and health has been done exactly this way.

Time

Since most investigators are working on jobs they are doing during the eight-hour workday from Monday through Friday, time for research needs to be taken from other places: lunch hour, late nights after family has gone to bed, weekends, holidays, vacations, and so forth.

Data

Various sources of data can be used to examine relationships between R/S and health: piggybacking on existing research of colleagues or mentors, using existing data sets (public or private), or identifying readily available sources of subjects. One of the best approaches is to piggyback onto planned or ongoing research projects by asking investigators to add a few questions on R/S involvement in one of their interviews. Adding the five-item Duke University Religion Index (see Chapter 13) to a baseline interview of a prospective study being done for other purposes can provide a rich source of longitudinal data on the effects R/S may be having on health outcomes or response to treatment. Another source of data is existing data sets, either those available to the public or private data sets with the permission of the primary investigator who owns the data. The one caveat is that the data sets need measures of R/S in them. Table 20.1 gives sources of public data sets and websites from which these data can be downloaded. Finally, original data can be collected from students (as part of their training on research methods), patients, or anyone who is willing to fill out a questionnaire (over the Internet, people waiting around at airports, etc.).

Statistical Skills

Without resources to pay a statistician, researchers must be able to analyze their own data, which requires basic knowledge about statistics, how to set up statistical analyses (correlations, chi-square, analysis of variance, regression), and how to run statistical programs such as SAS, SPSS, STATA, Epi-Info, and so on. Almost all colleges and universities have onsite classes or online courses on statistics, and it is worth the researcher's time to take one of these courses. Such exposure also provides some understanding of statistical language that one needs to use when writing up the results for publication (see chapters 14 and 15).

Ability to Write

Even if the researcher finds the time, obtains a data set, and learns how to analyze the data, he must also learn to write up the findings in a format and style that allows publication in an academic journal (see Chapter 19). Scientific writing is a skill that can be learned and must be practiced by writing and writing and writing. Such a skill is essential if R/S-health researchers expect to get their research findings published in the scientific literature. All four—time, data, statistical skills, and writing ability—are needed if an individual wants to do research without funding support (and they are also necessary for obtaining funding support).

TABLE 20.1.

Public Data Sets That Can Be Downloaded for Analysis

The Association of Religion Data Archives (ARDA), http://www.thearda.com/

U.S. Census Bureau (does not collect info on religion, but does provide other sources), http://www.census.gov/prod/www/religion.htm

Social Science Data on the Net (contains 156 sites that have numeric data ready to download), http://www.infochimps.com/datasets /social-science-data-on-the-net

Social Science Data Archives (contains 54 data libraries and data archives worldwide), http://www.socsciresearch.com/r6.html

Searchable Catalogues of Data (53 catalogs and lists of data from data libraries, archives), http://www.ifdo.org/scosci/clearinghouse.html

Social Science Data Sources, http://data.lib.uci.edu/ssda/datasources .html

National Archive of Computerized Data on Aging, http://www.icpsr .umich.edu/icpsrweb/NACDA/ssvd/variables?q=religion

National Center for Health Statistics Public-Use Data Files (includes NHANES, NHCS, etc.), http://www.cdc.gov/nchs/data_access /ftp_data.htm

Note: All information on number of sites or data archives were current as of the time of writing.

Funding Your Own Research

One way for researchers to financially support their research is to fund it on their own, which can be done in several different ways.

Setting Up a Research Fund

The researcher may approach her institution (usually the business office of her department) and ask that a special research fund code be set up. The researcher

> Time, data, statistical skills, and writing ability are needed if an individual wants to do research without funding support.

can then donate money or have a certain percent of her salary (10 percent) allocated to this fund, which may be used to support research—that is, pay interviewers, purchase computers, and so on. All donations are tax-deductible. The investigator may also choose to take on extra work for six months and contribute the earnings to this research fund, which could be used to support research for the next six months. Bear in mind that institutions often levy a "tax" of 10 to 15 percent on any donated contributions and may also tax money that is spent from such a research fund code (2 to 8 percent). In general, however, it is usually more cost-effective to pay for research out of such a fund code than to use private personal funds for research expenses.

> One way for researchers to financially support their research is to fund it on their own.

Setting Up a Nonprofit Foundation

An alternative to a research fund code at a university or medical center is for several investigators to set up a nonprofit research foundation completely separate from the primary institution. This foundation could then provide grants for conducting research to the investigators at their primary institution. An indirect cost rate, however, would likely have to be negotiated between the research foundation and the primary institution, which would serve as a kind of "tax" on each grant. The nonprofit might even specify that it does not allow any indirect rate to be charged to grants, as nonprofit foundations sometimes do. Conflict-of-interest issues may come into play, however, and would have to be sorted out.

Getting Family Involved

Research can also be a family affair. Investigators may convince a spouse, children, parents, or other relatives and friends to volunteer time to help run a research project. Missionaries often take their entire families to far-off places around the world to participate in mission work. The research project, too, might be considered a mission field, one that would not require travel, relocation, or pulling children out of school and separating them from their friends (who could also volunteer to work on the project).

National Institutes of Health

Table 20.2 lists various sources of external funding and Internet links for learning more about them. The NIH is the largest research funding organization in the world. In 2010 Congress appropriated $31 billion to NIH to fund research at its twenty-seven institutes and centers and their intramural and extramural research programs (plus $10.4 billion provided to NIH through the American Recovery and Reinvestment Act). In 2011 the director of NIH, Frances Collins, requested from Congress a budget of $32.1 billion.[3] Based on the latest data available in 2009, NIH gave out $3.7 billion in research grants, with a success rate of 20.6 percent for all applications and 17.6 percent for new applications. For example, the National Center for Complementary and Alternative Medicine (NCCAM) in 2009 gave out an estimated $100 million in funds for research grants, research training, research contracts, and miscellaneous kinds of extramural research activity;[4] a total of $76 million of that amount was specifically for external research grants ($22.5 million for new research grants, a 12.3 percent success rate). NCCAM is one of the institutes most receptive to grants related to R/S and health, and often R/S grants sent to other institutes are redirected to NCCAM. Unfortunately, NCCAM is not particularly interested in research focused on religion and health, and tends to favor Eastern forms of spirituality such as Buddhist-based mindfulness meditation.

NIH offers a variety of grant mechanisms that include career development awards for those within five years of their last degree (the K series provides five years of salary and research support), K99/R00 mentored "pathway to independence" grants (available to postdocs, multiyear support), small grants (R03, for young investigators, provides $50,000 in direct costs per year for two years), small research projects by students and faculty in health professional schools (R15, provides up to $100,000 direct costs per year for three years), early exploratory research grants (R21, provides $137,500 direct costs per year for two years), planning grants (R34, provides $150,000 direct costs per year up to three years for planning large projects), and the classic investigator-initiated grant (R01, provides $250,000 to $500,000 direct costs per year for three to five years, and is renewable).[5] NIH also provides grants for conferences or scientific meetings (R13), for small-business innovative research or technology (R41–R44), and for large research programs or centers (P series).

All of these grants are highly competitive. In 2009, for new grants, NCCAM funded 15.6 percent of R01s, 15.4 percent of R15s, and 10.7 percent of R21s (12.3 percent overall); NIA (National Institute on Aging) funded 16.7 percent of R01s, 7.2 percent of R03s, and 10.8 percent of R21s (14.7 percent overall); and NINR (National Institute of Nursing Research) funded 33.9 percent of R01s, 11.4 percent of R03s, and 10.6 percent of R21s (19.8 percent overall).[6] NCCAM, NIA, and NINR are the institutes *most* receptive to R/S grants.

TABLE 20.2.
Locating Sources of External Funding

NIH Office of Extramural Research, http://grants.nih.gov/grants/oer.htm (website contains basic information on NIH sources of funding) (free)
NIH Guide Archives, http://grants.nih.gov/grants/guide/index.html (website provides NIH program announcements and requests for proposals) (free)
Community of Science, http://fundingopps.cos.com (website provides a search of all nonfederal grants in the world; paid subscription; institutional access only)
Grantsnet, http://www.grantsnet.org (similar to Community of Science, but may pick up additional funding sources; free)
Illinois Researcher Information Service (IRIS), http://www.library.illinois.edu/iris/ (comprehensive search engine for grants; paid subscription)
GrantSelect, http://www.grantselect.com (comprehensive search engine for grants; paid subscription)
Foundation Center, http://fdncenter.org (comprehensive source of information on foundations and corporate giving programs; paid subscription to search Foundation Directory for grants)
Social Science Data on the Net (contains 156 sites that have numeric data ready to download), http://3stages.org/c/es2.cgi?search=getdata&file=/data/data.html&print=notitle&header=/header/data.header

Other Federal Government Sources

Other federal government sources of research support include the Centers for Disease Control (CDC), Centers for Medicare and Medicaid Services (CMS), and the Veterans Administration (VA). The CDC usually funds disease prevention research, through contracts on which they receive bids.[7] Although CDC advertises its contracts, anyone can submit unsolicited proposals for accomplishing the CDC's mission ("Collaborating to create the expertise, information, and tools that people and communities need to protect their health—through health promotion, prevention of disease, injury and disability, and preparedness for new health threats"). In 2009 the CDC set aside approximately $500 million for various contracts. Like the CDC, the CMS also advertises contracts and solicits competitive bids for those contracts, and in addition, provides research grants and engages in cooperative agreements. The purpose of CMS is to "support analyses, experiments, demonstrations and pilot projects in efforts to resolve major health care financing issues and to develop innovative methods for the administration of Medicare and Medicaid."[8] Grants range from $25,000 to $1 million (average $235,000).

For those employed by the VA (five-eighths time or more), the Merit Review Award Program could be an excellent source of support for R/S-health research projects.[9] This program supports investigator-initiated clinical research of disorders and diseases of importance to the health of veterans. Only fully trained VA investigators at VA medical centers or VA-approved sites are eligible. Amounts and duration of merit review awards depend on past award history and experience of the principal investigator, and can range from two to five years at $50,000 to $150,000 per year (excluding PI salary and equipment); these awards are renewable.[10] In the fall of 2009 a total of 431 proposals were reviewed, and 112 were awarded (26 percent success rate). The VA Office of Research and Development also offers other research grants for up to four years at up to $350,000 per year for a total budget of up to $1.1 million in most cases,[11] and offers program

> NCCAM, NIA, and NINR are the institutes *most* receptive to R/S grants.

> For those employed by the VA (five-eighths time or more), the Merit Review Award Program could be an excellent source of support for R/S-health research projects.

project grants for up to $600,000 per year for a maximum of four years.[12] Furthermore, the VA has a Career Development Award (CDA) Program that provides mentored research training awards at two levels. The CDA1 is for those within two years of clinical training (residency or clinical fellowship) or receipt of PhD, and provides two years of salary support to spend 75 percent of one's time devoted to research and training. The CDA2 is for those within five years of a doctorate degree (or clinical training), and provides salary support for three to five years of research training and mentorship and up to $50,000 for conducting research.[13]

The National Science Foundation (NSF) supports research in many areas, including the social and behavioral sciences.[14] NSF is an independent federal agency that receives a budget from Congress of about $6 billion per year ($6.9 billion FY 2010) and supports about 20 percent of all federally funded science research in the United States. It receives approximately forty thousand proposals each year for research, education, and training projects, of which about 28 percent are funded. NSF has provided research grants to support R/S-health research in the past (a doctoral dissertation on religion and well-being by Christopher G. Ellison at the University of Texas, and research on religion and mortality by Robert Hummer, also at the University of Texas). Investigators can search NSF's awards database to identify current and prior research on R/S and health for a sense of the kinds of grants given and the award amounts.[15]

> NSF has provided research grants to support R/S-health research in the past.

National Health Organizations

National Health Organizations include the American Federation on Aging Research (AFAR), American Federation for AIDS Research (AmFAR), Alzheimer's Association, American Cancer Society, American Diabetes Association, March of Dimes, and many similar groups. These organizations may provide grants of $20,000 to $50,000 per year for one to three years, which could be utilized to conduct pilot studies. For example, AFAR offers one- or two-year awards for up to $100,000 total for conducting aging-related research that may lead to more long-term research funding.

Industry/Corporations

Drug companies such as Lilly or Pfizer provide grants for research, and some pharmaceutical companies have provided grants specifically to support R/S-health research or related academic activity. For example, King Pharmaceuticals in Bristol, Tennessee (the world's thirty-ninth-largest drug company), provided support for R/S and health research conducted by the late David B. Larson at the National Institute for Healthcare Research. In October 2010, however, Pfizer acquired King Pharmaceuticals, and so may not be as receptive to R/S grant applications as King was. Another example of a pharmaceutical company supporting academic activity on R/S and health is the makers of the antidepressant Lexapro in Denmark, helped to support a book project on R/S and healing by a Danish theologian. The Lilly Endowment provides many grants for support of seminaries and theological schools to educate pastors and strengthen them in their capacities for excellence in ministry. Although Lilly does not typically support health-care projects and often restricts its grants to the state of Indiana, it has given grants for R/S and health-related research in select cases.

For-profit companies may be receptive to R/S-health research proposals if for no other reason than to improve their public image. These include the R.J. Reynolds Tobacco Company, which has its headquarters in Winston-Salem, North Carolina, and the Liggett & Myers Tobacco Company, headquartered in Durham, North Carolina. The Reynolds American Foundation provides one-year grants to communities where Reynolds' employees live and work. Although some R/S-health researchers may be reluctant to seek funding from such groups, other researchers may be more open to this. Personally, my ethical standards would permit this, and such research gives these companies a chance to give back and make up for some of the harm that they have caused as a result of their products.

> For-profit companies may be receptive to R/S-health research proposals if for no other reason than to improve their public image.

Health insurance companies might also provide support, especially since they are the ones most likely to benefit from the results of R/S-health research. If indeed R/S helps to keep the population healthy, then health insurance companies would receive a financial windfall as a result (e.g., less disease and illness, less payouts for health care). Among the major health insurers are Aetna, Cigna, Kaiser, AmeriHealth, Blue Cross–Blue Shield, Humana, Nationwide Health, Partners Health Plan, and United Healthcare. Contact these organizations directly to identify grant programs or related foundations that might provide support for research.

Local, Community, or State Grants

Funding for research on R/S and health may also be obtained from local sources. For example, churches and denominational offices may support small research projects. Likewise, hospital auxiliaries have small pots of money that could be requested for R/S-health research which might involve chaplain-related research projects at the hospital level. State departments of aging, health, and emergency management may also be sources of support for pilot projects that could lead to larger sources of funding related to population health at the state level. Although the amounts of support are limited, the grant applications are not as long or complex as those for NIH, VA, or NSF.

Institutional Grants

Universities and academic medical centers may have small institutional (intramural) grants available to faculty and students that provide support for pilot work. For example, when I was a geriatric medicine fellow at Duke University Medical Center, I received a $10,000 Mellon Foundation grant (administered by Duke) that was crucial in supporting my initial research on R/S and health. Likewise, the Duke Institute for Care at End of Life has an open competition for $20,000 grants to faculty and postdoctoral fellows who wish to conduct research on end-of-life care. Many universities

> Universities and academic medical centers may have small institutional (intramural) grants available to faculty and students that provide support for pilot work.

also have NIH-funded centers that focus on aging, diabetes, or cardiovascular disease, and these centers often provide small grants of $10,000 to $20,000 for pilot work that could lead to larger NIH grants that would benefit the center and the institution. The grants office at the researcher's university should have a list of institutional grant opportunities and deadlines for submission.

Private Foundations

Private foundations are one of the best sources of support for research on R/S and health. Foundations receptive to grant applications in this area include the Retirement Research Foundation, Arthur Vining Davis Foundation, Robert Wood Johnson Foundation, Greenwall Foundation, Samueli Institute, Institute of Noetic Sciences, Nathan Cummings Foundation, and possibly the Ford, McArthur, Kellogg, and Rockefeller foundations. The Fetzer Institute does not accept unsolicited grant proposals, but rather invites individuals and organizations to create and implement the institute's own projects (which focus on supporting research on the power of love, forgiveness, and compassion).

The largest supporter of R/S and health research in the world is the John Templeton Foundation (JTF). The foundation's mission is to serve as: a "philanthropic catalyst for discoveries relating to the Big Questions of human purpose and ultimate reality. We support research on subjects ranging from complexity, evolution, and infinity to creativity, forgiveness, love, and free will."[16] With an endowment of $1.6 billion, JTF made a total of $71 million in grant payouts in 2008.[17] This compares to the entire grant payout for NCCAM in 2009 ($76 million). The average grant size awarded by JTF in 2008 was $550,000,

> The largest supporter of R/S and health research in the world is the John Templeton Foundation (JTF).

although two-thirds of the grants awarded were under $250,000. In 2008, 130 grants were awarded, from the 1,486 proposals received (8.7 percent success rate). The foundation has five core funding areas: science and the big questions, character development, freedom and free enterprise, exceptional cognitive talent and genius, and genetics. The sciences and the big questions core (the largest of the five funding areas) is composed of five sub-fields: mathematical and physical sciences, life sciences, human sciences, philosophy and theology, and science in dialogue.[18] One of JTF's funding areas (under the human sciences sub-field) is spirituality and health.[19] Sir John Templeton's grandfather was a physician, and his son Jack Templeton (and current president of the foundation) is also a physician, so it is not surprising that the foundation provides support for research on R/S and health. Given that fewer than one in ten proposals are funded, however, those grants need to be at the NIH-quality level to stand a chance at support.

JTF has two submission cycles each year.[20] First, an online funding inquiry (letter of intent [LOI]) needs to be submitted using the foundation's format; the window for those inquiries are February 1–April 15 and August 1–October 15. After reviewing the LOI, the foundation lets the grant applicant know if the foundation is interested in a full proposal. The window for the full proposal submission is June 1–September 15 and December 1–March 15. Grant applicants are notified on December 22 or June 22 if the proposal is accepted for funding or rejected. Most R/S-health researchers come to this foundation first if they are looking for support for their research.

Individual Donors

R/S-health researchers should not underestimate the possibility of support from individual donors who are excited about the area and wish to help advance the field. This is exactly how David B. Larson identified and then inspired Sir John Templeton to support research in this area. There is usually no need for extensive pilot data or long grant applications. However, an individual must go through a process to obtain support from this source. First, the researcher should be committed to doing high-quality research on R/S and health, as well as to exciting everyone else about her vision. Second, the researcher needs a thoughtful, innovative, and well-developed proposal ready to show to anyone who may be interested. Third, the researcher should develop a personal relationship with the donor, and make sure that it is genuine—way beyond simply getting that person to fund research, which is deceitful and manipulative. The researcher will likely have common interests with the donor (at least interests in R/S) that both can share openly and passionately. Fourth, the researcher should publicize her need for funding support, which may be done by writing an article in the newspaper (or a letter to the editor), talking about it on TV or radio, or describing it on a personal or a university's website. The researcher should put out the word about her research idea that could impact community health and individual well-being. The only thing holding progress up is a little funding.

Fifth, conduct a formal fund-raising campaign. The researcher may hold a dinner in a nice place, invite a dozen potential donors, give an inspiring talk at the dinner about the research and its importance, and present ideas about specific projects and the funding required for each. Better yet, the researcher may convince the development office of a university or hospital to assign a development officer to keep an eye open for donors with special interests in R/S and health who might be approached for a donation. Still better, if seed money is available, hire a professional fund-raiser to develop and execute a fund-raising plan, *but* be careful to select a fund-raiser who is personally committed to the R/S-health area, since otherwise the researcher may lose the seed money and have nothing to show for it. Finally, once a donor has been identified, get that person involved in the research. Encourage him to volunteer to perform project tasks that would utilize his skills. The fact is that the connection of R/S and health is close to the hearts of many people, and in my opinion, there is no better way to leave a legacy than to support a study that could make a real difference in people's health and spiritual lives.

SUMMARY AND CONCLUSIONS

Lack of external funding support should not stop anyone from doing R/S and health research. Much research can be done without funding or with resources provided by the researcher and those whom he knows. No doubt, it takes a lot to get external research funding. However, while it is hard to get, it is not impossible. Many sources of external funding are available, from government sources to private foundations to individual donors. The key to getting support is having an exciting research question, developing a solid proposal for addressing that question, and acquiring some encouraging pilot data (usually done without support). The investigator then needs to publicize the need for support and shop the proposal around, doing so with enthusiasm and tenacious commitment. In the next chapter, I describe how to put together a successful grant application.

> The key to getting support is having an exciting research question, developing a solid proposal for addressing that question, and acquiring some encouraging pilot data.

Writing a Grant

IN THIS CHAPTER I describe how to write a grant. Grant writing is brutal and scary business, but essential for any sustained research program. The presentation should be logical, rational, and tell a story. Sections should be clear with distinct headings. The format is similar for most funding agencies (FA), and grants can be submitted to more than one FA at a time. If the grant is returned from the FA with reviewers' comments, the researcher should read the comments carefully and respond to every one of them, altering the protocol as reviewers suggest. NIH now allows only one resubmission, and many foundations allow only the initial proposal. For this reason, the first submission must be the best one. If writing the grant has to be rushed to make a submission deadline, then slow down and wait for the next cycle.

Preliminary Steps

Several preliminary steps should be taken when preparing a grant for submission.

1. **Have an innovative research question and a solid research design** (chapters 4–8 should help with this).

2. **Be sure the applicant's time frame (for submission and execution of the research) is on the same time frame as that of the funding agency.** Funding agencies have specific deadlines for grant submissions (usually two or three times per year) and often only fund research projects for a certain time period (typically two to five years). There is no flexibility in submission deadlines.

3. **Learn about the funding agency and its priorities.** Does the funding agency support R/S and health research? Many government agencies and private foundations do not. If not, there is no reason to make the effort and pay the postage to submit a grant to them. Congress hands its funding priorities down to NIH, and therefore NIH often announces a request for proposals (RFP) in a certain research area. Private foundations likewise have priorities that are often established by the president and other officers of the foundation, and these priorities may be outlined in the foundation's charter.

4. **Prepare a one-page summary of the grant proposal** (two or three paragraphs single-spaced, 12-point type, one-inch margins throughout). In this summary include the research questions, why the research is important, the proposed research design (along with a brief description of the sample), time frame, and brief description of the budget. The summary should

capture the essence of the project. It should be easy to read and quickly understood in two minutes or less. This summary, then, will serve as the primary document for discussing the research with colleagues, co-investigators, consultants, and especially, program staff at funding agencies.

5. **Contact program staff at the funding agency and discuss the project with them.** Identify the person in charge of the particular area under which the research falls by calling the agency's general number. Find out if that person communicates by e-mail, and if so obtain their e-mail address. Contact the person via e-mail, attaching a copy of the one-page summary and schedule a time to speak with him on the phone (or arrange a personal visit if that is easy, convenient, and possible). During the contact, review the proposal briefly with the program officer and listen carefully to the feedback. Does the funding agency support research of this kind, what similar projects have the agency supported previously, and what is the level of enthusiasm for the present proposal? Maintain contact with that person while writing the grant. At NIH, the project officer's endorsement has nothing to do with the score the grant will receive from the review section, although the project officer will likely be in the room when the grant is discussed and scored (without contributing to that discussion), and so can provide feedback after the review.

6. **Review successful grant applications.** The purpose is to determine the form and structure of a grant likely to be funded, to avoid duplication, and to gauge priories of the FA. Most institutions' office of research support can acquire successful grant applications for the applicant to review. At NIH, the Freedom of Information coordinator can get copies of NIH grants (or at least parts of them) for a processing and copying fee.[1] Another source of successful grant submissions is the Research Portfolio Online Reporting Tool (RePORT), which contains key information on all NIH-funded grants.[2] For example, using the search term "religion" provides the following on relevant funded grants: the title of the grant, the abstract, the principal investigator (PI), the university receiving the grant, the fiscal year awarded, the NIH institute, and the amount of the award per year. When I did this search using the word "religion," 346 different grants came up

in the results. To acquire successful grants submitted to private foundations, contact the foundation for a list of recently funded grants and contact the PI directly.

7. **Contact the office of research support at your institution and find out whether workshops are held on developing grants, submitting grants, or identifying sources of funding.** Besides obtaining information in these areas that will be important for developing a successful grant application, attending such a seminar will provide contacts with knowledgeable people in one's institution who can serve as a resource as the grant is being developed.

8. **Find out as much as possible about the reviewers on the study section who will likely review the grant application.** For NIH, go to the Centers for Scientific Review website, which has the names and affiliations of everyone on the study section likely to review the grant. For foundations, go to their website and identify members of the board of directors, foundation staff, and advisory board (e.g., see the Templeton Foundation);[3] these are often the people who review grants submitted to these foundations. For the persons thus identified, use Google or another Internet search engine to find out information about them— their areas of interest, research focus, prior positions, and so forth. This information may help to craft the grant in a way that will be attractive to reviewers.

9. **Try to understand the reviewers' perspective.** They are intelligent, know a lot about research methods, and have a broad fund of scientific knowledge. However, they may have very little knowledge about research in religion/spirituality (R/S) and health. They are also likely to be busy clinical researchers reviewing research proposals on borrowed time, time they have taken away from their own projects. Thus, they want to quickly scan the proposal to get the general idea and then read certain sections more carefully. For this reason, give them what they want and where they want it (see grant structure below). The application should be highly focused, concise, and conceptually clear. Make the significance of the research question crystal clear, but don't overstate. Avoid jargon, especially theological jargon that is not commonly understood. Avoid abbreviations except for standard ones (reviewers get irritated when they have to search

the application to find what abbreviations stand for). Reviewers will not look up references so make sure they don't have to. The proposal should be completely self-contained within the main text (don't refer reviewers to an appendix, which may not even arrive with the application). At most, reviewers will spend two hours on an application (even the primary reviewer who has to present the proposal to the review section).

10. From the very start, **stress the significance of the study—that is, what contribution it is making to the existing body of knowledge, and how it will advance the field and alleviate human disease and suffering.** Express the significance in quantitative terms (i.e., in percentages and numbers). Show innovation and creativity, and paint a clear picture of the impact the proposed study will have in terms of creating a paradigm shift. The significance should be stated in a way that is readily apparent to those outside the field of R/S and health.

11. **Always consult a statistician early on in the course of grant writing.** As noted in chapters 14 and 15, the statistician is almost always the person with the most influence over other members of the grant review section. Therefore, don't bring a statistician onto the grant at the last moment, but rather include her from the start in the development of the study design, plan for data management, analysis plans, power calculations, and other aspects of the grant. The statistician reviewing the proposal can recognize the extent to which a statistician has been involved during the grant development process.

12. **Obtain the guidelines for writing the proposal for the particular FA and follow the rules exactly.** Failure to do so may result in the grant being returned without being reviewed or with a low-priority score. Follow carefully the instructions regarding font size, margin width, format, and content. Grammatical and spelling errors bother reviewers, because they indicate sloppiness on the grant applicant's part. The reviewers will naturally conclude that the research itself will also be done in a sloppy manner, which will adversely affect the priority score.

13. Always **leave plenty of time for preview of the grant by others and for revision of the grant in response to their comments**, which requires completing the application at least six to eight weeks before the deadline. Ask colleagues, consultants,

and experienced investigators to preview the application and give them at least two to four weeks to do so. Also allow several weeks to refine the budget and get the application through the institution's grants office. Allow time for obtaining letters of support from consultants and other key individuals controlling access to subjects or other resources. Again, if feeling rushed as the grant deadline approaches, slow down and wait for the next cycle.

14. Finally, **three key references can be of great assistance to the grant applicant:** (1) the *Grant Application Writer's Handbook,*[4] which details the process of organizing and structuring a grant application; (2) a short article published in the *Annals of Internal Medicine* that reports the results of a survey of grant reviewers on the most common errors they found in grant applications;[5] and (3) an NIH tutorial on grant writing.[6]

Having carefully considered and followed the previous fourteen steps, the grant applicant is now ready to start writing or re-revising a grant.

Grant Structure

The grant structure is essential since, as noted earlier, grant reviewers get upset if things are not where they expect them. Reviewers read dozens of similar grants and look for specific things in specific sections of the grant. If the information is not found where it belongs, the reviewers have to search the grant for that information or assume it has been left out. As irritation goes up, the applicant's priority score gets worse and worse.

I now describe each section of a grant and comment on its content, referring when appropriate to concerns mentioned by grant reviewers in the *Annals of Internal Medicine* article referred to above. Although the placement of sections in the grant application may vary depending on the particular FA, the content of those sections is pretty constant.

As I review the grant structure, bear in mind that the sections of the grant that reviewers scrutinize most carefully are the specific aims/hypotheses, the methods, the preliminary studies, and the abstract.

Abstract

The first portion of the grant that reviewers read, and which is crucial for creating a good first impression, is the abstract. In fact, this may be all that many of the reviewers who will be scoring the application read. Therefore, the abstract must engage reviewers' interest immediately. The following should be highlighted: (a) the nature of the problem, (b) the need for the research, (c) the hypotheses to be tested (specific aims), (d) the methods to be used (50 to 70 percent of the abstract), (e) the significance and relevance to public health, and (f) the unique features of the study. An NIH application abstract should be around four hundred to five hundred words (about half a page, single spaced). Sentences should be short, concise, and clear. The flow of thought should be logical and progressive. I encourage grant applicants to write the abstract early on, and then revise it throughout the grant writing process.

> The sections of the grant that reviewers scrutinize most carefully are the specific aims/hypotheses, the methods, the preliminary studies, and the abstract.

> The first portion of the grant that reviewers read, and which is crucial for creating a good first impression, is the abstract.

Research Team

Sometimes called "key personnel," the research team consists of the principal investigator (PI), two to four co-investigators, a statistician, and one to three consultants (from outside the PI's institution). A letter of support is required from each of the key personnel (except the PI). This letter describes the person's contribution and time commitment to the project, and it is often helpful if the PI writes a draft of each of these letters of support (to ensure that what is in those support letters is what is needed). Also required is a CV for each of the key personnel. NIH requires a biosketch and other support, which are presented in a specific format and limited to four pages. Research staff is not included in this section. For NIH grants, there may be more than one PI, especially if more than one institution is involved (e.g., a multisite study).

Budget and Budget Justification

Find out the maximum funding support that can be asked for under the particular funding mechanism (e.g., R03, R21) and ask for that amount. There is no credit for asking for less than the maximum. If less funds are needed to complete the research, then seek a different funding mechanism. When developing the budget, be sure that the funds requested are sufficient to cover the costs of the research, and keep in mind considerations such as inflation, yearly personnel and staff raises, vacations, holidays, sick days, and unexpected price increases for equipment. Keep a cushion of about 5 percent in the budget each year for such costs. Reviewers are almost always asked if the budget is appropriate for the proposed project, so attention to detail is important here. The budget for the project should be developed with the researcher's department business office, since people in the office know the salary levels and rules about what can and cannot be charged to a grant. The principal investigator can usually ask for 10 to 30 percent salary support, and salary support for co-investigators is typically about half of that. Somewhere between five thousand and ten thousand dollars should be included for each consultant in order to demonstrate that they are contributing substantial effort to the project.

> Find out the maximum funding support that can be asked for under the particular funding mechanism (e.g., R03, R21) and ask for that amount.

Understand the differences between direct costs (DC) and indirect costs (IDC). DC represents how much the researcher needs to complete the research project, whereas IDC represents what the researcher's institution receives for allowing the project to take place there. IDC may vary from 0 percent to 75 percent of the total DC, depending on the institution's IDC rate and what the funding agency will allow (institutions negotiate an IDC rate with NIH; private foundations set their own IDC rate).

Justify every dollar that is requested, as this helps prevent under- and overbudgeting. Provide as much detail as possible, since this is not included in the page limits for most grant applications. Follow the rules for federal grants (no administrative support, computers, etc.), although grants from private foundations (like Templeton) may allow what NIH excludes. Reviewers often focus on this section, since how well the applicant justifies expenses provides clues on how experienced the applicant is and whether the proposed project can be done within the budget requested. Describe exactly what each key personnel and member of the research staff will do and how much time it will take, all in order to justify the amount of salary support being requested. The same is true for supplies and equipment. Again, the department's business office or grant specialist can help with this.

RESOURCES AND ENVIRONMENT

The researcher needs to describe in this section the kinds of resources that are already in place to carry out the project. This includes working space for research personnel, computers and other equipment, administrative support, the availability of a biostatistics laboratory, and so forth. Matching resources should also be described in this section, including time contributed to the research project at no cost from key personnel and any funding support that the applicant's institution or other grants will provide. Matching resources are especially important for grants submitted to foundations like Templeton.

> **Matching resources are especially important for grants submitted to foundations like Templeton.**

Also include here a description of sources of subjects for the study, agreements with those who control access to those subjects (letters of support), and alternative sources of subjects if needed. The purpose of this section is to convince reviewers that the applicant's research environment is ideal for successfully carrying out the proposed study and that everything is already in place ready to begin.

RESEARCH PLAN

The research plan is the heart of the grant. There is usually a page limit for this section (six to twelve pages for NIH, ten pages for Templeton), requiring that applicants provide a brief, focused, yet sufficiently detailed description of what is being proposed.

> **The research plan is the heart of the grant.**

First Paragraph

The first paragraph should be a concise overview of the research project, and include the study design, sample size, study groups if a clinical trial, sample description if an observational study, and primary outcomes.

Specific Aims

The specific aims are the most important part of the research plan and come right after the introductory paragraph. There should be a maximum of three or four aims. *The first aim (primary research question) must sell the grant to the reviewers and FA,* and any secondary aims must be directly related to and naturally flow from the first aim (see Chapter 4). Include a two- or three-sentence description for each specific aim, and state what the researcher expects to find (i.e., a hypothesis). Be sure that the background section (coming up) justifies the hypothesis. Make the specific aims simple, clear, and short (see page W31 in the *Annals of Internal Medicine* article cited earlier). The most common complaints of reviewers regarding applicants' specific aims were that they were poorly focused, underdeveloped, or overly ambitious.

> The most common complaints of reviewers regarding applicants' specific aims were that they were poorly focused, underdeveloped, or overly ambitious.

Background

The background section of the research plan should provide the current state of knowledge concerning the specific aims, identify the gaps in knowledge, and show how the proposed project fills those gaps by building on previous work. The focus should be on the specific aims and the need for the proposed study. Provide a theoretical framework and describe it with a figure. The background section should tell a story that leads reviewers to conclude that the proposed study is the next logical, most important step necessary to advance knowledge in the field. Explicitly state how each point made in the background section is related to the proposed study. This section should conclude with a paragraph that summarizes the current status of the work in the field and explain how the proposed study will make the next key contribution, although don't overstate its significance. Reviewers tend to pay less attention to the background section, which should make up no more than 25 percent of the research plan. The most common complaints from reviewers about the background section are that the applicant did not justify the need for the study, provided too much extraneous information not related to the specific aims, and overstated the study's significance.

The most common complaints from reviewers about the background section are that the applicant did not justify the need for the study, provided too much extraneous information not related to the specific aims, and overstated the study's significance.

Preliminary Studies

When authors of the *Annals of Internal Medicine* article surveyed grant reviewers, 41 percent said that this grant section was the one most commonly lacking—that is, pilot data were not included or not sufficient. This section describes the research team's previous work that is directly linked to the proposed study. The research team includes the PI, co-investigators, and possibly consultants. For any work cited in this section, the names of one or more of those on the research team need to be among the authors. The applicant must convince reviewers that the research team has the experience and expertise to do the work, that the work is feasible, and that suitable groundwork for the proposed study has been done. Preliminary studies should demonstrate experience with the proposed methods (i.e., study design, intervention, assessment tools, enrollment strategies), evidence of past successes, evidence that the research team can work together, evidence of access to subjects, and evidence of ability to publish the results. Here, more is better, but only if it can help convince reviewers that the proposed project is the natural next step in the applicant's research program. The most common complaints about the preliminary studies section were that the pilot work was lacking, the pilot work was not adequately described, or no clear link to the proposed study was apparent.

The most common complaints about the preliminary studies section were that the pilot work was lacking, the pilot work was not adequately described, or no clear link to the proposed study was apparent.

Methods and Procedures

After the specific aims, this is the most important section of the grant and is considered the heart of the research plan (and should make up at least 50 percent of it). After inadequate preliminary studies, the most common criticism by reviewers of research proposals was that the methods were underdeveloped. Therefore, the applicant must describe the procedures in detail from A to Z. Every aspect of logic must be explained; make no assumptions about what reviewers might know.

Design, Setting, and Sample

State whether the study is observational (qualitative, cross-sectional, or prospective) or experimental (with or without a control group), and describe the setting in which the research will take place (the community, outpatient or inpatient, or other setting).

Describe the method of sample selection (systematic, random, through advertisements, referral, etc.). Then outline the inclusion and exclusion criteria, justifying each one as it relates to the proposed study, addressing the potential biases that may result, and explaining how those biases will be handled. This section is also a place to assure reviewers that there will be sufficient subjects to recruit from various sources to meet the targeted sample size; the best evidence for this assertion comes from previous pilot work.

Data Collection

Describe the data collection procedures in detail. Provide information about the qualifications of the interviewers, how the interviewers will be trained and retrained, and how assessments will be standardized. Describe the screening and enrollment procedures for study subjects, the method of randomization (if a clinical trial), and the baseline assessment and follow-up procedures.

Independent and Dependent Variables

Describe the control variables and independent variables and provide information on validity and reliability for each measure. Discuss alternative measures that might have been chosen and why the proposed measures were chosen over them. List all of the study variables in a table (see pages W-32 and W-33 in the *Annals of Internal Medicine* article).

Fully describe and define the primary and secondary outcomes and how they will be measured, along with information on validity and reliability of the measures. Describe the procedures to be taken to ensure that those assessing the outcome will be blinded to previous responses (in an observational study) or to treatment group (in an intervention study), and how that blinding will be maintained throughout the study.

Intervention

Describe the intervention in detail and how it will be standardized (i.e., through a manual of procedures), so that other investigators in other settings can replicate the intervention. Describe the qualifications and credentials of those delivering the intervention and the additional training that will be required. Provide a plan on how adherence to the intervention will be monitored and the quality of the intervention maintained (quality assurance plan). Describe how contamination will be measured (i.e., other treatments that those in the intervention or control groups might be receiving which may affect study outcomes), and how this contamination will be handled. The applicant must convince reviewers that the intervention is sufficiently powerful to have an effect on the outcomes, that it will be delivered in a consistent fashion, and that unblinded administration of the intervention will not lead to biases in assessment that would invalidate the study's findings.

Data Management

Provide a plan to ensure the quality of the data collected and its safety. Data management procedures should include double entry of data, regular error and validity checks, and the training of staff who handle the data.

Statistical Plan

This section should describe the approach to statistical analyses.

Obtain Statistical Help

As emphasized in chapters 14 and 15, the applicant should not write the statistical analysis section, but instead hire a statistician to do so. The statistician on the review panel will be looking for the fluent use of statistical language in this part of the grant, so be sure it is present. The statistician should describe the statistical analysis for each specific aim, with a separate section and bolded heading for each aim. The most attention should be paid to the first specific aim or primary research question. Each method of analysis chosen should be described and cited, along with alternative statistical methods and an explanation of why the present statistical approach is being taken and not the alternative ones. In observational studies, describe how confounders, mediators, and moderators will be handled (see Chapter 16). For prospective studies or clinical trials, this is also the section in which a plan for handling missing data and losses to follow-up will be described.

> The applicant should not write the statistical analysis section, but instead hire a statistician to do so.

Power Analysis

A power analysis (see definition below) will be done for the first specific aim to determine the number of subjects in the sample that are needed to detect the effects of predictor variables or interventions on the outcome. In addition, it is helpful to provide a sensitivity table that gives the power of the study to detect the effect at varying sample sizes, so that reviewers can see how failure to achieve the targeted sample size will affect the study's ability to detect significant effects.

Power is the probability of rejecting the null hypothesis (or confirming the study's hypothesis) when the real effect is equal to the predicted effect size. The standard convention is that power should be at least 80 percent or higher to detect an effect of size "X" at a significance level of 0.05. As power increases, there is an increased likelihood of detecting an effect if there really is an effect (i.e., to minimize Type II error). A power analysis, then, determines the smallest sample size necessary to detect an effect at a particular statistical level. The effect size (strength of the relationship between predictor and outcome variables, or size of an intervention's effect on the outcome compared to controls) is often the major unknown in doing a power analysis. The effect size is usually obtained either from pilot data or from published studies in the literature. The Cohen's d is one of the most common measures of effect size (especially for clinical trials),[7] and it is simply the difference between the mean of the outcome in the intervention group (M_1) and the mean of the outcome in the control group (M_2) divided by the average of the combined standard deviations of the intervention (σ_1) and control (σ_2) groups [$M_1 - M_2 / \sigma_{pooled}$, where $\sigma_{pooled} = (\sigma_1 + \sigma_2) / 2$]. The effect size can also be guessed at, although this is not the best way, unless there are no other options. A trivial effect size is a Cohen's d of < 0.1, a small effect size is 0.1–0.3, a moderate effect size is 0.3–0.5, and a large effect size is > 0.5.[8]

For example, the researcher doesn't know how many subjects need to be included in a randomized clinical trial to determine the effects of a religious intervention vs. a standard intervention on reducing depressive symptoms. Let's say the investigator hasn't any pilot data and can't locate a study in the literature that has examined the effect of a religious intervention vs. a standard intervention on depressive symptoms. Therefore, she hypothesizes (guesses) that the religious intervention will have a moderate effect on depressive symptoms compared to the standard intervention (e.g., Cohen's d = 0.40). If she wants to achieve a power of 80 percent to detect that effect size at a p-value of 0.05, then she can simply plug these numbers into a sample size calculator.[9] The result of such a calculation would be the minimal sample size needed for such a study. For this example, that minimal sample size would be 156 (78 in each group) for a one-tailed hypothesis. By "one-tailed hypothesis," I mean that the investigator is assuming that the religious intervention will be more effective than the standard intervention; if this were not assumed (i.e., the standard intervention might be more effective than the religious intervention), then she would be testing a two-tailed hypothesis, which would require a sample of 200 persons (100 in each group). If, however, she only has enough resources to recruit and conduct the clinical trial on 70 subjects (perhaps this is a pilot study), then she would have to report that the power of her study to detect a moderate effect size of 0.40 (Cohen's d) at a p-value of 0.05 is only 45 percent for a one-tailed test and 33 percent for a two-tailed test.[10] Each of these examples is called a *power analysis.*

The most common complaints by reviewers concerning the statistical analysis section were that the analytic approach was not adequately described, there was inadequate control for potential confounders, there was insufficient description of how to handle missing data and study dropouts, and for intervention studies, an intention-to-treat (vs. per-protocol) analytic strategy was not employed.

Timeline

A simple, visual timeline should be provided, where time zero indicates the beginning of the grant period, followed by a couple months for hiring and training of personnel; time for recruitment of subjects; the intervention (if a clinical trial); the follow-up (prospective study or clinical trial); and time for cleaning the data, performing the statistical analysis, and writing research papers on the results.

Final Paragraph

The research plan should end with a summary paragraph that discusses the strengths and weaknesses of the proposal, explains how the weaknesses will affect the validity of the results, and speculates about the implications of the work for advancing scientific knowledge or clinical practice. The aim of the applicant is to convince reviewers that the limitations (which are always present in every study) will not invalidate the results.

HUMAN SUBJECTS CONSIDERATIONS

Grant applications also require that applicants consider the potential risks and benefits of the research they are proposing. Before beginning, all research studies need to receive Institutional Review Board (IRB) approval to ensure that risks to subjects are minimized (although IRB approval is not usually required for a grant submission).

Risks and Dangers

The risks and dangers of a research study depend to some extent on the study design. For experimental studies or clinical trials, investigators need to consider the potential risks of the intervention. What are the side effects of the intervention? An R/S intervention might induce negative emotional reactions such as an exacerbation of guilt, fear, or sudden realization of deeply suppressed memories. What effects of subjects' medical or psychiatric condition might become evident during the study? Subjects in research examining R/S interventions in depression, posttraumatic stress disorder, or substance abuse might be at risk for suicide. They might stop their antidepressants or other medications that could adversely affect mental or physical health. Another concern might be how safe it is for subjects in the control group to go without treatment (if a no-treatment control arm). Can investigators expect subjects not to seek other treatments during the study (i.e., prayer from others, visits by ministers, or spiritual counseling)?

For observational studies, what are the risks of simply observing and not intervening in subjects who are diagnosed with severe depression, anxiety, or dangerous patterns of substance abuse? Can subjects be safely observed without intervention or referral for treatment? What do investigators do when subjects report to interviewers that they are suicidal? These kinds of risks must be considered when proposing a study, and the human subjects section of every grant prompts investigators to think about them and develop a plan to minimize those risks.

Benefits

Applicants must also describe the potential benefits that subjects (or patients more broadly) might experience as a result of their being in the study. In an intervention study, participants may receive benefits from the intervention. In observational and intervention studies, the benefit might be learning new information about predictors of disease or effectiveness of interventions. Even though subjects themselves may or may not benefit, the information learned might benefit others. Some judgment also needs to be made about whether the benefits outweigh the risks of study participation.

Plan to Minimize Risks

Applicants need to describe a plan to minimize the risks to the study's subjects. For example, in an observational study or a clinical trial involving subjects with depressive disorder, the applicant would need to come up with a suicide prevention plan that might involve screening for suicidal thoughts and then protecting subject safety and referral for treatment if certain minimal criteria are met. Intervention studies, especially those testing new drugs or new procedures, may need a data safety monitoring board (DSMB) to monitor the results of the study and to stop the clinical trial early if either dangerous side effects emerge or if results from the intervention are so effective that no further data need be collected. For clinical trials involving R/S interventions, a DSMB is usually not required. Nevertheless, all grant applications for intervention studies submitted to NIH must address whether a DSMB is needed and provide clear justification if plans for one are not included.

Inclusion of Women, Children, Minorities

All NIH/NSF grant applications must include plans to recruit women, children, and minorities into the study. If any one of these groups is not included, applicants need to justify why not. If a study concerns research questions that are clearly applicable only to adults or to the elderly, then excluding children can be justified on scientific grounds. However, justification for excluding women or minorities is much more difficult, and the applicant should usually develop a plan to include adequate numbers of women, African Americans, and Hispanics in a study. This requirement, however, does not usually apply to foundation or other nonfederal sources of funding support.

OTHER MATTERS

References

The applicant needs to include citations throughout the research plan, and a special section at the end of the grant usually lists the full references. Citations should be recent (published within the last ten years), although may include a few earlier classic studies or those that have made seminal contributions to the field. There is usually no page limit to this section, but all references must be relevant to the specific aims of the study.

Appendices

In general, applicants should avoid the use of appendices except for supporting materials such as questionnaires or intervention manuals. The grant should stand alone; all material necessary to make a decision on the application should be contained within the body of the grant. Appendices are often lost, and even if not lost, reviewers don't usually read them.

Submitting the Application

Applicants should be crystal clear about grant deadlines and know where to send the applications (both NIH and Templeton now require online application). For NIH applications, include a letter with the application that contains instructions on which NIH institute should review the grant and whether the application should be assigned to other institutes for funding. If the application is relevant to more than one NIH institute, then this should be specified and dual or triple assignment requested. The reason for doing so is that if the grant is awarded, more than one institute may be asked to fund the study, which could increase the likelihood of getting the full amount of support requested.

> Applicants should be crystal clear about grant deadlines and know where to send the applications (both NIH and Templeton now require online application).

Summary and Conclusions

Grant writing is difficult and time consuming, but necessary for sustaining a research program. Know what preliminary steps need to be taken before starting to write a grant, and follow the grant structure that the funding agency requires. Make the grant easy to read, using a plain and direct writing style with simple short sentences, and consider having a professional editor work on the proposal before submission. Give grant reviewers what they expect when they expect it (content, detail, length). Make applications easy to scan or selectively read by outlining wherever possible. Include a table of contents with page numbers, frequent subject headings, and lots of white space throughout the application. Anticipate every question and possible critique. Admit study weaknesses or limitations and describe how you will address them. The *Annals of Internal Medicine* article has a grant checklist that can help to ensure that applicants cover all the important bases when writing a grant. Finally, don't be discouraged or overwhelmed when writing a grant. Just address one piece at a time and do it well.

Final Thoughts

THE GREATEST NEED of the religion/spirituality (R/S) and health field today is for well-trained investigators in academic positions with programs of sustained research. In other words, we need talented individuals to build research teams, to design research studies, get those studies funded, execute and manage them successfully, analyze the data correctly, and publish the findings—and do this in a sustained manner over decades. The results of this research will inform educators in medicine, psychology, nursing, social work, and the allied health-care sciences, who will form the practitioners of the future.

Why are we doing this? The ultimate goal of such research is to enhance human health and improve health care so that disease is prevented, diagnosed early, and managed successfully in a holistic manner that considers physical, emotional, social, and spiritual needs. Improving our understanding of the relationship between R/S and health will partially help achieve this goal. Is there a causal relationship between R/S and health? Does R/S enhance health and promote human flourishing? What aspects of R/S do so? What aspects lead to worse health and a more restricted and inhibited life? Scientific research can help to answer these questions. Getting the training to do such high-quality research is important for those interested in contributing to this endeavor. All the medical and technological advances that science brings us will not in the end create lives that are full, happy, and meaningful. Those advances can only reverse disease and extend life, and as

> The greatest need of the religion/spirituality (R/S) and health field today is for well-trained investigators in academic positions with programs of sustained research.

> The ultimate goal of such research is to enhance human health and improve health care so that disease is prevented, diagnosed early, and managed successfully in a holistic manner that considers physical, emotional, social, and spiritual needs.

important as that is, if life is only about physical survival, then for some it may not be worth it. Consider the millions in good physical health who commit suicide because life has become a torturous, meaningless existence.

Research is rapidly increasing on the connections between R/S and health (see Figure 1.1). The qualitative reports from patients themselves and the sheer force of rational logic testify to there being some kind of R/S-health relationship. Therefore, it should not be surprising that a growing number of new investigators are now publishing in this area, from academic institutions across the United States and around the world. Many reports come from PhD dissertations of young investigators who are just beginning their academic careers. The purpose of this book has been to provide tips, suggestions, and tools to help these researchers be more successful in conducting studies on R/S and health, as well as to assist senior investigators who wish to move their research into this area. The topics covered have spanned the very basics of study design to the more technical aspects of mechanisms and statistical modeling to the challenges of getting funding support. These chapters have been sprinkled with ideas and tips that I've gathered over twenty-five years of doing R/S-health research and from analyzing and synthesizing the research of hundreds of others in two editions of the *Handbook of Religion and Health*.

> The need for specialized training in this area is underscored by the sheer complexity of the relationships between R/S and health.

The need for specialized training in this area is underscored by the sheer complexity of the relationships between R/S and health. Admittedly, many of the research findings on R/S and health are weak or only moderate in strength, and investigators do not always report the same results. However, the fact that researchers can identify *any* kind of consistent relationship here testifies to the strength of the underlying connections. Consider the following barriers that confront us in the domains of measurement, methodology, statistical analysis, relationship complexity, and practical challenges:

Measurement

1. Lack of agreement on definitions of religion and spirituality
2. Confounding and contamination of R/S measures
3. Contamination in health measures (i.e., indicators of R/S in health measures)
4. Lack of precision even in the best R/S measures
5. Failure of subjects to accurately report R/S beliefs and activities

Methodology

6. Less involvement in research studies by those who are not R/S
7. Failure in most studies to consider lifetime exposure to R/S

Statistical Analysis

8. Failure to correctly model R/S variables in their relationship to health
9. Failure to consider indirect effects of R/S through other variables

Relationship Complexity

10. Subtle effects of psychosocial factors on physiological outcomes
11. Genetic and environmental influences on R/S and health outcomes
12. Constantly changing nature of R/S and health (two moving targets)
13. Bidirectional effects of R/S and health on each other over time

Practical Challenges

14. Lack of funding to design and execute high-quality studies on R/S and health
15. Difficulty executing even well-designed studies due to necessary compromises
16. Limits of the scientific method in studying such a subjective, fluid topic

All of the above factors, and probably many others not mentioned, add variability and error to R/S predictors, control variables, mediators, and health outcomes, making it difficult to identify relationships and effects. Consequently, what we have discovered thus far is probably only the tip of the iceberg, and much, much more research is needed before any true understanding of the relationship between R/S and health is arrived at.

> **What we have discovered thus far is probably only the tip of the iceberg, and much, much more research is needed before any true understanding of the relationship between R/S and health is arrived at.**

The bottom line is that this research area is wide open and filled with opportunity for young, motivated investigators wanting to make a contribution, or for seasoned researchers willing to use their talents and experience to advance scientific knowledge in this area. So, dive in and join the group of pioneers who are pushing forward the frontiers of knowledge in this new and exciting field. There is plenty of room and plenty at stake.

Notes

Introduction

1. Information about the Duke summer research workshops can be obtained from http://www.spiritualityhealthworkshops.org/. The workshop has also been given in several other countries, including Switzerland and Australia and plans are now being made to give it in South America and Saudi Arabia.

Chapter 1—Overview of the Research

1. Pew Forum (2007). U.S. religious landscape survey. See http://religions. pewforum.org/; The Gallup Poll (2009). State of the States: Importance of Religion. See http://www.gallup.com/poll/114022/state-states-impor- tance-religion.aspx.
2. Koenig HG, McCullough ME, Larson DB (2001). *Handbook of Religion and Health*, 1st ed. New York: Oxford University Press; Koenig HG, King DE, Carson VB (2012). *Handbook of Religion and Health*, 2nd ed. New York: Oxford University Press.
3. Lopez AD, Murray CC (1998). The global burden of disease, 1990–2020. *Nature Medicine 4*, 1241–43.
4. Murray C, Lopez A (1996). *The Global Burden of Disease*. Cambridge, MA: Harvard University Press.
5. Steffens DC, Skoog I, Norton MC, Hart AD, Tschanz JT, Plassman BL, Wyse WB, Welsh-Bohmer KA, Breitner JC (2000). Prevalence of depression and its treatment in an elderly population: The Cache County Study. *Archives of General Psychiatry 57*, 601–7.
6. Bostwick JM, Pankratz VS (2000). Affective disorders and suicide risk: A re-examination. *American Journal of Psychiatry 157*, 1925–32.
7. Hawton K, van Heeringen K (2009). Suicide. *Lancet 373*(9672), 1372–81.
8. Reese, TJ (2007). No atheists in foxholes. *Washington Post*, May 31. See http://newsweek.washingtonpost.com/onfaith/panelists/thomas_j_ reese/2007/05/no_atheist_in_fox_holes.html (phrase first coined during World War II).
9. House JS, Landis KR, Umberson D (1988). Social relationships and health. *Science 241*, 540–45; Uchino BN (2009). Understanding the links between social support and physical health. *Perspectives on Psychological Science 4*(3), 236–55.
10. Rolfe, RE (2006). Social cohesion and community resilience: A multi-disci- plinary review of the literature for rural health research. See http://citese- erx.ist.psu.edu/viewdoc/download?doi=10.1.1.129.9571&rep=rep1&type=

pdf (accessed October 2, 2010); Koh HK, Cadigan RO (2008). Disaster preparedness and social capital. In Kawachi I, Subramanian SV, Kim D (eds.), *Social Capital and Health*, 273–85. New York: Springer.

Chapter 2—Strengths, Weaknesses, and Challenges

1. Strawbridge WJ, Cohen RD, Shema SJ, Kaplan GA (1997). Frequent attendance at religious services and mortality over 28 years. *American Journal of Public Health 87*, 957–61.
2. McCullough ME, Friedman HS, Enders CK, Martin LR (2009). Does devoutness delay death? Psychological investment in religion and its association with longevity in the Terman sample. *Journal of Personality and Social Psychology 97*, 866–88.
3. Hill AB (1965). The environment and disease: Association or causation? *Proceedings of the Royal Society of Medicine 58*, 1217–19.
4. Sloan RP, Bagiella E, Powell T (1999). Religion, spirituality, and medicine. *Lancet 353*(9153), 664–67; Sloan RP (2006). *Blind Faith: The Unholy Alliance of Religion and Medicine.* New York: St. Martin's Press.
5. VanderWeele TJ, Hawkley LC, Thisted RA, Cacioppo JA (2011). A marginal structural model analysis for loneliness: Implications for intervention trials and clinical practice. *Journal of Consulting and Clinical Psychology 79*(2), 225–35.

Chapter 3—A Research Agenda for the Field

1. Dew RE, Daniel SS, Koenig HG (2008). A pilot study on religiousness/spirituality and ADHD. *International Journal of Adolescent Health and Medicine 19*(4), 507–10.
2. Bowen R, Baetz M, D'Arcy C (2006). Self-rated importance of religion predicts one-year outcome of patients with panic disorder. *Depression and Anxiety 23*(5), 266–73.
3. Kaufman Y, Anaki D, Binns M, Freedan M (2007). Cognitive decline in Alzheimer's disease: Impact of spirituality, religiosity, and QOL. *Neurology 68*(18), 1509–14
4. Knoops KT, de Groot, LC, Kromhout D, Perrin AE, Moreiras-Varela O, et al. (2004). Mediterranean diet, lifestyle factors, and 10-year mortality in elderly European men and women: The HALE project. *Journal of the American Medical Association 292*, 1433–39; Khaw, KT, Wareham N, Bingham S, Welch A, Luben R, Day N (2008). Combined impact of health behaviours and mortality in men and women: The EPIC-Norfolk Prospective Population Study. *PLOS Medicine 5*(1), 39–47; Ford ES, Bergmann MM, Kroger J, Schienkiewitz A, Weikert C, Boeing H. (2009). Healthy living is the best revenge: Findings from the European prospective investigation into cancer and nutrition-Potsdam study. *Archives of Internal Medicine 169*, 1355–62; Kvaavik E, Batty GD, Ursin G, Huxley R, Gale CR (2010). Influence of individual and combined health behaviors on total and cause-specific mortality in men and women: The United Kingdom Health and Lifestyle Survey. *Archives of Internal Medicine 170*, 711–18.
5. Idler EL (1995). Religion, health, and nonphysical senses of self. *Social Forces 74*, 683–704.

6. Wachholtz AB, Pargament KI (2008). Migraines and meditation: Does spirituality matter? *Journal of Behavioral Medicine 31*(4), 351–66.

7. Koenig, HG, Cohen HJ, George LK, Hays JC, Larson, DB, Blazer DG (1997). Attendance at religious services, interleukin-6, and other biological indicators of immune function in older adults. *International Journal of Psychiatry in Medicine 27*, 233–50.

8. Masters KS, Hill RD, Kircher JC, Lensegrav Benson TL, Fallon JA (2004). Religious orientation, aging, and blood pressure reactivity to interpersonal and cognitive stressors. *Annals of Behavioral Medicine 28*(3), 171–78.

9. Epel ES, Blackburn EH, Lin J, Dhabhar FS, Adler NE, Morrow JD, Cawthon RM (2004). Accelerated telomere shortening in response to life stress. *Proceedings of the National Academy of Sciences 101*, 17312–15; Miller L, Weissman M, Gur M, Greenwald S (2002). Adult religiousness and history of childhood depression: Eleven-year follow-up study. *Journal of Nervous & Mental Disease 190*(2), 86–93.

10. Lissoni P, Messina G, Balestra A, Colciago M, Brivio F, Fumagalli L, Fumagalli G, Parolini D (2008). Efficacy of cancer chemotherapy in relation to synchronization of cortisol rhythm, immune status and psychospiritual profile in metastatic non-small cell lung cancer. *In Vivo: International Institute of Anticancer Research 22*(2), 257–62; Lissoni P, Messina G, Parolini D, Balestra A, Brivio F, Fumagalli L (2008). A spiritual approach in the treatment of cancer: Relation between faith score and response to chemotherapy in advanced non-small cell lung cancer patients. *In Vivo: International Institute of Anticancer Research 22*(5), 577–82.

11. Marucha PT, Kiecolt-Glaser JK, Favagehi M (1998). Mucosal wound healing is impaired by examination stress. *Psychosomatic Medicine 60*, 362–65; Kiecolt-Glaser JK, Marucha PT, Malarkey WB, Mercado AM, Glaser R (1996). Slowing of wound healing by psychological stress. *Lancet 346*(8984), 1194–96.

12. Oxman TE, Freeman DH, Manheimer ED (1995). Lack of social participation or religious strength and comfort as risk factors for death after cardiac surgery in the elderly. *Psychosomatic Medicine 57*, 5–15.

13. Contrada RJ, Goyal TM, Cather C, Rafalson L, Idler EL, Krause TJ (2004). Psychosocial factors in outcomes of heart surgery: The impact of religious involvement and depressive symptoms. *Health Psychology 23*(3), 227–38.

14. Catanzaro AM, Meador KG, Koenig HG, Kuchibhatla M, Clipp EC (2007). Congregational health ministries: A national study of pastors' views. *Public Health Nursing 24*(1), 6–17.

15. Frieden J (2005). Incremental changes key to health care reform. *Clinical Psychiatry News 33*(4), 86.

16. Koenig HG, Larson DB (1998). Use of hospital services, church attendance, and religious affiliation. *Southern Medical Journal 91*, 925–32.

17. Koenig HG, George LK, Titus P, Meador KG (2004). Religion, spirituality, and acute care hospitalization and long-term care use by older patients. *Archives of Internal Medicine 164*(14), 1579–85.

18. Phelps AC, Maciejewski PK, Nilsson M, Balboni TA, Wright AA, Paulk ME, Trice E, Schrag D, Peteet JR, Block SD, Prigerson HG (2009). Religious coping and use of intensive life-prolonging care near death in patients with

advanced cancer. *Journal of the American Medical Association 301*(11), 1140–47.

19. Balboni TA, Paul ME, Balboni MJ, Phelps AC, Loggers ET, Wright AA, Block SD, Lewis EF, Peteet JR, Prigerson HG (2010). Provision of spiritual care to patients with advanced cancer; Associations with medical care and quality of life near death. *Journal of Clinical Oncology 28*, 445–52.

20. King DE, Pearson WS (2003a). Religious attendance and continuity of care. *International Journal of Psychiatry in Medicine 33*, 377–89; Spiritual Assessment. Joint Commission for the Accreditation of Hospital Organizations. See http://www.jointcommission.org/standards_information/jcfaqdetails.aspx?StandardsFaqId=290&ProgramId=1 (accessed December 21, 2010).

21. Koenig HG (2007). *Spirituality in Patient Care*, 2nd ed. Philadelphia: Templeton Press.

22. Puchalski C, Ferrell B (2010). *Making Health Care Whole: Integrating Spirituality into Patient Care*. Philadelphia: Templeton Press.

23. Curlin F, Chin MH, Sellergren SA, Roach CJ, Lantos JD (2006). The association of physicians' religious characteristics with their attitudes and self-reported behaviors regarding religion and spirituality in the clinical encounter. *Medical Care 44*, 446–53.

24. Kristeller JL, Rhodes M, Cripe LD, Sheets V (2005). Oncologist Assisted Spiritual Intervention Study (OASIS): Patient acceptability and initial evidence of effects. *International Journal of Psychiatry in Medicine 35*(4), 329–47.

25. Curlin F, Chin MH, Sellergren SA, Roach CJ, Lantos JD (2006). The association of physicians' religious characteristics with their attitudes and self-reported behaviors regarding religion and spirituality in the clinical encounter. *Medical Care 44*, 446–53.

26. Cadge W, Freese J, Christakis NA (2008). The provision of hospital chaplaincy in the United States: A national overview. *Southern Medical Journal 101*, 626–30.

27. Staffing for Quality Chaplaincy Care Services: A position paper of the APC Commission on Quality in Pastoral Services. See http://www.professionalchaplains.org/uploadedFiles/pdf/ChaplainToPatientRatios.pdf (accessed December 22, 2010).

28. Vandecreek L, Siegel K, Gorey E, Brown S, Toperzer R (2001). How many chaplains per 100 inpatients? *Journal of Pastoral Care 55*, 289–301

29. Koenig HG, Hooten EG, Lindsay-Calkins E, Meador KG (2010). Spirituality in medical school curricula: Findings from a national survey. *International Journal of Psychiatry in Medicine*, 40(4), 391–98.

30. Krucoff MW, Crater SW, Gallup D, Blankenship JC, Cuffe M, Guarneri M, et al. (2005). Music, imagery, touch, and prayer as adjuncts to interventional cardiac care: The Monitoring and Actualisation of Noetic Trainings (MANTRA) II randomised study. *Lancet 366*(9481), 211–17; Benson H, Dusek JA, Sherwood JB, Lam P, Bethea CF, Carpenter W, et al. (2006). Study of the Therapeutic Effects of Intercessory Prayer (STEP) in cardiac bypass patients: A multicenter randomized trial of uncertainty and certainty of receiving intercessory prayer. *American Heart Journal 151*(4), 934–42.

Chapter 4—Identifying a Research Question

1. This is an example only. I would not encourage anyone to conduct a double-blinded intercessory prayer study to answer such a research question, since it is not a feasible one (see Chapter 3).

2. Inouye SK, Fiellin DA (2005). An evidence-based guide to writing grant proposals for clinical research. *Annals of Internal Medicine 142*, 274–82, w31–w36.

3. Be aware that there is some disagreement among experts on whether the hypothesis should be highly focused as described here, or whether it should be a broader statement of what the investigator expects to find (even broader than the specific aim).

Chapter 5—Choosing a Research Design

1. Hulley SB, Cumming SR, Browner WS, Grady DG, Newman TB (2006). *Designing Clinical Research*, 3rd ed. Philadelphia: Lippincott, Williams & Wilkins.

2. Kenny DA (1979). *Correlation and Causality*. New York: Wiley-Interscience.

3. Strictly speaking, phenomenology is more a theoretical perspective, not a method. Grounded theory (the most common approach to qualitative data analysis) refers to a method for developing theory, but one can also use ethnographic methods to achieve this, so they aren't necessarily distinct. Qualitative research also comes from a variety of theoretical perspectives that researchers take toward collecting and interpreting qualitative data, including positivism, interpretive (symbolic interactionism, phenomenology, hermeneutics), critical theory, feminism, and postmodernism. With regard to religion and health research, what we really need to know are the most common approaches for collecting qualitative data, which are in-depth interviews, field observations (participant/nonparticipant), and maybe content analysis. One of the biggest challenges that qualitative religion-health researchers face is the task of rigorously and systematically reducing the huge amount of interview and observation data usually collected. The unique strengths of qualitative research, however, are its validity, thick and detailed descriptions of process, and theory development, compared to the complementary strengths of quantitative research that are reliability, theory testing, and generalization.

Chapter 6—Selecting a Sample

1. Denzin NK, Lincoln YS (eds.) (2005). *The Sage Handbook of Qualitative Research*, 3rd ed. Thousand Oaks, CA: Sage.

2. Inclusion (and exclusion) criteria are also important for defining the sample for observational studies. For both observational and experimental studies, those criteria need to be detailed and rigorously defined.

Chapter 7—Qualitative Research

1. Taylor SJ, Bogdan R (1998). *Introduction to Qualitative Research Methods*. New York: John Wiley.

2. Denzin NK, Lincoln YS (eds.) (2005). *The Sage Handbook of Qualitative Research*, 3rd ed. Thousand Oaks, CA: Sage.

3. Streubert Speziale HJ, Carpenter DR (2003). *Qualitative Research in Nursing: Advancing the Humanistic Perspective*, 3rd ed. Philadelphia: Lippincott.

4. As I compare qualitative and quantitative methods in this chapter, I emphasize the extremes in order to distinguish the two. For example, many quantitative researchers call those who are involved in the study "participants" rather than "subjects." Furthermore, quantitative research is almost never "context" free, i.e., the interests and research questions of quantitative researchers always develop in some context. The reality is that quantitative and qualitative methods really exist on a continuum, and many individual researchers may not function at the ends of the continuum.

5. Glaser BG, Strauss A (1967). *Discovery of Grounded Theory: Strategies for Qualitative Research*. Chicago: Aldine Publishing Co.

6. Busha C, Harter SP (1980). *Research Methods in Librarianship: Techniques and Interpretations*. New York: Academic Press.

7. Taylor-Powell E, Renner M (2003). Analyzing qualitative data. For a short summary article on this topic see http://learningstore.uwex.edu/assets/pdfs/g3658-12.pdf (accessed October 16, 2010).

8. QDA Software. See http://sophia.smith.edu/~jdrisko/qdasoftw.htm (accessed January 9, 2011).

9. May C (1996). More semi than structured? Some problems with qualitative research methods. *Nurse Education Today 15*, 189–92, 191.

Chapter 8—Observational Research

1. Gallemore JL, Wilson WP, Rhoads JM (1969). The religious life of patients with affective disorders. *Diseases of the Nervous System 30*, 483–86.

2. Friedlander Y, Kark JD, Stein Y (1986). Religious orthodoxy and myocardial infarction in Jerusalem—a case-control study. *International Journal of Cardiology 10*, 33–41.

3. Visser PS, Krosnick JA, Marquette J, Curtin M (1996). Mail surveys for election forecasting? An evaluation of the Colombia Dispatch Poll. *Public Opinion Quarterly 60*, 181–227.

4. Keeter S, Kennedy C, Dimock M, Best J, Craighill P (2006). Gauging the impact of growing nonresponse on estimates from a national RDD telephone survey. *Public Opinion Quarterly 70*(5), 759–79.

5. Holbrook A, Krosnick J, Pfent A (2007). The causes and consequences of response rates in surveys by the news media and government contractor survey research firms. In Lepkowski JM, Tucker NC, Brick JM, De Leeuw ED, Japec L, Lavrakas PJ, Link MW, Sangster RL (eds.), *Advances in Telephone Survey Methodology*. New York: Wiley.

6. The researcher can also test for nonrandom attrition by predicting the odds of dropping out from baseline to follow-up. If attrition is random, it doesn't matter how many participants are lost to follow-up.

7. First MB, Spitzer RL, Gibbon M, Williams JBW (1996). *Structured Clinical Interview for DSM-IV Axis I Disorders*, Nonpatient ed. (SCID-I/NP, Version 2.0), Biometrics Research Department, New York State Psychiatric Institute, New York.

8. Keller M, Lavori P, Friedman B, Nielson E, Endicott J, McDonald-Scott P, Andreasen N. The longitudinal interval follow-up evaluation: A comprehensive method for assessing outcome in prospective longitudinal studies. *Archives of General Psychiatry 44*, 540–48.

9. Frank E, Prien RF, Jarrett RB, Keller MB, Kupfer DJ, Lavori PW, Rush AJ, Weissman MM (1991). Conceptualization and rationale for consensus definitions of terms in major depressive disorder: Remission, recovery, relapse, and recurrence. *Archives of General Psychiatry 48*, 851–55.

10. Guyatt GH, Nogradi S, Halcrow S, Singer J, Sullivan MJJ, Fallen EL (1989). Development and testing of a new measure of health status for clinical trials in heart failure. *Journal of General Internal Medicine 42*, 101–7.

11. Jaeschke R, Singer J, Guyatt GH (1989). Measurement of health status: Ascertaining the minimal clinically important difference. *Controlled Clinical Trials 10*, 407–15.

Chapter 9—Clinical Trials

1. Amberson JB, McMahon BT, Pinner M (1931). A clinical trial of sanocrysin [sodium gold-theosulfate] in pulmonary tuberculosis. *American Review of Tuberculosis 24*, 401–35.

2. Ho PM, Peterson PN, Masoudi FA (2008). Evaluating the evidence: Is there a rigid hierarchy? *Circulation 118*, 1675–84.

3. By "random," I don't mean just some principle of assignment that does not seem systematic. Rather, I mean the participant is assured of an equal probability of assignment to treatment and control group by using a random number generator, coin flip, random numbers table, or other similar method. Therefore, there can be no causal factors other than chance associated with group membership. The other important distinction to make is that this assignment has to be made on an individual basis, not randomly assigning groups (hospital A gets the treatment and hospital B gets the control).

4. Bear in mind that many researchers and statisticians would disqualify a study from being an RCT if it had a nonrandomized control group. The same applies to historical controls and withdrawal controls.

5. In nonexperimental studies, self-selection (e.g., the subject deciding whether to participate in a study) introduces what is called *selection bias*. Selection bias also arises in experimental studies if the investigator nonrandomly assigns subjects to intervention or control groups, leading to noncomparable groups.

6. Statisticians differ on recommendations here. If subjects are randomly assigned to treatment groups, there is no need to use a repeated measures analysis. Most researchers would typically only make between-subjects comparisons at posttest (while checking to make sure there were no differences at pretest). When preexisting differences do exist (especially in studies with nonrandomized concurrent controls, historical controls, or withdrawal controls), then investigators might use ANCOVA, in which pretest scores are used as a covariate to statistically equate the groups initially. This approach is sometimes said to have greater statistical power than a mixed factorial analysis, although some additional assumptions are required (e.g., homogeneous slopes of change).

7. Shen D, Lu Z (2006). Randomization in clinical trial studies. See http://www.lexjansen.com/pharmasug/2006/posters/po06.pdf (accessed October 23, 2010).

Chapter 10—Clinical Trials with Religious Interventions

1. Propst LR (1980). The comparative efficacy of religious and nonreligious imagery for the treatment of mild depression in religious individuals. *Cognitive Therapy and Research 4*, 167–78.

2. Propst LR, Ostrom R, Watkins P, Dean T, Mashburn D (1992). Comparative efficacy of religious and nonreligious cognitive-behavior therapy for the treatment of clinical depression in religious individuals. *Journal of Consulting and Clinical Psychology 60*, 94–103.

3. Azhar MZ, Varma SL (1995). Religious psychotherapy in depressive patients. *Psychotherapy & Psychosomatics 63*, 165–73.

4. Azhar MZ, Varma SL (1995). Religious psychotherapy as management of bereavement. *Acta Psychiatrica Scandinavica 91*, 233–35.

5. Azhar MZ, Varma SL, Dharap AS. (1994). Religious psychotherapy in anxiety disorder patients. *Acta Psychiatrica Scandinavica 90*, 1–3.

6. Razali SM, Aminah K, Khan UA (2002). Religious-cultural psychotherapy in the management of anxiety patients. *Transcultural Psychiatry 39*(1), 130–36.

7. Zhang Y, Young D, Lee S, Li L, Zhang H, Xiao Z, Hao W, Feng Y, Zhou H, Chang DF (2002). Chinese Taoist cognitive psychotherapy in the treatment of generalized anxiety disorder in contemporary China. *Transcultural Psychiatry 39*(1), 115–29.

8. Koenig HG, King MB, Robins C, Pearce M, Dolor R, deLeon D, Nelson B, Berk L, Bellinger D, Cohen HJ (2011). Conventional vs. religious psychotherapy for major depression in patients with chronic illness (in progress).

9. The exception here is about two dozen double-blinded intercessory prayer studies that are neither scientifically nor theologically credible (see Chapter 3).

10. Diane Becker, DSc, is a nurse and clinical trials expert who is the recipient of two Presidential Awards for her community-based clinical trials research.

11. Pennington MB (1980). *Centering Prayer: Renewing an Ancient Christian Prayer Form*. Garden City, NY: Doubleday.

12. Florell JL (1973). Crisis-intervention in orthopedic surgery: Empirical evidence of the effectiveness of a chaplain working with surgery patients. *Bulletin of the American Protestant Hospital Association 37*(2), 29–36.

13. Gartner JG, Lyons JS, Larson DB, Serkland J, Peyrot M (1990). Supplier-induced demand for pastoral care services in the general hospital: A natural experience. *Journal of Pastoral Care 44*, 266–70.

14. Iler AL, Obenshain D, Camac M (2001). The impact of daily visits from chaplains on patients with chronic obstructive pulmonary disease (COPD): A pilot study. *Chaplaincy Today 17*(1, summer), 5–11.

15. Bay PS, Beckman D, Trippi J, Gunderman R, Terry C. (2008). The effect of pastoral care services on anxiety, depression, hope, religious coping, and religious problem solving styles: A randomized controlled study. *Journal of Religion & Health 47*(1), 57–69.

16. Boelens PA, Reeves RR, Replogle W, Koenig HG (2009). A randomized trial of the effect of prayer on depression and anxiety. *International Journal of Psychiatry in Medicine 39*(4): 377–92.

17. Brown CG, Mory SC, Williams R, McClymond MJ (2010). Study of the therapeutic effects of proximal intercessory prayer (STEPP) on auditory and visual impairments in rural Mozambique. *Southern Medical Journal 103*(9), 864–69.

18. Paul-Labrador M, Polk D, Dwyer JH, Velasquez I, Nidich S, Rainforth M, et al. (2006). Effects of a randomized controlled trial of Transcendental Meditation on components of the metabolic syndrome in subjects with coronary heart disease. *Archives of Internal Medicine 166*(11), 1218–24.

19. Barnes VA, Treiber FA, Johnson MH (2004): Impact of Transcendental Meditation on ambulatory blood pressure in African-American adolescents. *American Journal of Hypertension 17*(4), 366–69.

20. Schneider RH, Alexander CN, Staggers F, Orme-Johnson DW, Rainforth M, Salerno JW, et al. (2005). A randomized controlled trial of stress reduction in African Americans treated for hypertension for over one year. *American Journal of Hypertension 18*(1), 88–98.

21. Castillo-Richmond A, Schneider RH, Alexander CN, Cook R, Myers H, Nidich S, et al. (2000). Effects of stress reduction on carotid atherosclerosis in hypertensive African Americans. *Stroke 31*(3), 568–73.

22. Davidson RJ, Kabat-Zinn J, Schumacher, J, Rosenkranz M, Muller D, Santorelli SF, Urbanowski F, Harrington A, Bonus K, Sheridan JF (2003). Alterations in brain and immune function produced by mindfulness meditation. *Psychosomatic Medicine 65*, 564–70.

23. Granath J, Ingvarsson S, von Thiele U, Lundberg U (2006). Stress management: A randomized study of cognitive behavioural therapy and yoga. *Cognitive Behavioral Therapy 35*(1), 3–10.

24. Tekur P, Singphow C, Nagendra HR, Raghuram N. (2008). Effect of short-term intensive yoga program on pain, functional disability and spinal flexibility in chronic low back pain: A randomized control study. *Journal of Alternative and Complementary Medicine 14*(6), 637–44.

Chapter 11—Definitions

1. Koenig HG, King DE, Carson VB (2012). *Handbook of Religion and Health*, 2nd ed. New York: Oxford University Press. See Chapter 2.

2. Carrette J, King R (2004). *Selling Spirituality: The Silent Takeover of Religion*. London: Routledge.

3. Sheldrake P (2007). *A Brief History of Spirituality*. Boston: Blackwell Publishing; Sheldrake P (2010). Spirituality and healthcare. *Practical Theology 3*, 367–79.

4. Figures 11.1–11.3 were originally published in the *Journal of Nervous & Mental Disease 196*(5), 349–55.

5. Koenig HG (2008). Concerns about measuring "spirituality" in research. *Journal of Nervous & Mental Disease 196*(5), 349–55.

6. Salander P (2006). Who needs the concept of "spirituality"? *Psycho-Oncology 15*(7): 647–49; Tsuang MT, Simpson JC, Koenen KC, Kremen WS, Lyons MJ (2007). Spiritual well-being and health. *Journal of Nervous and Mental Disease 195*, 673–80; Tsuang MT, Simpson JC, Tsuang MT, Simpson JC (2008).

Commentary on Koenig (2008): "Concerns about measuring 'spirituality' in research." *Journal of Nervous & Mental Disease 196*(8), 647–49; Koenig HG (2008). Concerns about measuring "spirituality" in research. *Journal of Nervous & Mental Disease 196*(5), 349–55; Krause NM (2008). *Aging in the Church: How Social Relationships Affect Health.* West Conshohocken: Templeton Foundation Press. See Introduction.

7. Brady MJ, Peterman AH, Fitchett G, Mo M, Cella D (1999). A case for including spirituality in quality of life measurement in oncology. *Psycho-Oncology 8*, 417–28.

8. Spirituality in Cancer Care: Standardized Assessment Measures. National Cancer Institute. See http://www.cancer.gov/cancertopics/pdq/supportivecare/spirituality/HealthProfessional/allpages#Section_29 (accessed November 6, 2010).

9. Cella DF, Tulsky DS, Gray G, Sarafian B, Linn E, Bonami P, et al. (1993). The Functional Assessment of Cancer Therapy Scale: Development and validation of the general measure. *Journal of Clinical Oncology 11*(3), 570–79.

10. Underwood LG, Teresi JA (2002). The daily spiritual experience scale: Development, theoretical description, reliability, exploratory factor analysis, and preliminary construct validity using health-related data. *Annals of Behavioral Medicine 24*(1), 22–33.

11. Piedmont R (1999). Does spirituality represent the sixth factor of personality? Spiritual transcendence and the five-factor model. *Journal of Personality 67*(6), 985–1013.

12. Paloutzian RF, Ellison CW (1982). Loneliness, spiritual well-being, and the quality of life. In Peplau LA, Perlman D (eds.), *Loneliness: A Sourcebook of Current Theory, Research and Therapy*, 224–34. New York: John Wiley & Sons.

Chapter 12—Measurement I

1. Glock CY, Stark R (1966). *Christian Beliefs and Anti-Semitism.* New York: Harper & Row.

2. Allport GW, Ross JM (1967). Personal religious orientation and prejudice. *Journal of Personality & Social Psychology 5*, 432–43.

3. Hays JC, Meador KG, Branch PS, George LK (2001). The Spiritual History Scale in four dimensions (SHS-4): Validity and reliability. *Gerontologist 41*(2), 239–49.

4. Krause N (1999). Religious support. In *Multidimensional Measurement of Religiousness/Spirituality for Use in Health Research: A Report of the Fetzer Institute/National Institute on Aging Workshop Group*, 57–63. Kalamazoo, MI: Fetzer Foundation. See http://www.fetzer.org/images/stories/pdf/MultidimensionalBooklet.pdf (accessed November 7, 2010).

5. Hood R (1975). The construction and preliminary validation of reported mystical experience. *Journal for the Scientific Study of Religion 14*, 29–41.

6. Underwood LG, Teresi JA (2002). The daily spiritual experience scale: Development, theoretical description, reliability, exploratory factor analysis, and preliminary construct validity using health-related data. *Annals of Behavioral Medicine 24*(1), 22–33.

7. Levin JS, Kaplan B (2010). The Sorokin Multidimensional Inventory of Love Experience (SMILE): Development, validation, and religious determi-

nants. *Review of Religious Research 42*(3), 277–93; Rosmarin DH, Pirutinsky S, Pargament KI (2010). A brief measure of core religious beliefs for use in psychiatric settings. *International Journal of Psychiatry in Medicine 41* (3), 253–61.

8. Rowatt WC, Kirkpatrick LA (2002). Two dimensions of attachment to God and their relation to affect, religiosity, and personality constructs. *Journal for the Scientific Study of Religion 41*(4), 637–51; Beck R, McDonald A (2004). Attachment to God: The Attachment to God Inventory, tests of working model correspondence, and an exploration of faith group differences. *Journal of Psychology and Theology 32*(2), 92–103.

9. Stark R, Glock C (1970). *American Piety: The Nature of Religious Commitment*. Berkeley: University of California Press.

10. King MB (1967). Measuring the religious variable: Nine proposed dimensions. *Journal for the Scientific Study of Religion 6*, 173–85.

11. Batson CD (1976). Religion as prosocial agent or double agent? *Journal for the Scientific Study of Religion 15*, 29–45, 32.

12. Koenig HG, Futterman A (1995). Religion and health outcomes: A review and synthesis of the literature. Background paper, published in proceedings of *Conference on Methodological Approaches to the Study of Religion, Aging, and Health*, sponsored by the National Institute on Aging and the Fetzer Institute. March 16–17.

13. Ben-Meir Y, Kedem P (1979). Index of religiosity of the Jewish population of Israel. *Megamot 24*, 353–62.

14. Rosmarin DH, Pargament KI, Krumrei EJ, Flannelly KJ (2009). Religious coping among Jews: development and initial validation of the JCOPE. *Journal of Clinical Psychology 65*, 670–83.

15. Islamic religiosity: Measures and mental health. (2007/2008). *Journal of Muslim Mental Health 2*(2), 109–217; *3*(1), 1–88.

16. Thorson JA (1998). Religion and anxiety: Which anxiety? Which religion? In Koenig HG (ed.), *Handbook of Religion and Mental Health*, 147–59. San Diego: Academic Press.

17. Bhushan LI (1971). Religiosity scale. *Indian Journal of Psychology 45*, 335–42.

18. Hassan MK, Khalique A (1981). Religiosity and its correlates in college students. *Journal of Psychological Researches 25*, 129–36.

19. Tarakeshwar N, Pargament KI, Mahoney A (2003). Initial development of a measure of religious coping among Hindus. *Journal of Community Psychology 31*(6), 607–28.

20. Emavardhana T, Tori CD (1997). Changes in self-concept, ego defense mechanisms, and religiosity following seven-day Vipassana meditation retreats. *Journal for the Scientific Study of Religion 36*, 194–206.

21. Granqvist P, Hagekull B (2001). Seeking security in the new age: On attachment and emotional compensation. *Journal for the Scientific Study of Religion 40*, 527–45.

Chapter 13—Measurement II

1. Idler EL, Musick MA, Ellison CG, George LK, Krause N, Ory MG, et al. (2003). Measuring multiple dimensions of religion and spirituality for

health research: Conceptual background and findings from the 1998 General Social Survey. *Research on Aging, 25*(4), 327–65.

2. Fetzer Institute can be contacted by e-mail (info@fetzer.org) or telephone (616-375-2000). A copy of the full, long version of the Multidimensional Measure of Religiousness/Spirituality (with the BMMRS and norms from GSS survey located in the back of the booklet) can be downloaded from http://www.fetzer.org/images/stories/pdf/MultidimensionalBooklet.pdf (accessed November 7, 2010).

3. Allport GW, Ross JM (1967). Personal religious orientation and prejudice. *Journal of Personality & Social Psychology 5*, 432–43.

4. Donahue MJ (1985). Intrinsic and extrinsic religiousness: Review and meta-analysis. *Journal of Personality and Social Psychology 48*, 400–419.

5. Hoge DR (1972). A validated intrinsic religious motivation scale. *Journal for the Scientific Study of Religion 11*, 369–76; Koenig HG, Smiley M, Gonzales J (1988). *Religion, Health, and Aging*, 171–87. Westport, CT: Greenwood Press.

6. Koenig HG, Meador K, Parkerson G. (1997). Religion index for psychiatric research: A 5-item measure for use in health outcome studies. *American Journal of Psychiatry 154*, 885–86.

7. Koenig HG, Bussing A (2010). The Duke Religion Index: A brief measure for use in epidemiological studies. *Religions 1*, 78–85, doi:10.3390/rel1010078.

8. Francis LJ, Stubbs T (1987). Measuring attitudes towards Christianity: From childhood to adulthood. *Personality and Individual Differences 8*, 741–43.

9. Francis LJ, Greer E, Gibson M (1991). Reliability and validity of a short measure of attitude toward Christianity among secondary school pupils in England, Scotland, and Northern Ireland. *Collected Original Resources in Education 15*(3), Fiche 2, G09.

10. Lewis CA, Cruise SM, McGuckin C, Francis LJ (2006). Temporal stability of the Francis Scale of Attitude toward Christianity among 9- to 11-year-old English children: Test-retest data over six weeks. *Social Behavior and Personality 34*(9), 1081–86.

11. Batson CD (1976). Religion as prosocial agent or double agent? *Journal for the Scientific Study of Religion 15*, 29–45, 44.

12. Paloutzian RF, Ellison CW (1982). Loneliness, spiritual well-being, and the quality of life. In Peplau LA, Perlman D (eds.), *Loneliness: A Sourcebook of Current Theory, Research and Therapy*, 224–34. New York: John Wiley & Sons.

13. Brady MJ, Peterman AH, Fitchett G, Mo M, Cella D (1999). A case for including spirituality in quality of life measurement in oncology. *Psycho-Oncology 8*, 417–28.

14. Cloninger CR, Svrakic DM, Przybeck TR (1993). A psychobiological model of temperament and character. *Archives of General Psychiatry 50*, 975–90.

15. Reed PG (1986). Developmental resources and depression in the elderly. *Nursing Research 35*(6), 368–74.

16. Hood R (1975). The construction and preliminary validation of reported mystical experience. *Journal for the Scientific Study of Religion 14*, 29–41.

17. Piedmont R (1999). Does spirituality represent the sixth factor of personality? Spiritual transcendence and the five-factor model. *Journal of Personality 67*(6): 985–1013.

18. Piedmont R (1999, 2004). Spiritual transcendence scale: Short form. See http://evergreen.loyola.edu/rpiedmont/www/stsr.htm (accessed November 8, 2010).

19. Underwood LG, Teresi JA (2002). The daily spiritual experience scale: Development, theoretical description, reliability, exploratory factor analysis, and preliminary construct validity using health-related data. *Annals of Behavioral Medicine 24*(1), 22–33.

20. Levin JS, Kaplan B (2010). The Sorokin Multidimensional Inventory of Love Experience (SMILE): Development, validation, and religious determinants. *Review of Religious Research 42*(3), 277–93.

21. Rosmarin DH, Pargament KI, Mahoney A (2009). The role of religiousness in anxiety, depression and happiness in a Jewish community sample: A preliminary investigation. *Mental Health Religion and Culture 12*(2), 97–113.

22. Rosmarin DH, Pirutinsky S, Pargament KI (2010). A brief measure of core religious beliefs for use in psychiatric settings. *International Journal of Psychiatry in Medicine*, in press.

23. Rowatt WC, Kirkpatrick LA (2002). Two dimensions of attachment to God and their relation to affect, religiosity, and personality constructs. *Journal for the Scientific Study of Religion 41*(4), 637–51.

24. Beck R, McDonald A (2004). Attachment to God: The Attachment to God Inventory, tests of working model correspondence, and an exploration of faith group differences. *Journal of Psychology and Theology 32*(2), 92–103.

25. Pargament KI, Koenig HG, Perez LM (2000). Comprehensive measure of religious coping: Development and initial validation of the RCOPE. *Journal of Clinical Psychology 56*, 519–43.

26. Pargament KI, Smith BW, Koenig HG, Perez L (1998). Patterns of positive and negative religious coping with major life stressors. *Journal for the Scientific Study of Religion 37*(4), 710–24.

27. Koenig HG, Cohen HJ, Blazer DG, Pieper C, Meador KG, Shelp F, Goli V, DiPasquale R (1992). Religious coping and depression in elderly hospitalized medically ill men. *American Journal of Psychiatry 149*, 1693–1700.

28. Ibid.

29. Krause N (1999, October). Religious support. In *Multidimensional Measurement of Religiousness/Spirituality for Use in Health Research: A report of the Fetzer Institute-National Institute on Aging working group*, 57–63. Kalamazoo, MI: Fetzer Institute; see http://www.fetzer.org/images/stories/pdf/MultidimensionalBooklet.pdf (accessed November 7, 2010).

30. Hays JC, Meador KG, Branch PS, George LK (2001). The Spiritual History Scale in four dimensions (SHS-4): Reliability and validity. *Gerontologist 42*, 239–49.

31. George LK (1999, October). Religious/spiritual history. In *Multidimensional Measurement of Religiousness/Spirituality for Use in Health Research: A Report of the Fetzer Institute-National Institute on Aging Working Group*, 65–69. Kalamazoo, MI: Fetzer Institute; see http://www.fetzer.org/images/stories/pdf/MultidimensionalBooklet.pdf (accessed November 7, 2010).

32. Ellison CE (1999, October). Religious preference. In *Multidimensional Measurement of Religiousness/Spirituality for Use in Health Research: A Report of the Fetzer Institute-National Institute on Aging Working Group*, 81–84. Kalamazoo, MI: Fetzer Institute; see http://www.fetzer.org/images/stories/pdf/MultidimensionalBooklet.pdf (accessed November 7, 2010).

33. Hill P, Hood R (1999). *Measures of Religiosity*. Birmingham, AL: Religious Education Press.

34. Hoge DR (1972). A validated intrinsic religious motivation scale. *Journal for the Scientific Study of Religion 11*, 369–76.

35. Koenig HG, Meador K, Parkerson G (1997). Religion Index for Psychiatric Research: A 5-item measure for use in health outcome studies. *American Journal of Psychiatry 154*, 885–86.

36. Koenig HG, Bussing A (2010). The Duke Religion Index: A brief measure for use in epidemiological studies. *Religions 1*, 78–85, doi:10.3390/rel1010078.

37. *Multidimensional Measurement of Religiousness/Spirituality for Use in Health Research: A Report of the Fetzer Institute-National Institute on Aging Working Group*. Kalamazoo, MI: Fetzer Institute. See http://www.fetzer.org/images/stories/pdf/MultidimensionalBooklet.pdf (accessed November 12, 2010).

38. Masters KS, Carey KB, Maisto SA, Caldwell PE, Wofe TV, Hackney HL (2009). Psychometric examination of brief multi-dimensional measure of religiousness/spirituality among college students. *International Journal for the Psychology of Religion 39*, 106–20.

39. Pargament K (2007). *Spiritually Integrated Psychotherapy: Understanding and Addressing the Sacred*. New York: Guilford Press

40. Idler EL, Boulifard DA, Labouvie E, Krause TJ, Contrada RJ, Chen YY (2009). Looking inside the black box of "attendance at services": New measures for exploring an old dimension in religion and health research. *International Journal for the Psychology of Religion 19*(1), 1–20.

41. Krause N (2002). A comprehensive strategy for developing closed-ended survey items for use in studies of older adults. *Journal of Gerontology 57B*(5), S263–S274.

Chapter 14—Statistics I

1. CDC Epi Info Version 3.5.1. Available for free download at http://wwwn.cdc.gov/epiinfo/html/downloads.htm (accessed November 27, 2010).

2. Harrell F (2010). Practical stats: Is Excel an adequate statistics package? See http://www.practicalstats.com/xlsstats/excelstats.html (accessed April 14, 2011).

3. STATA: Data Analysis and Statistical Software. See http://www.stata.com/ (accessed November 27, 2010).

4. Available at https://www.acponline.org/atpro/timssnet/products/tnt_products.cfm?action=long&primary_id=330351060.

5. A Type I error involves detecting a significant association when there is really no association present. Technically, however, the Type I error rate is that out of *all hypotheses* tested when the null hypothesis is true (e.g., there is no relationship between two variables), 5 percent will be significant due to chance alone. There is often a misunderstanding that 5 percent of *all significance tests* will be incorrect or significant in error. Assuming half of the hypotheses researchers really test in the population are true (although who knows?), this would mean that only 2.5 percent of all significant results are in error (one-half of 5 percent). Thus, if 100 statistical tests are done, then 2.5 of those tests will be significant by chance alone, not 5 as I said earlier. In contrast to Type I error, a Type II error is when a

significant relationship is present in reality, but either the sample size is not large enough, the statistical test is too insensitive, or the measures are not accurate enough for the significant effect to be detected.

6. Another issue sometimes comes up when respondents round their answers when estimating, for example, the number of days or miles to the doctor, using whole numbers more frequently than exact numbers. Because this leads to odd-looking response distributions, the tendency is often to categorize the responses into an ordinal scale. Statisticians recommend using the appropriate level of categorization at the point of data collection, e.g., providing in the questionnaire the response categories that the investigator actually plans to analyze. This can also save time and other headaches that arise when respondents are not sure what metric to use. Studies show that there is no real harm in using the original data even though some individuals are rounding and others are being more exact. One can also make the case that once a question has at least five ordinal response options, the researcher does not gain too much in precision by using the exact numbers, at least with data that are roughly normally distributed. So, as long as the researcher uses pretty equally spaced ordinal categories and uses five or more, there is not likely to be a lot of harm by recategorizing (or precategorizing).

7. MacCallum RC, Zhang S, Preacher KJ, Rucker DD (2002). On the practice of dichotomization of quantitative variables. *Psychological Methods* 7, 19–40.

8. Some researchers will include the confounders (age, gender, education, etc.) in the statistical model first and then add the R/S variable; it doesn't make much difference. However, if confounders are entered first in the model, then the researcher will not know what the uncontrolled bivariate association is between the R/S variable and the health outcome.

9. Since the term "affect" here is being used to describe relationships in observational studies, it should not be interpreted as indicating a causal relationship, which only a randomized clinical trial can do. The same applies to the word "predict" as I use it here. With regard to providing evidence toward causal inferences, the order of variable entry does not contribute much.

10. This may require adjusting the significance level (p-value) down a bit for multiple comparisons, but I think it's worth it.

11. Perneger PV (1998). What is wrong with Bonferroni adjustments? *British Medical Journal 316*, 1236.

12. Olejnik S, Li J, Supattahum S, Huberty CJ (1997). Multiple testing and statistical power with modified Bonferroni procedures. *Journal of Educational and Behavioral Statistics 22*, 389–406.

13. Kantardzic M (2003). *Data Mining: Concepts, Models, Methods, and Algorithms*. Hoboken, NJ: Wiley-Interscience, IEEE Press.

Chapter 15—Statistics II

1. Admittedly, use of terms such as "parametric" and "nonparametric" vary among statisticians. Some statisticians use the term "parametric" only to refer to tests used to analyze data from large samples where estimates of population parameters (not variables) have normal distributions, and use the term "nonparametric" to refer to tests used to analyze data

from smaller samples that have fewer assumptions about the population distribution.

2. Labovitz S (1970). The assignment of numbers to rank order categories. *American Sociological Review 35*, 515–24.

3. Myers JL, Well AD (2003). *Research Design and Statistical Analysis*, 2nd ed. Mahwah, NJ: Lawrence Erlbaum Associates.

4. Borgatta EF, Bohrnstedt GW (1980). Level of measurement: Once over again. *Sociological Methods & Research 9*(2), 147–60; Newsom JT (2011). Basic longitudinal analysis approaches for continuous and categorical variables. In Newsom JT, Jones RN, Hofer SM (eds.), *Longitudinal Data Analysis: A Practical Guide for Researchers in Aging, Health, and Social Sciences*, 144. New York: Routledge.

5. From a purist's perspective, the χ^2 statistic only tests whether there is a relationship, not the strength of the relationship, which requires a *phi contingency coefficient* or *Cramer's V*.

6. Delucchi KL (1983). The use and misuse of chi-square: Lewis and Burke revisited. *Psychological Bulletin 94*, 166–76.

7. I am using "risk factor," "exposure," and "predictor" synonymously here, and by "risk" factor, I mean a characteristic that either increases risk of a disease or is protective.

8. Cohen J (1988). *Statistical Power Analysis for the Behavioral Sciences*, 2nd ed. Hillsdale, NJ: Lawrence Erlbaum Associates.

9. A parameter coefficient or regression coefficient is also called a "B" (or "b"). This is the unstandardized regression coefficient. A parameter coefficient may also be expressed as a "beta" (or β), which is a standardized regression coefficient that allows the parameter coefficients for each covariate to be compared in size (regardless of a covariate's metric or scale of units). Further explanation of these terms is provided in the Glossary.

10. In case-control studies, the predictor is often called a "risk factor"; the risk factor can either increase risk or decrease risk (i.e., be a protective factor).

11. Cohen J, Cohen P (1983). *Applied Multiple Regression/Correlation Analysis for the Behavioral* Sciences, 2nd ed., 56. Hillsdale, NJ: Lawrence Erlbaum Associates.

12. Agresti A (2002). *Categorical Data Analysis*. New York: Wiley Interscience.

13. Card NA, Selig JP, Little T (2008). *Modeling Dyadic and Interdependent Data in the Developmental and Behavioral Sciences*. New York: Routledge Academic.

14. Newsom JT (2011). Basic longitudinal analysis approaches for continuous and categorical variables. In Newsom JT, Jones RN, Hofer SM (eds.), *Longitudinal Data Analysis: A Practical Guide for Researchers in Aging, Health, and Social Sciences*. New York: Routledge, pp. 143–180.

15. Ibid., 157.

16. I am only considering changes in a sample over time here, not examining predictors or covariates

17. Rasch G (1961). On general laws and the meaning of measurement in psychology. In Neyman J (ed.), *Proceedings of the 4th Berkeley Symposium on Mathematics, Statistics, and Probability*, 4:321–33. Berkeley: University of California Press.

18. Cook WL, Kenny DA (2005). The actor-partner interdependence model

of bidirectional effects in developmental studies. *International Journal of Behavioral Development 29*(2): 101–9.

19. Koenig HG, Cohen HJ (2002). *The Link between Religion and Health: Psycho-neuroimmunology and the Faith Factor*. New York: Oxford University Press; Koenig HG, King DE, Carson VB (2011). *Handbook of Religion and Health*, 2nd ed. New York: Oxford University Press.

20. Propst LR, Ostrom R, Watkins P, Dean T, Mashburn D. (1992). Comparative efficacy of religious and nonreligious cognitive-behavior therapy for the treatment of clinical depression in religious individuals. *Journal of Consulting and Clinical Psychology 60*, 94–103; Wachholtz AB, Pargament KI (2008). Migraines and meditation: Does spirituality matter? *Journal of Behavioral Medicine 31*(4), 351–66; Koenig HG, King MB, Robins C, Pearce M, Dolor R, deLeon D, Nelson B, Berk L, Bellinger D, Cohen HJ (2011). Conventional vs. religious psychotherapy for major depression in patients with chronic illness (in progress).

21. Application of a treatment to a single group, however, is not always considered an experiment and depends on how one defines "experiment." Technically speaking, one has to distinguish between introduction of a treatment in a single group and a true within-subjects experiment in which there is complete control over the treatment with no potential confounders (including maturation or external events that occur simultaneously). Generally, the true within-subjects experiment would involve a counterbalanced group, e.g., half of the sample (subsample A) would get the treatment first, while the other half (subsample B) serves as the control, and then treatment status is switched so that subsample B receives the treatment while subsample A serves as the control group. This would be true experimental manipulation.

22. If the outcome is a binary categorical response (e.g., sick vs. well), it doesn't make sense to adjust for baseline status since in an RCT all subjects are sick ("not recovered") at recruitment; this is not the case for continuous and ordinal outcomes (see below) where illness is being assessed using a continuous or ordinal variable and subjects are recruited with a range of values on the outcome at baseline that need to be equalized between treatment and control groups.

23. Wothke W (2010). *Introduction to Structural Equation Modeling*. See http://www.smallwaters.com/Courses%20and%20Presentations/Structural%20Equation%20Modeling/Introduction%20to%20SEM%20with%20Proc%20Calis/Introduction%20to%20SEM%20(Webinar%20Slides).pdf (accessed December 7, 2010).

24. Demidenko E (2004). *Mixed Models: Theory and Application*. New York: John Wiley & Sons.

25. Acock AC, Li F (date unknown). Latent growth curve analysis: A gentle introduction. See http://oregonstate.edu/dept/hdfs/papers/lgcgeneral.pdf (accessed December 6, 2010).

26. Includes hierarchical modeling, multilevel modeling, individual growth curve assessments, random regression models, latent growth curves, etc.

27. DanielSoper.com Statistics Calculations. See http://www.danielsoper.com/statcalc/ (accessed December 9, 2010).

28. See Chapter 20 for more in-depth discussion of power analyses with examples.

29. This is my opinion. Many statisticians would disagree with this statement

and the recommendations I've made in this section. They would empha-size the need to always involve a statistician early in the design of a study and have the oversight of a statistician throughout its execution.

Chapter 16—Confounders, Explanatory Variables, and Moderators

1. Sloan RP (2006). *Blind Faith: The Unholy Alliance of Religion and Medicine.* New York: St. Martin's Press, 96–97.
2. Not all studies show that people who attend religious services more fre-quently are physically healthier and more mobile than those who attend less frequently. For example, one of the best and longest prospective stud-ies of religious attendance and survival—Strawbridge and colleagues' twenty-eight-year follow-up of an original cohort of 5,286 persons from 1965 to 1994 in Alameda County, California—found that participants with mobility limitations were actually *more likely* to frequently attend religious services compared to those without such health problems (35.3 percent of mobility-impaired individuals attended religious services weekly vs. 24.8 percent of the nonimpaired, OR = 1.66, 95% CI 1.22–2.25). Further analy-ses revealed that despite their worse physical mobility at the start of the study, frequent attendees at religious services were 36 percent more likely to be alive after twenty-eight years of follow-up, and this effect remained after controlling for confounders such as age, gender, ethnicity, education, and religious group (RH = 0.64, 95% CI 0.53–0.77), and barely changed after controlling for baseline health conditions (see Strawbridge WJ, Cohen RD, Shema SJ, Kaplan GA [1997]. Frequent attendance at religious services and mortality over 28 years. *American Journal of Public Health 87*, 957–61).
3. "Explanatory variable" is sometimes an alternative term for "predictor," and so is not necessarily specific to mediation or suppression; here, how-ever, I use this term only to refer to variables that research and common sense suggest are on the causal pathway between predictor and outcome.
4. Baron RM, Kenny DA (1986). The moderator-mediator variable distinction in social psychological research: Conceptual, strategic and statistical con-siderations. *Journal of Personality and Social Psychology 51*, 1173–82.
5. There has been considerable discussion of the four steps that Baron and Kenny originally proposed, and there are some exceptions to these rules; that discussion, however, is beyond the present text. For a thorough and accessible update, see MacKinnon DP (2008). *Introduction to Statistical Mediation Analysis.* Mahwah, NJ: Erlbaum.
6. By splitting the sample in two or three, however, stratification loses a great deal of power and precision when exploring the nature of the interaction. Simple slope analysis uses the full sample size to explore the nature of the interaction and has several other advantages (for details, see Cohen J, Cohen P, West SG, Aiken LS [2003]. *Applied Multiple Regression/Correlation Analysis for the Behavioral Sciences*, 3rd ed. Hillsdale, NJ: Erlbaum).
7. Sloan RP, Bagiella E, Powell T (1999). Religion, spirituality, and medicine. *Lancet 353*(9153), 664–67.
8. Bagiella E, Hung V, Sloan RP (2005). Religious attendance as a predictor of survival in the EPESE cohorts. *International Journal of Epidemiology 34*, 443–51.

9. Clark KM, Friedman HS, Martin LR (1999). A longitudinal study of religiosity and mortality risk. *Journal of Health Psychology 4*, 381–91.

10. Gillum RF, King DE, Obisesan TO, Koenig HG (2008a). Frequency of attendance at religious services and mortality in a U.S. national cohort. *Annals of Epidemiology 18*(2), 124–29.

11. Of course, given the observational nature of the research in both studies above, investigators could not prove that either self-rated religiosity or religious attendance caused the greater longevity since unmeasured, poorly measured, or unknown confounders may have accounted for the relationships (as would be true for any observational study).

12. Christenfeld NJS, Sloan RP, Carroll D, Greenland S (2004). Risk factors, confounding, and the illusion of statistical control. *Psychosomatic Medicine 66*, 868–75.

13. With cross-sectional data, there is no certain way to distinguish among confounding relationships and mediational relationships. Indeed, MacKinnon and colleagues describe how one cannot statistically distinguish confounders and mediators in the absence of experimental or longitudinal data (MacKinnon DP, Krull JL, Lockwood CM [2000]. Equivalence of the mediation, confounding, and suppression effect. *Prevention Science 1*, 173–81).

14. Rothman KJ, Greenland S (1998). *Modern Epidemiology*. Philadelphia: Lippincott-Raven.

15. Christenfeld NJS, Sloan RP, Carroll D, Greenland S (2004). Risk factors, confounding, and the illusion of statistical control. *Psychosomatic Medicine 66*, 868–75.

16. Ibid., 872, 2nd column.

17. Desmond SA, Morgan KH, Kikuchi G (2010). Religious development: How (and why) does religiosity change from adolescence to young adulthood? *Sociological Perspectives 53*(92), 247–70.

18. Wink P, Dillon M (2001). Religious involvement and health outcomes in late adulthood: Findings from a longitudinal study of women and men. In Plante TG, Sherman AC (eds.) (2001). *Faith and Health: Psychological Perspectives*, 75–106. New York: Guilford Press.

19. McCullough ME, Enders CK, Brion SL, Jain A (2005). The varieties of religious development in adulthood: A longitudinal investigation of religion and rational choice. *Journal of Personality and Social Psychology 89*, 78–89.

20. As previously acknowledged, this statement and the paragraph that follows assume that all possible confounding variables have been statistically controlled and that they have been perfectly measured. To the extent that confounders are measured with error or not fully measured, then they cannot be fully controlled or their influence removed entirely from the relationship. This problem, however, is characteristic of *all* observational studies, and explains why only a randomized clinical trial can establish causality.

Chapter 17—Models and Mechanisms

1. Koenig HG, King DE, Carson VB (2012). *Handbook of Religion and Health*, 2nd ed. New York: Oxford University Press (original source for this model).

2. The original source of figures 17.1–17.3 is the *Handbook of Religion and Health*, 2nd ed. (2012).

3. Kudel I, Cotton S, Szaflarski M, Holmes WC, Tsevat J (2011). Spirituality and religiosity in patients with HIV: A test and expansion of a model. *Annals of Behavioral Medicine* 41(1), 92–103.

4. Bjorck JP, Thurman JW (2007). Negative life events, patterns of positive and negative religious coping, and psychological functioning. *Journal for the Scientific Study of Religion* 46(2), 159–67.

5. Pargament KI, Koenig HG, Tarakeshwar N, Hahn J (2001b). Religious struggle as a predictor of mortality among medically ill elderly patients: A two-year longitudinal study. *Archives of Internal Medicine* 161, 1881–85.

6. Israel S, Lerer E, Shalev I, Uzefovsky F, Riebold M, Laiba E, Bachner-Melman R, Maril A, Bornstein G, Knafo A, Ebstein RP (2009). The oxytocin receptor (OXTR) contributes to prosocial fund allocations in the dictator game and the social value orientations task. *Plos One* 20; 4(5)e5535; Ebstein RP (2006). The molecular genetic architecture of human personality: beyond self-report questionnaires. *Molecular Psychiatry* 11(5), 427–45.

7. Weiss A, Bates TC, Luciano M (2008). Happiness is a personal(ity) thing: The genetics of personality and well-being in a representative sample. *Psychological Science* 19(3), 204–10.

8. Karg K, Murmeister M, Shedden K, Sen S (2011). The serotonin transporter promoter variant (5-HTTLPR), stress, and depression meta-analysis revised: Evidence of genetic moderation. *Archives of General Psychiatry* 68(1), January 3 online version.

9. Haas BW, Mills D, Yam A, Hoeft F, Bellugi U, Reiss A (2009). Genetic influences on sociability: Heightened amygdala reactivity and event-related responses to positive social stimuli in Williams syndrome. *Journal of Neuroscience* 29, 1132–39.

10. Levinson DF (2006). The genetics of depression: A review. *Biological Psychiatry* 60(2), 84–92.

11. Browner WS, Kahn AJ, Ziv E, Reiner AP, Oshima J, Cawthon RM, Hsueh WC, Cummings SR (2004). The genetics of human longevity. *American Journal of Medicine* 117(1), 851–60.

12. Hamer D (2004). *The God Gene: How Faith Is Hardwired into Our Genes*. New York: Doubleday.

13. Caspi A, Hariri AR, Homes A, Uher R, Moffitt TE (2010). Genetic sensitivity to the environment: The case of the serotonin transporter gene and its implications for studying complex diseases and traits. *American Journal of Psychiatry* 167, 509–27.

14. Bachner-Melman R, Dina C, Zohar AH, Constantini N, Lerer E, et al. (2005). *AVPR1a* and *SLC6A4* gene polymorphisms are associated with creative dance performance. *PLoS Genetics* 1(3), e42. doi:10.1371/journal.pgen.0010042.

15. Levin JS, Wickramasekera IE, Hirschberg C (1998). Is religiousness a correlate of absorption? Implications for psychophysiology, coping, and morbidity. *Alternative Therapies in Health and Medicine* 4(6), 72–77.

16. Lorenzi C, Serretti A, Madelli L, Tubazio V, Ploia C, Smeraldi E (2005). 5-HT1A polymorphism and self-transcendence in mood disorders. *American Journal of Medical Genetics Part B* (*Neuropsychiatric Genetics*) 137B, 33–35.

17. Borg J, Andree B, Soderstrom H, Farde L, Borg J, Andree B, et al. (2003). The serotonin system and spiritual experiences. *American Journal of Psychiatry 160*(11), 1965–69.

18. Comings DE, Gonzales N, Saucier G, Johnson JP, MacMurray JP (2000). The DRD4 gene and the spiritual transcendence scale of the character temperament index. *Psychiatric Genetics 10*(4), 185–89.

19. Kendler KS, Myers J. (2009). A developmental twin study of church attendance and alcohol and nicotine consumption: A model for analyzing the changing impact of genes and environment. *American Journal of Psychiatry 166*(10), 1150–55.

20. Davis EP, Glynn LM, Dunkel C, Schetter CH, Chicz-Demet A, Sandman CA (2007). Prenatal exposure to maternal depression and cortisol influences infant temperament. *Journal of the American Academy of Child & Adolescent Psychiatry 46*, 737–46.

21. Thomas A, Chess S, Birch HG (1970). The origin of personality. *Scientific American 223*, 102–9.

22. Hall L (2010). Epigenetics, early development, and adult disease. National Institute of Environmental Health Sciences. See http://www.niehs.nih.gov/news/newsletter/2010/june/science-epigenetics.cfm (accessed November 20, 2010).

23. Hicks BM, South SC, DiRago AC, Iacono WG, McGue M (2009). Environmental adversity and increasing genetic risk for externalizing disorders. *Archives of General Psychiatry 66*(6), 640–48.

24. Sing CF, Stengard JH, Kardia SLR (2003). Genes, environment, and cardiovascular disease. *Arteriosclerosis, Thrombosis, and Vascular Biology 23*, 1190–96.

Chapter 18—Statistical Modeling

1. A path model is the result of a path analysis, which is an extension of the regression model that looks at the correlations or paths that link the different variables being analyzed. This allows the researcher to determine both the direct effects of the primary predictor on the outcome and indirect effects of the predictor on the outcome through other variables. A path model is usually depicted in a circle-and-arrow figure in which single-headed arrows indicate direction of causation.

2. Murphy PE, Ciarrocchi JW, Piedmont RL, Cheston S, Peyrot M, Fitchett G. (2000). The relation of religious belief and practices, depression, and hopelessness in persons with clinical depression. *Journal of Consulting & Clinical Psychology 68*(6), 1102–6.

3. Admittedly, there is no way to determine whether level of hope is a mediator or a confounder, since these are cross-sectional data (see Chapter 15); the hypothesis that having religious belief increases hope and hope decreases depression, however, is not unreasonable.

4. Steffen PR, Masters KS (2005). Does compassion mediate the intrinsic religion-health relationship? *Annals of Behavioral Medicine 30*(3), 217–24.

5. Clark L, Leedy S, McDonald L, Muller B, Lamb C, Mendez T, et al. (2007). Spirituality and job satisfaction among hospice interdisciplinary team members. *Journal of Palliative Medicine 10*(6), 1321–28.

6. Kogan SM, Luo Z, Murry VM, Brody GH (2005). Risk and protective factors

for substance use among African American high school dropouts. *Psychology of Addictive Behaviors 19*(4), 382–91.

7. Kudel I, Cotton S, Szaflarski M, Holmes WC, Tsevat J (2011). Spirituality and religiosity in patients with HIV: A test and expansion of a model. *Annals of Behavioral Medicine 41*(1), 92–103.

8. Koenig HG (2004). Religion, spirituality, and medicine: Research findings and implications for clinical practice. *Southern Medical Journal 97*, 1194–1200.

9. Again, by "effect" I mean to infer a hypothetical causal relationship.

10. In this particular case, EWB will probably act as a suppressor variable since the product of the indirect effects is likely to be negative (−), either suppressing a negative direct effect between RWB and depression or, as in the earlier example presented in this chapter, actually reversing the negative direct effect and converting it to a positive one.

11. This applies both to linear regression and to logistic regression (although regression coefficients need to be standardized for logistic regression).

12. MacKinnon DP (2008). *Introduction to Statistical Mediation Analysis.* Mahwah, NJ: Erlbaum.

13. MacKinnon DP, Warsi G, Dwyer JH (1995). A simulation study of mediated effect measures. *Multivariate Behavioral Research 30*, 41–62.

14. Kenny DA (2008). Mediation with dichotomous outcomes. See http://www.davidakenny.net/cm/mediate.htm.

15. Clogg C, Petkova E, Haritou A (1995). Statistical methods for comparing regression coefficients between models. *American Journal of Sociology 100*, 1261–93.

16. There appears to be some disagreement on whether the total effect is determined with or without confounders in the model. There appears to be no strict convention here. However, if the total effect is interpreted as the true nonspurious, nonmediated association between the religious predictor and the health outcome, then it must be calculated *with* confounders in the model.

17. MacKinnon DP, Krull JL, Lockwood CM (2000). Equivalence of the mediation, confounding, and suppression effect. *Prevention Science 1*, 173–81.

Chapter 19—Publishing Results

1. Strunk W, White EB (1918, 2008). *The Elements of Style.* New York: Longman.

2. Flesch R (1951). *How to Write Better.* Chicago: Science Research Associates.

3. Flesch R (1949). *The Art of Readable Writing.* New York: Harper & Row.

4. Flesch R (1964). *The ABC of Style.* New York: Harper & Row.

5. Flesch–Kincaid readability test. Wikipedia. See http://en.wikipedia.org/wiki/Flesch%E2%80%93Kincaid_readability_test (accessed December 10, 2010).

6. The impact factor (IF) of a journal is the average number of citations to articles published in that journal and is frequently used to indicate the relative importance of the journal within its field. Higher impact factors indicate more important journals. For example, the journal with the highest IF is *CA: A Cancer Journal for Clinicians* (IF = 87.925), whereas a number of journals have an IF of 0.000 (i.e., nobody ever cites papers in these journals).

7. Trade publishers typically don't send books out for peer review, but university presses and academic presses (American Psychological Association Press or American Psychiatric Association Press) often do.

8. Carnoy D (2010). How to self-publish an e-book. See http://news.cnet.com/8301-17938_105-20010547-1.html (accessed December 11, 2010).

Chapter 20—Funding for Research

1. Between 2002 and 2010 we had a one- to two-year postdoctoral research fellowship program at Duke supported by the John Templeton Foundation; however, in 2010 we closed this program and replaced it with our summer research workshops. The David B. Larson Fellowship in Health and Spirituality provides independent study fellowships (six to twelve months) involving concentrated use of the collections of the Library of Congress through full-time residency in the Library's John W. Kluge Center. The fellowship provides a monthly stipend, but does not provide research training, mentorship, or support for conducting research studies.

2. Inouye SK, Fiellin DA (2005). An evidence-based guide to writing grant proposals for clinical research. *Annals of Internal Medicine 142*, 274–82, 276.

3. NIH FY 2011 Budget Request. See http://www.nih.gov/about/director/budgetrequest/fy2011testimony.pdf (accessed November 25, 2010).

4. FY 2009 Budget, NIH, NCCAM. See http://officeofbudget.od.nih.gov/pdfs/FY08/FY08%20COMPLETED/NCCAM.pdf (accessed November 25, 2010).

5. Types of Grant Programs, Office of Extramural Research, NIH. See http://grants1.nih.gov/grants/funding/funding_program.htm (accessed November 26, 2010).

6. NIH Success Rates. See http://report.nih.gov/success_rates/index.aspx (accessed November 26, 2010).

7. Contracts—doing business with the CDC. See http://www.cdc.gov/od/pgo/funding/contracts/dobiz_main.shtm (accessed November 26, 2010).

8. Centers for Medicare and Medicaid Services (CMS) Research, Demonstrations and Evaluations. See http://www.educationmoney.com/prgm_93.779_hhs.html (accessed November 26, 2010).

9. Merit Review Program. See http://www.research.va.gov/programs/csrd/merit_review.cfm (accessed November 26, 2010).

10. VHA Handbook. Merit Review Award Program for the Biomedical Laboratory Research and Development (BLR&D) and Clinical Science Research and Development (CSR&D) services. See http://www1.va.gov/resdev/resources/policies/docs/1202_Merit_Review_Handbook_JIT.doc (accessed November 26, 2010).

11. Program announcement. HSR&D priorities for investigator-initiated research. See http://www.research.va.gov/funding/solicitations/docs/HSRD-IIR-Priorities-2011.pdf.

12. Program Project Award. See http://www.research.va.gov/funding/default.cfm (accessed November 26, 2010).

13. VA Career Development Program. See http://www.research.va.gov/funding/cdp.cfm (accessed November 26, 2010).

14. National Science Foundation: Social, Behavioral, and Economic Sciences (SBE). See http://www.nsf.gov/dir/index.jsp?org=sbe (accessed November 26, 2010).

15. NSF Award Search. See http://www.nsf.gov/awardsearch/ (accessed November 26, 2010).

16. John Templeton Foundation: Mission. See http://www.templeton.org /who-we-are/about-the-foundation/mission (accessed November 26, 2010).

17. John Templeton Foundation: Foundation at a Glance. See http://www.templeton.org/who-we-are/about-the-foundation/foundation-at-a-glance (accessed November 26, 2010).

18. John Templeton Foundation: Overview of Core Funding Areas. See http:// www.templeton.org/sites/default/files/overview-cfa_0.pdf (accessed November 26, 2010).

19. John Templeton Foundation: How Does Spirituality Promote Health. See http://www.templeton.org/what-we-fund/funding-priorities/how-does-spirituality-promote-health (accessed November 26, 2010).

20. John Templeton Foundation: Our Grant Making Process. See http:// www.templeton.org/what-we-fund/our-grantmaking-process (accessed November 26, 2010).

Chapter 21—Writing a Grant

1. NIH Freedom of Information Coordinators. See http://www.nih.gov/icd /od/foia/coord.htm (accessed November 26, 2010).

2. NIH RePORTER. See http://projectreporter.nih.gov/reporter.cfm (accessed November 26, 2010).

3. John Templeton Foundation: Who We Are. See http://www.templeton.org/ who-we-are (accessed November 26, 2010).

4. Reif-Lehrer L (2004). *Grant Application Writer's Handbook*. Sudbury, MA: Jones & Bartlett Learning.

5. Inouye SK, Fiellin DA (2005). An evidence-based guide to writing grant proposals for clinical research. *Annals of Internal Medicine 142*, 274–82.

6. NIH Grant Writing Tutorial. See http://funding.niaid.nih.gov/research-funding/grant/pages/aag.aspx (accessed November 27, 2010).

7. Cohen J (1988). *Statistical Power Analysis for the Behavioral Sciences*, 2nd ed. Hillsdale, NJ: Lawrence Erlbaum.

8. Power Analysis, Statistical Significance, & Effect Size: My Environmental Education Evaluation Research Assistant (MEERA). See University of Michigan website, http://meera.snre.umich.edu/plan-an-evaluation /plonearticlemultipage.2007-10-30.3630902539/power-analysis-statistical-significance-effect-size (accessed January 7, 2011).

9. DanielSoper.com Statistics Calculations. Free statistics calculators. See http://www.danielsoper.com/statcalc/calc47.aspx (accessed December 9, 2010).

10. Ibid., http://www.danielsoper.com/statcalc/calc49.aspx (accessed December 9, 2010).

Glossary of Technical Terms

B. An unstandardized regression coefficient from a statistical model that indicates the strength of the relationship between an independent variable and dependent variable. Let's say that the B of an independent variable (such as R/S) is 0.35 in a regression model examining a dependent variable (such as a health outcome). This means that for one unit increase in the independent variable, the dependent variable would increase by .35 units (using the original metric for the independent variable and for the dependent variable).

Beta (β). A regression coefficient from a statistical model that indicates the strength of the relationship between an independent variable and a dependent variable, where the unstandardized B coefficient is standardized using a formula based on its standard deviation so that the effect can be compared with the effects of other independent variables measured using different metrics. More specifically, the standardized beta (β) is the estimated standard deviation difference in the dependent variable (regardless of scale used to measure the dependent variable) for every one standard deviation increase on the independent variable (regardless of scale used to measure the independent variable).

Bias. A term used to describe the tendency of a researcher to want to find a particular outcome.

Bivariate. The relationship between two variables in a statistical analysis (without controlling for other variables).

Blinding. The researcher evaluating a subject's health outcome in a study does not know whether the subject is in the intervention group or the control group.

Case-control. A study design that matches controls to cases with a particular disease and then examines what is uniquely different about cases (compared to controls) that might explain why they have the particular disease.

Categorical variable. A variable or subject characteristic that is measured in terms of categories which cannot be ranked as higher or lower than one another (e.g., race, gender). Also called a *nominal variable.*

Causality. The establishing of whether one variable or characteristic of a subject (independent variable) causes or results in changes of another characteristic (dependent variable).

Cognitive behavioral therapy (CBT). A type of psychotherapy in which therapists help patients think more positively and realistically about their situations and engage in behaviors that produce positive emotions and a sense of well-being.

Community-based sample. Subjects in a research study who live in the community (as opposed to those who are hospitalized or institutionalized).

Confidence interval (CI). A range of values within which the "true" value of a statistic lies; this usually refers to the 95 percent confidence interval (e.g., there is a 95 percent chance that the true value lies within this interval).

Confounder. A variable that is not on the causal path between a predictor and an outcome that partially or fully explains the relationship between the two.

Contamination. When a measure of an independent variable contains indicators of the dependent variable, assuring a relationship between the independent and dependent variable.

Continuous variable. A variable or subject characteristics that can be measured on a continuous basis from low to high with equal space between measurements (e.g., age, blood pressure, longevity).

Control group. Refers to subjects who do not receive the intervention in a clinical trial; their outcomes are compared to those who receive the intervention.

Controls. In observational studies, refers to variables that may influence the relationship between one variable and another; statistical methods (such as a regression analysis) are used to remove the effects that controls have on such a relationship in order to determine whether that relationship is independent of those control variables.

Cross-sectional. A study that assesses variables and examines relationships at a single point in time with no follow-up.

Data. Responses to research questions (depressive symptoms, religiosity, etc.) or results from measures taken on subjects such as blood pressure, immune function, etc.

Dependent variable. The outcome (often a health outcome such as depression or mortality) that is being predicted by other subject characteristics (such as age, race, religiosity, etc., known as *independent variables*).

Direct effects. Effects that a predictor variable has on an outcome after control variables have been accounted for.

Epidemiology. The scientific field that focuses on quantitative observational studies.

Epigenetics. Effects that environment has on gene expression that results in various diseases.

Experimental study. A type of study design where the researchers intervene in the lives of subjects in some way and then assess the resulting outcomes; in contrast to *observational studies*, where subjects are simply being observed.

Explanatory variable. Another name for a mediator, i.e., a variable that mediates or explains how one variable affects another.

External validity. Indicates the ability of a study design to produce findings that are generalizable to other persons besides those immediately participating in the study (see also *internal validity*).

Hypothesis. What the researcher expects to find from the research, i.e., the answer to the primary or secondary research question.

Impact factor. The average number of times that articles in a journal are cited by others; an indicator of the journal's prestige or rank in the field.

Independent variable. The characteristic of subjects that is thought to predict or influence a health outcome (dependent variable). Independent variables can be predictors, confounders, moderators, mediators, or suppressor variables.

Index. A series of questions that measures different characteristics of an individual and are not meant to be added up to produce a total score; this contrasts with questions that make up a scale that is designed to measure a specific subject characteristic.

Indirect effects. Effects that a predictor variable has on an outcome because of its effects on other variables that affect the outcome.

Institutional Review Board (IRB). A group of researchers, clinicians, and ethicists who review a research study and determine whether the research is ethical, does not cause excessive risk, and respects the rights of subjects who are involved.

Internal validity. The ability of a study design to determine the causal nature of a relationship between independent and dependent variables (also see *external validity*).

Mechanism. How a variable or characteristic of a subject affects another characteristic of the subject, i.e., describes the pathway by which this occurs.

Mediator (explanatory variable). The variable that lies on the causal path between one variable and another, partially or completely explaining the effect that one variable has on the other.

Model. A detailed description of how one variable or characteristic of a subject (i.e., an independent variable such as religiosity) affects another characteristic of the subject (i.e., a dependent variable such as a health outcome); in statistics, this refers to a statistical equation that relates the independent variables to the dependent variable.

Moderator. A variable that influences the relationship of one variable to another in that the latter variables are more strongly related at one level of the moderator; for example, religiosity is more strongly related to depression in persons who experience high stress levels (i.e., stress level moderates the relationship between religiosity and depression); this is also called an "interaction" (i.e., the moderator interacts with an independent variable in its relationship to a dependent variable).

Multivariate. The relationship between two variables (independent and dependent) in a statistical analysis controlling for the effects of other independent variables.

Nominal variable. A level of measurement of a variable that involves discrete, nonordered categories of response; examples include gender, race, etc. Also called a *categorical variable.*

Observational study. A type of study design in which the researchers observe what naturally happens to subjects without intervening in any way.

Ordinal variable. A variable or subject characteristic that is measured in categories that can be ordered or ranked (i.e., subjective health—poor, fair, good, very good).

Ordinary least squares (OLS). A type of regression; a more specific term for linear regression or multiple regression; all three terms (OLS, linear regression, and multiple regression) generally mean the same thing.

Outcome. Same as the dependent variable (and in R/S-health research is usually some indicator of health).

Peer review. The review of articles submitted for journal publication; the article is sent out to experts in the field (peers) to determine whether the study's methods are appropriate and findings important enough to merit journal publication.

Population-based (probability sample). Refers to a random sample of the general population using a specific sampling method.

Power (power analysis). The ability of a study as designed to detect an effect of a certain size of one variable on another (or of an intervention on an outcome) at a statistically significant level.

Predictor. An independent variable that is being examined in its ability to predict the level of a dependent variable or health outcome.

Prospective (longitudinal or cohort) study. A study that follows subjects over time, often examining the effects that baseline predictors have on health outcomes assessed during follow-up.

Qualitative. Focusing on descriptive self-reports from participants' life experiences.

Quantitative. Measures of predictors and outcomes, and associations between them in terms of numbers.

Randomize. As it applies to assigning subjects to an intervention or a control group, this method assures that each subject has an equal chance of ending up in one or the other group.

Retrospective. A study that depends on subjects' reports of their past experiences.

Scale. A series of questions measuring a particular characteristic of a subject, the answers to which are often added up to produce a score that reflects how much of the characteristic the subject has.

Significance. When referring to statistical significance, an indicator that the relationship is strong enough so that it is not thought to be due to chance alone; a "p-value" indicates the level of statistical significance or the strength of the relationship.

Specific aim. The primary research question to which the researcher is seeking the answer.

Standard deviation (SD). A measure used to indicate how widely individuals in a group vary: if individual observations vary greatly from the group mean, the SD is large; if they vary only a little, the SD is small. The SD is an index of the variability of the data points.

Standard error (SE). The standard error is a measure of the variability of a statistic or regression coefficient. The SE reflects the variability of the mean values, as if the study were repeated a large number of times. The SE is used in constructing 95% confidence intervals (CIs), which indicate a range of values within which the "true" value lies.

Suppressor variable. A variable that serves a similar role as a mediator, except that when a suppressor is controlled in a statistical model, a significant relationship may emerge between predictor and outcome (a relationship that was suppressed by the suppressor variable before it was controlled).

Type I error. An error involving the detection of an effect or an association between two variables when the effect or association is actually not present, i.e., the finding is due to chance alone (due to multiple statistical comparisons or biased assessments).

Type II error. Failure to detect an effect or an association between two variables when the effect or association is really present (due to too small a sample size or measures that are not sensitive enough to detect the effect).

Variable. A measurable characteristic of a subject, i.e., age, race, religiousness, social support, depressive symptoms, longevity, etc.

Index

anxiety
    intercessory prayer study, 183–84
    mental health, 174–76
    negative emotions, 18
Archives of Internal Medicine, 362
Arthur Vining Davis Foundation,
    381
The Art of Readable Writing
    (Flesch), 350
atheists, 32, 150–51, 201
Attachment/Relationship to God
    Scales, 225–26
Azhar, M. Z., 173–74

B coefficient (unstandardized),
    285, 297, 341, 342, 433
Baptists, 39–40, 82–83, 98
Barnes, V. A., 185–86
Barnes & Noble, 365
Baron, R. M., 293
baseline physical health, 8
Batson, Daniel, 215, 222
Bay, P. S., 182–83
Baylor University, 225
BDI. *See* Beck Depression Inven-
    tory
Beck, Richard, 226
Beck Depression Inventory (BDI),
    172–73, 335
Becker, Diane, 177–79
belief or orthodoxy, 211
bell curve, 256
Ben-Meir, Y., 216
bereavement, 173–74
beta (β) coefficient (standard-
    ized), 255, 341, 433
between subjects experimental
    studies, statistical analyses
    categorical outcomes, 280
    continuous outcomes, 280–81
    ordinal outcomes, 281–82
bias, 433
    investigators', 41
    personal, 195
    preexisting, 125
    randomization and, 163
    subjects, 167
    volunteer, 151–52
Bible, 197, 222
    Jewish, 315
    New Testament, 315

BiomedCentral.com, 363
Biostatistics: The Bare Essentials
    (Norman/Streiner), 240
bivariate, 433
    categorical observational stud-
        ies, 261–62, 267–68
    continuous observational stud-
        ies, 264–65
    correlation, 334
    multivariate, continuous obser-
        vational studies, 269
    ordinal observational studies,
        265–66
blinding, 433
    double-blind, 69, 167
    in RCTs, 166–68
    single-blind, 166–67
    triple-blind, 167–68
    unblinded, 166
blocked randomization, 164–65
blood pressure (BP), 185–87
Blue Cross–Blue Shield, 380
BMMRS. *See* Brief MMRS
Boelens, P. A., 183–84
Bonferroni correction, 249
book chapter contributions, 364
book writing, 364–65
BP. *See* blood pressure
Brahman, 319
Brief MMRS (BMMRS), 220,
    230–31
Brigham Young University, 336
Brown, C. G., 184–85
Buddha, 196, 319
Buddhists, 7, 217
budget, in grant writing, 392–93
burying findings, 42

CABG. *See* coronary artery bypass
    graft surgery
CAM. *See* Complementary Alter-
    native Medicine
Cambridge Theological Federa-
    tion, 197
cancer, 179
    American Cancer Society, 23, 378
    breast cancer, 177–78
    in children, 76
    Duke University research, 237,
        239
    malignant melanoma, 179

religious growth, 215
religious history, 213
religious knowledge, 214
religious motivation, 212
religious quest, 215
religious support, 213
religious well-being, 212
subjective religiousness, 211
direct cost (DC), 392
direct effects, 36, 295, 435
  computer programs, 339
  regression models, 340–41
  statistical modeling and, 339–42
discourse analysis, 120
discussion, for research report, 356
distorter variable, 330
distortion, 295, 330
Divine, 196, 319
donors, for research funding, 382–83
double-blind blinding, 69, 167
double-blinded distant intercessory prayer studies, 69
double-entry, 143
dredging data, 42, 240–41
drift, 139
dropouts, 140–41
drug abuse, 18. *See also* substance abuse disorders
DSE. *See* Daily Spiritual Experiences Scale
DSMB. *See* data safety monitoring board
Duke University, 94, 177, 208, 221, 229–31
  cancer research, 237, 239
  grants, 380
  Institute for Care at End of Life, 381
Duke University Religion Index (DUREL), 208, 221, 229–31

Eastern meditation, 56, 176, 180, 185, 189. *See also* Hindu yoga; Kundalini yoga; Mindfulness Meditation; Transcendental Meditation
Eastern Model, 319–20
Einstein, Albert, 115
The Elements of Style, 350

Ellison, C. W., 212, 378
Emavardhana, T., 217
emergency room, 63
emotional disorders, 49–50. *See also* negative emotions
emotional well-being, 331. *See also* positive emotions
endocrine dysfunction, 22, 25, 188
end-of-life care, 64–65
engagement, 195
environmental influences, 323–24
EPESE. *See* Established Populations for Epidemiologic Studies in the Elderly
epidemiology, 208, 298–99, 362, 435
epigenetic influences, 324–25
epigenetics, 59–60, 324–25, 435
Epi-Info, 372
Established Populations for Epidemiologic Studies in the Elderly (EPESE), 298–99
ethics, 5, 79–80
ethnography, 119–20
EWB. *See* existential well-being
Excel, 238–39
exclusion criteria. *See* inclusion and exclusion criteria
exercise, 22, 61, 131, 186, 189
existential well-being (EWB), 295, 328–33
experimental design, 91, 92, 278
experimental studies, 31, 435
  between subjects design, 279–82
  overview, 276–77
  sampling methods, 111–14
  single group, 278
  statistical tests for, 276–82
  within subjects design, 277–79
explanatory variables, 8, 293–94, 435
  confounders and, 297–300
  controlling for, 304–5
  critics' response, 301–3
  multiple, 9
  path analysis with multiple, 340
  path analysis with single, 340
  recommendations for handling, 303–5

intercessory prayer studies, 183–85

intergenerational transmission, 59–60

intermediate outcomes, 160

internal validity, 150, 270, 278, 436

International Journal of Psychiatry in Medicine, 362

International Journal of the Psychology of Religion, 363

Internet, 354. *See also* websites
publishing research for fee, 363–64

interval level variable, 257

interventions. *See also* chaplain interventions; clinical trials with R/S interventions; R/S interventions
prayer intervention study, 177–78
research plan, 397
standardization of, 155

interviewer, 142
administered scales, 7, 209

interviews
open-ended, 125
SCID, 144

Intrinsic Religiosity Scale (IR), 208, 221, 229–31

introduction, for research report, 354–55

Intuitive Biostatistics (Motulsky), 240

inverse probability of treatment weighting, 39

investigative groups, 32

investigators. *See also* research team
bias, 41
experience in research design, 93
feasibility of time, 78
lack of trained, 43
PI, 386, 391
R/S health research, 116
subject recruitment, 78

IR. *See* Intrinsic Religiosity Scale

IRB. *See* Institutional Review Board

Islam, 173

JAMA, 287, 362

Jehovah's Witnesses, 216

Jesus, 222

Jews, 7, 216, 315, 363

JTF. *See* John Templeton Foundation

job satisfaction, 337–38

John Templeton Foundation (JTF), 81, 370, 381–82

Johns Hopkins, 3, 177

Joint Commission for the Accreditation of Hospital Organizations, 66

Jones, R. N., 240

Journal for the Scientific Study of Religion, 363

Journal of Consulting & Clinical Psychology, 287, 362

Journal of Family Practice, 362

Journal of General Internal Medicine, 362

Journal of Gerontology, 287

Journal of Healthcare Chaplaincy, 363

Journal of Muslim Mental Health, 217, 363

Journal of Nervous & Mental Disease, 362

Journal of Pastoral Care, 363

Journal of Psychology and Christianity, 363

Journal of Psychology and Theology, 363

Journal of Religion, Spirituality & Aging, 363

Journal of Religion and Health, 363

Journal of the American Geriatrics Society, 362

Journal on Jewish Aging, 363

Journals of Gerontology, 362

journals
recommended journals, 361–62
statisticians for, 287
writing for, 355

k-1 binary variables, 255

Kabat-Zinn, J., 189–90

Kaiser, 380

Kedem, P., 216

Kellogg Foundation, 381

Kendall rank order correlation, 266

National Science Foundation (NSF), 42, 81, 378
National Survey of Black Americans, 98
Nationwide Health, 380
natural history, 143
NCCAM. *See* National Center for Complementary and Alternative Medicine
negative emotions
  alcohol use and abuse, 18, 51, 63, 113, 152, 300
  anxiety, 18
  depression, 17
  drug abuse, 18
  suicide, 17
neurological diseases, 50, 57
New Age, 7, 218
New Age Orientation Scale, 218
New England Journal of Medicine, 362
Newsom, J. T., 240, 271, 276
NHANES. *See* National Health and Nutrition Examination Survey
NIA. *See* National Institute on Aging
NIH. *See* National Institutes of Health
NINR. *See* National Institute of Nursing Research
noise in measurement, 159
nominal variable, 254–55, 434, 437
nonorganizational religiosity, 215–16
nonparametric statistical tests, 257
nonparticipants, 109–10, 135–36, 142
nonprobability sampling methods, 101. *See also* probability sampling methods
  convenience nonprobability sample, 101–4
  purposive nonprobability sample, 101
  quota nonprobability sample, 101
  referral nonprobability sample, 101
  snowball, 101
nonprofit foundation, setup, 374

nonrandomized concurrent control groups, 156
nonreligious persons, 199
nonrespondents, 142
Norman, Geoffrey, 240
Northwestern Memorial Hospital, 181
novelty (concerning research question), 79
NSF. *See* National Science Foundation

objectivity in research
  accuracy and, 7, 210, 218
  concerns, 70
  illusion, 76
  in quantitative research, 117, 126
observational research (in general), 30–31, 437
  conducting, 141–43
  convenience nonprobability sample, 101–4
  cross-sectional studies, 130–36
  historical research, 120
  longitudinal studies, 136–38
  overview, 129–30
  prospective cohort studies, 138–41
  purpose of, 130
  qualitative research, 86–88
  quantitative research, 88–91
  research design, 6, 86–91
  sampling methods, 101–11
  study example, 144–46
  summary and conclusions, 146–47
observational studies, dependent samples (statistical methods)
  bivariate, categorical, 267–68
  bivariate and multivariate, continuous, 269
  multivariate, categorical, 268
  overview, 267
  statistical tests for, 267–70
observational studies, independent samples (statistical methods)
  bivariate, categorical, 261–62
  bivariate, continuous, 264–65
  bivariate, ordinal, 265–66
  multivariate, categorical, 262–64

submission to journals, 358–61
summary and conclusions,
366–67
tenure achievement, 349
writing skills, 350–52
purposive nonprobability sample,
101
p-value, 83, 439
adjustments, 249
calculating, 258
lowering or reducing, 240, 249
role, 102
significance, 241

QOL. *See* quality of life
qualitative research, 6, 438
approaches, 118–21
characteristics, 117
criticisms of, 127
data analysis, 122–24
data generation, 122–23
description, 116–17
discourse analysis, 120
ethnography, 119–20
grounded theory, 119
importance, 116
literature review, 121
negative perceptions, 125
observational research, 86–88
open-ended interviews, 125
overview, 115–16
participants, 118, 121
phenomenology, 118
problems, 124–25
quantitative research *vs.*, 70,
117–18
research agenda, 70
role of, 86
sample, 121–22
setting, 121–22
standards, 125
strengths, 124
triangulation, 120–21
when appropriate, 87
quality of life (QOL), 331, 333–34
quality of measures, 39–40
quantitative measurement, 7
quantitative research, 30, 438
case-control, 88–89
cross-sectional design, 6, 33,
86, 89

longitudinal studies, 89–90
objectivity, 117, 126
observational research, 88–91
problems with, 126
prospective cohort designs,
90–91
qualitative research *vs.*, 70,
117–18
retrospective cohort designs,
90–91
summary and conclusions,
126–27
well-being, 15
Quest Scale, 222
quota nonprobability sample, 101,
107
Qur'an, 174, 314

R. J. Reynolds Tobacco Company,
379
RA. *See* religious attendance
randomization
bias and, 163
blocked, 164–65
consent after, 161–63
consent before, 161
in RCTs, 163–66
role of, 163
simple, 164
stratified, 165
unequal, 165–66
randomize, 438
randomized clinical trials (RCTs),
6–7, 37, 92, 139, 280–81
analysis of results, 168–69
blinding, 166–68
consent, 161–63
control groups, 155–59
feasibility, 150–51
features, 154–55

hierarchy in strength of evidence, 150
I/E criteria, 152
importance, 150
outcomes, 160
randomization in, 163–66
research team, 153
standardization of intervention,
155
subject selection, 159–60

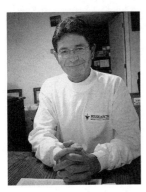

Harold G. Koenig, MD, completed his undergraduate education at Stanford University, his medical school training at the University of California at San Francisco, and his geriatric medicine, psychiatry, and biostatistics training at Duke University Medical Center. He is on the faculty at Duke as professor of psychiatry and behavioral sciences and associate professor of medicine. Dr. Koenig is also director of the Center for Spirituality, Theology, and Health at Duke University Medical Center and is distinguished adjunct professor at King Abdulaziz University in Jeddah, Saudi Arabia. Dr. Koenig has published extensively in the fields of mental health, geriatrics, and religion, with over 350 scientific peer-reviewed articles and book chapters and nearly 40 books in print or in preparation. He has given invited testimony to both the U.S. Senate and the U.S. House of Representatives on the role of religion in public health.